Intellectual Disabilities: Health and Social Care Across the Lifespan

W0043649

Fintan Sheerin • Carmel Doyle
Editors

Intellectual Disabilities: Health and Social Care Across the Lifespan

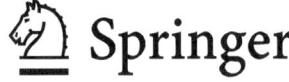 Springer

Editors
Fintan Sheerin 🆔
School of Nursing & Midwifery
Trinity College Dublin
Dublin, Ireland

Carmel Doyle 🆔
School of Nursing & Midwifery
Trinity College Dublin
Dublin, Ireland

ISBN 978-3-031-27495-4   ISBN 978-3-031-27496-1   (eBook)
https://doi.org/10.1007/978-3-031-27496-1

© The Editor(s) (if applicable) and The Author(s), under exclusive license to Springer Nature Switzerland AG 2023
This work is subject to copyright. All rights are solely and exclusively licensed by the Publisher, whether the whole or part of the material is concerned, specifically the rights of translation, reprinting, reuse of illustrations, recitation, broadcasting, reproduction on microfilms or in any other physical way, and transmission or information storage and retrieval, electronic adaptation, computer software, or by similar or dissimilar methodology now known or hereafter developed. The use of general descriptive names, registered names, trademarks, service marks, etc. in this publication does not imply, even in the absence of a specific statement, that such names are exempt from the relevant protective laws and regulations and therefore free for general use.
The publisher, the authors, and the editors are safe to assume that the advice and information in this book are believed to be true and accurate at the date of publication. Neither the publisher nor the authors or the editors give a warranty, expressed or implied, with respect to the material contained herein or for any errors or omissions that may have been made. The publisher remains neutral with regard to jurisdictional claims in published maps and institutional affiliations.

This Springer imprint is published by the registered company Springer Nature Switzerland AG
The registered company address is: Gewerbestrasse 11, 6330 Cham, Switzerland

Introduction

The past decades have seen much change in the demographics of intellectual disability and in the responses of states and professionals to the needs and wishes of people with intellectual disabilities. There has been a move from institutionalisation to community living, from congregated services to person-focused supports, and an increased grounding in human rights. Such developments require professionals to think in different ways and to work together with people with intellectual disabilities in new and innovative ways. This interdisciplinary book offers nursing, health and social care professionals evidence-based material to assist them to respond in this new reality, so that they can support individuals with intellectual disabilities and their families throughout the lifespan. It also provides a basis for professionals to develop partnership with individuals and their families in order to facilitate and support meaningful daily living.

This book is unique as it has brought together a diverse array of international authors from the fields of nursing, social care, social work, sociology, education, policy, psychology, psychiatry, and pharmacology, as well as family perspectives. Many of these authors are writing together for the first time, thus allowing for a rich exploration of topics, drawing on a variety of viewpoints.

There are three main parts to the book, each comprising a number of chapters. These are structured to provide readers with an in-depth understanding of the topic in question, and, through the use of reflective exercises, vignettes and reader activities, afford potential users further learning opportunities.

Part I: Introduction to Key Concepts

The first part presents the *Key Concepts* which form a basis for the remaining parts. As such, it is foundational and also provides an important context for understanding the issues that have and continue to inform provision of service and supports to people with intellectual disabilities. The history of service provision is discussed in *Chapter 1: Foundations of Intellectual Disability* with some consideration of how that history has continued to play out despite the significant changes in recent decades. Models of care and support are explored, with some focus on recent instances where those models broke down. The philosophies that underpin current provision are discussed as well as the relationship between service and social perceptions. *Chapter 2: Communication as a Basis for Person-Centred Support* focuses on one of the central concepts of service provision, person-centredness and considers the role of communication in supporting the voices of people with intellectual disabilities to be heard and become the driving force in their lives. The role of formal and informal caregivers in achieving this is explored in the context of self-advocacy and active listening. The chapter is strongly grounded in a rights-based perspective of intellectual disability. Furthermore, it progresses from an understanding that care and support are now being approached from an interdisciplinary context. *Chapter 3: Care and Support in a Multi/Interdisciplinary Context* considers the different ways that professionals can work together and, even more importantly, how they can include people with intellectual disabilities and their families in planning services that are responsive on an individual level. Two national case studies are presented, one from Norway and the other from Australia, which explore the difference between multidisciplinary and interdisciplinary approaches. Part I concludes with a chapter focused on behaviour. *Chapter 4: Attachment, Cognitive Dissonance and Reciprocation in Intellectual Disability Care Provision*, moves away from the traditional behaviourist approach and, instead, explores a number of psychological mechanisms that may underly some of the behaviours that people with intellectual disabilities and other human beings may display. The authors uncover important perspectives and provide an understanding of behaviour that will assist readers to consider the reasons for certain behaviours and develop more meaningful responses to them.

Part II: From Birth to Adolescence

The second part, *From Birth to Adolescence*, focuses on the causative factors underlying intellectual disability. An initial introduction to the prevalence of intellectual disability and the main causes is addressed in *Chapter 5: The Nature of Intellectual Disability*. This also explores the effect of receiving a diagnosis of intellectual disability on parents. That is further considered in the next chapter which examines the impact of intellectual disability on the child and family. This is addressed in *Chapter 6: Children and Adolescents with Intellectual Disability*. In this, the authors also explore the range of key supports that should be available in the health, social, and educational domains. *Chapter 7: Intellectual and Developmental Disabilities and Rare Diseases* and *Chapter 8: Other Neurodevelopmental Conditions* provide the reader with an in-depth understanding of the aetiology, presenting features and management strategies pertinent to some of the most frequently encountered causes of intellectual disability. This is accompanied by a detailed explanation of, where relevant, the genetic or other bases for intellectual disability. Co-occurring autism and autistic spectrum disorder is also discussed. The impact of intellectual disability in childhood and adolescence, on the person with intellectual disability and their family, is explored through vignettes and case studies.

Part III: From Adulthood to Older Age

The third part explores the area of *Adulthood to Older Age*, comprising three individual chapters relating to health care needs, ageing, and mental health of people with intellectual disability. Specific health care needs of those with an intellectual disability are considered in *Chapter 9: Chronic Health Among Those with an Intellectual Disability*. The most prevalent chronic health conditions experienced by individuals are explored including epilepsy, musculoskeletal conditions focusing on osteoporosis, cardiovascular disease, respiratory disease, gastrointestinal disease, and sensory impairments. Contributing factors to chronic health conditions are outlined and factors to consider in addressing chronic health conditions are also identified, an important step in promoting a healthy lifestyle. With growth in the ageing population of people with intellectual disability, concerns about health, changes in function, potential for loneliness, possible feelings of isolation alongside unwanted transitions are all areas addressed in *Chapter 10: Ageing and Intellectual Disability*. These are considered in this part with an examination of the meaning of growing older successfully, ageing in place and exercising self-determination. International perspectives and longitudinal data are presented on such things as prevention of early ageing and health promotion. Challenges around service changes required in ageing are identified and specific areas explored, such as palliative care and dementia. The concept of mental health, quality of life for people with intellectual disability and its relationship with mental health disorders and problem behaviours are contemplated in *Chapter 11: Intellectual Disability, Mental Health and Mental Disorders*. Within this chapter, the prevalence, classification, and assessment of mental health disorders in people with intellectual disabilities is also examined. With services developing in this area of care, access is explored and the importance of recognition and management of common mental disorders. The recovery model in supporting the person with intellectual disability and a mental health condition is also studied.

Part IV: Integrating Health and Social Perspectives

The fourth and final part explores the Integration of Health and Social Perspectives addressing such issues as supporting and enabling families, education, employment, and sexuality and relationships. This part of the textbook comprises five chapters all providing key information for the reader. The sociological basis for care is considered in *Chapter 12: The Social Contract of Care for People with an Intellectual Disability*. This chapter considers the responsibility of care provision for people with intellectual disabilities and places the spotlight on social policies and the impact of deinstitutionalisation and de-congregation on caregiving. Changing family structures are also examined in the context of care giving in family homes. Enabling individuals to live a life of their choosing is considered in *Chapter 13: Enabling Families to Support Adults with an Intellectual Disability to Live a Life of their Choosing*. Appreciation is given to the role of family in the lives of people with intellectual disability, and how this impacts care and support over the life course. Key supports that enable people with intellectual disability to remain living with family, if they choose, are also assessed. *Chapter 14: Social Integration and Inclusion* considers the importance of integration and inclusion in facilitating people with intellectual disabilities to become part of their communities. Governmental inclusive policies and the tenets of inclusive education are explored with the rights of individuals with intellectual disability to the fore. As people with intellectual disabilities experience a variety of transitions over their life course, the concept of transition and underpinning theories are examined in *Chapter 15: Supporting Transitions*. Research evidence regarding transitions across the lifespan is presented and detail offered on the supports required to enable effective transitions. The final chapter, *Chapter 16: Sexuality, Gender Identity and Relationships*, considers the importance of relationships in the lives of people with intellectual disabilities across the lifespan. A historical context of relationships and sexuality for people with intellectual disabilities is introduced with key terms identified. A discussion on diversity of sexual identity and binary understandings of gender in the lives of people with intellectual disabilities is presented. Challenges for society and services are addressed, and exemplars of best practices and approaches in sexual health are proffered.

Overall, we hope that this book will provide a rich source of information for readers and will encourage them to embed the concepts encountered in their practice, whether in the professions of health or social care, thus embellishing the lives of people with intellectual disabilities and those of their families.

Dublin, Ireland   Fintan Sheerin
Dublin, Ireland   Carmel Doyle

Contents

Part I

Introduction to Key Concepts

Foundations of Intellectual Disability

Ruth Northway and Edward Oloidi

Chapter Topics

At the end of this chapter, the reader should:

- Be able to discuss the definitions and constructions of intellectual disability.
- Understand the historical perspectives on care and support for people with intellectual disabilities.
- Know the changing models of care and support across the lifespan.
- Be able to explain the relationship between societal perceptions of intellectual disability and care and support.

Introduction

The aim of this chapter is to provide a foundation and context for the other chapters in this book. It will first explore definitions of intellectual disability, and then move to examine how intellectual disability has been understood historically in diverse ways, and how it continues to be understood differently across cultures. Patterns of service provision, care, and support will then be discussed before drawing conclusions.

Current Definitions and Terminology

The terminology used in this chapter is 'intellectual disability' since this is currently most widely used internationally. However, differing terminology is used in different countries. For example, in the UK the term 'learning disabilities' is used, whereas in the USA, this refers to those with specific learning difficulties such as dyslexia. In several countries reference is made to those with 'intellectual and developmental disabilities' that encompasses individuals with impairments such as autism and cerebral palsy that may or may not be accompanied by intellectual disabilities.

It is also important to acknowledge that terminology has changed over the centuries and decades. Previous terminology has included terms such as idiot, feebleminded, mentally defective, mentally subnormal and mentally retarded. Each of these terms is now considered derogatory, but in this chapter, it will be necessary to use them when making historical references.

Current definitions vary their detail, but most agree that for an individual to be considered to have an intellectual disability, three criteria must be satisfied:

R. Northway (✉) · E. Oloidi
University of South Wales, Pontypridd, UK
e-mail: ruth.northway@southwales.ac.uk;
edward.oloidi@southwales.ac.uk

© The Author(s), under exclusive license to Springer Nature Switzerland AG 2023
F. Sheerin, C. Doyle (eds.), *Intellectual Disabilities: Health and Social Care Across the Lifespan*,
https://doi.org/10.1007/978-3-031-27496-1_1

- The individual must have significant impairment of intellectual functioning.
- The individual must have significant impairment of social functioning.
- These impairments must have been evident during the developmental period.

Impairment of intellectual functioning is often clinically determined by an intelligence quotient (IQ) score, with a score of 70 or less being viewed as meeting the criterion. What this means for an individual is that they may have difficulties with learning new or complex information and they may have difficulties with processing and retaining information. In relation to social functioning, an individual may require support with everyday tasks such as meeting their nutritional and hygiene needs, with budgeting and financial management and with other aspects of daily living. The criterion of the impairment occurring during the developmental period distinguishes intellectual disability from acquired brain injury occurring later in life. Whilst some definitions define the developmental period as being up to the age of 16, others extend this to age 25.

Whilst these criteria appear straightforward, critical examination is required. First, the term 'intellectual disability' encompasses people with diverse strengths and support needs. Some may live independently with little or no external support, whilst others may require full assistance with activities of daily living. It is therefore common to refer to people as having 'mild', 'moderate', 'severe' or 'profound' intellectual disabilities. However, given that intellectual disability encompasses such diverse needs, it then gives rise to a second key issue, namely, the boundary between those with mild intellectual disabilities and those considered not to have intellectual disabilities.

As noted above the criterion for 'diagnosis' or assessment is often taken as being an IQ score of 70 or less. However, does someone with an IQ score of 70 have dissimilar needs to someone with an IQ score of 71? This highlights that the concept of intellectual disabilities is a social construct since the boundary of intellectual disability is socially created. Indeed, as was noted earlier,

terminology used over the centuries has changed, and Jarrett and Tilley (2022) caution against assuming that people we refer to today as having intellectual disabilities comprise a fixed, unchanging, group that has simply had a different term applied to them. The scope of who is deemed to 'fit' into such a category can both expand and constrict according to the 'values, priorities and preoccupations of different societies' (Jarrett and Tilley 2022:134).

This gives rise to a third consideration of why it is deemed important to categorise people in this way. A primary reason is that access to key services and support is usually dependent upon a 'diagnosis'. From the perspective of service providers, it is thus a mechanism for ensuring that services are targeted on those for whom they are primarily intended. However, where a dividing line is drawn between those who are eligible (meet the diagnostic criteria) and those who are not, there will always be those who are at the border (e.g. have an IQ of 72) who may still have significant support needs.

Another reason for identifying people as having intellectual disabilities is that by doing so it enables policymakers and service providers to better plan services to meet current and anticipated need. It also facilitates identification of disparities between those who have an intellectual disability and the wider population (e.g. in relation to health). However, despite these positive reasons for identification, it also needs to be acknowledged that some individuals may not wish to be identified as having an intellectual disability and that stigma may accompany the application of such a label particularly within some cultures.

It is difficult to provide accurate statistics as to how many people within a given population have intellectual disabilities. For example, looking at data from England, Hatton et al. (2016) estimate that the overall prevalence of intellectual disabilities is 2.5% of the population. However, they also note that the prevalence drops from 2.5% amongst children receiving education to 0.6% amongst young adults (20–29 years). This reflects the reality that individuals who require additional support during their education may not transfer to adult services either due to problems of transition or due to not meeting the eligibility criteria for adult services.

It is also important to note that people with intellectual disability are not a homogenous group and that intellectual disability is only one aspect of their identity. An intersectional approach (Bjornsdottir and Traustadottir 2010) that acknowledges that the lives of people with intellectual disabilities are shaped by a wide range of personal factors such as race, age, gender, culture and social class is thus required.

Historical Understandings of Intellectual Disability

Ryan and Thomas (1987) argue that the history of people with intellectual disabilities has been shaped by how their differences have been defined by wider society with such differences usually been viewed negatively. Their lives have thus always been defined by others rather than through self-definition. This view has recently been restated, as Jarrett and Tilley (2022) argue that the very nature of intellectual disabilities means that it is difficult for people so labelled to leave their own historical account. They also observe that whilst other historically marginalised groups (such as those from minority ethnic communities and those identifying as LBGTQ+) have started to claim their own histories as part of a wider process of liberation, such progress has been more limited for people with intellectual disabilities.

People with intellectual disabilities have always existed within society, but historical data prior to the end of the eighteenth century is limited. However, from what is known, it is evident that they had variously been viewed as being a gift from God, as changelings, as a punishment for the sins of parents and as immoral being of a distinct species (Ryan and Thomas 1987). This reflects what Wolfensberger (1972) identified as the historic roles into which groups of people viewed by society as being 'deviant' have been cast. These include being viewed as subhuman, as a menace, as an unspeakable object of dread, as an object of pity, as a holy innocent, as a dis-

eased organism, as an object of ridicule and as an eternal child.

Whilst some roles identified by Wolfensberger (1972) might be thought of as being relatively benign, it is important to critically examine the impact of others perceiving individuals in this manner. For example, if someone is viewed as an eternal child, then they will never be supported to take on adult roles and relationships. Other roles perhaps have more overt negative connotations; if an individual is seen as a menace, then others will seek to control them, and if they are also viewed as subhuman, then the way such control is exerted will not be questioned. It is not possible here to explore all the ways in which people with intellectual disabilities have historically been viewed, but key examples will be provided to illustrate changing perceptions over time.

During the 1800s Edward Seguin, a French physician and educationalist, proposed a method of educating 'idiots' (the terminology of the time) comprising physical activity, education of the senses and moral treatment (Trent 1994). In contrast to previous perceptions, he argued that 'idiots' could be educated and, based on his work, educational institutions were established in several countries.

The original intention of such institutions was to educate individuals and then return them to live with their families. However, society was changing, employment was becoming more industrialised, and families often had to move for employment. Therefore, rather than returning to their families, the numbers within institutions grew and this failure was often 'attributed to the hopeless nature of the idiots themselves' (Ryan and Thomas 1987:102). The institutions started to come under medical control and interest grew in studying the causes and types of idiocy (Ryan and Thomas 1987).

Also, towards the end of the nineteenth century, wider social concerns regarding society's ills (such as poverty, crime and immorality), coupled with a growing interest in genetics, led to the rise of the eugenics movement. Broadly, the aim of this movement was to improve the overall 'quality' of the population through promoting desirable characteristics amongst the population (positive eugenics) and through reducing characteristics deemed to be undesirable (negative eugenics) (Kevles 1999). Those deemed to be 'feebleminded' were viewed as undesirable, as being responsible for a range of social ills, and to be reproducing at a rate that was causing a threat to social resources and social stability (Kevles 1999).

The growing number of the 'feebleminded' and 'idiots' in institutions was viewed as evidence of an actual increase in the numbers of such people within the population, and institutions became places that could protect society by segregating them from the wider population and by controlling behaviour within the institutions. For example, men and women were segregated within these settings and not allowed to mix (to prevent them from reproducing).

In 1896, in the UK, the National Association for the Care and Control of the Feebleminded was established to campaign for the lifetime segregation of those considered to be feebleminded and to prevent them from reproducing (feeblemindedness being viewed as being inherited) (Ryan and Thomas 1987). The 1913 Mental Deficiency Act made provision for compulsory certification of those admitted to institutions, but slow progress led the Wood Committee to argue in 1929 that the mentally defective (as they were then known) posed a continuing threat and that action was needed to prevent the 'racial disaster of mental deficiency' (Ryan and Thomas 1987). This view of people we now refer to as having intellectual disabilities posing a threat to society was not, however, confined to the UK: in the 1920s and 1930s, eugenic sterilisation legislation was passed in the USA, Canada and Sweden (Kevles 1999). Whilst compulsory segregation and sterilisation may be thought to be distant history, Sweden was found to still be carrying out compulsory sterilisation in the 1970s.

Some commentators argue that rather than disappearing, eugenic perceptions and practices remain but that the form they take has evolved. For example, Shakespeare (1998) distinguishes between the 'hard' eugenics of the past and the 'soft' eugenics of the present, whereby prenatal screening programmes are provided by govern-ments to identify certain impairments and to enable parents to choose whether they wish to terminate a pregnancy should an impairment be identified. He argues that such programmes place a negative value on the lives of people with certain conditions. What is interesting, however, is that people with intellectual disabilities themselves are beginning to challenge such perceptions and practices as evidenced by the recent High Court case in which Heidi Crowther, a woman with Down syndrome, sought to prevent the practice of late termination of foetuses with Down syndrome on the basis that it is discriminatory and did not value her life (BBC News On-Line 2021). Whilst this case was lost, it indicates that people with intellectual disabilities are now seeking to challenge perceptions and to self-assert their human rights.

Cross-Cultural Understandings of Intellectual Disability

It has been argued that how people reason, recall events and experiences and express their thoughts differs across cultures (D'Andre 1995). Moreover, despite a well-documented correlation between ethnicity and culture, research has shown that groups from similar ethnic backgrounds often differ in terms of their social use of language, lifestyle and culture (Keogh et al. 1997).

In their discussion of cross-cultural understandings of quality of life for persons with intellectual disabilities, Schalock et al. (2002) noted that how intellectual disability is understood varies from country to country and across states, cultures and geographical locations within a country. Similarly, in their cross-cultural review of inclusion and intellectual disabilities, Taub and Foster (2020) noted that disability is increasingly recognised as a culturally constructed phenomenon.

Given such cross-cultural differences, understanding sociocultural perceptions of intellectual disabilities is crucial to understanding intellectual disabilities and cultural diversity, and it is impossible to generate understanding of individuals with intellectual disabilities in isolation from sociocultural environmental practices (Keogh et al. 1997). What is deemed desirable and important in different cultures is thus sensitive to cultural needs and meaning making about intellectual disabilities. This has implications for prognosis and beliefs held in specific cultures about the cause of intellectual disabilities (Venkatesan 2017). For example, in cultures where the medical model remains influential, intellectual disabilities continue to be understood as 'situated in the person', whereas cultures that embrace social model of disability view disability as 'situated outside' the person (Venkatesan 2017: 53).

Research has linked the absence of a commonly agreed definition and/or understanding of intellectual disabilities to the disparities in economic and social opportunities that exist within and across geographical locations (Ajuwon and Brown 2012). For example, the disparities between people with intellectual disabilities in high-income economies, such as the USA and Europe, and low- and middle-income economies such as Africa and Asia are associated with sociocultural values held towards intellectual disabilities within those countries.

In low- and middle-income countries, such as sub-Saharan Africa, inequalities often interact with factors like religious and social beliefs concerning people with intellectual disabilities (Ajuwon and Brown 2012). Knowledge concerning such interactions is still evolving (Ajuwon and Brown 2012), but cultural and ethical challenges for provision of care and support arise (Aniek van Herwaarden et al. 2021).

Despite the international drive for disabled people's social inclusion, human rights and fundamental freedoms (United Nations 1975), people with intellectual disability continue to experience challenges to their realisation (Capri et al. 2018). As seen above, societal perceptions of intellectual disability have varied historically, but differing views across cultures continue. Thompson et al. (2011) explain that sociocultural norms (including local attitudes) interact with meaning making at personal, organisational and structural levels within a specific society. Furthermore, cross-cultural research has demonstrated that, internationally, culture-specific norms dictate service provision for people with

intellectual disabilities, contribute to a lack of agreed 'nomenclature' for understanding disability and underpin the general lack of accepted terms to describe the phenomenon (Venkatesan 2017; Opoku et al. 2021).

It can thus be concluded that local 'history, culture, context and social processes' shape understanding of intellectual disability experiences (Starke et al. 2016).

Models of Service, Care and Support

Institutional and Congregate Settings

An earlier section of this chapter detailed the origins of institutional care for people with intellectual disabilities as illustrated by the rise in large scale long-stay institutions in many countries. Whilst such large institutions have closed in many countries, some institutional care remains.

The European Coalition for Community Living (2013) described institutional/congregated care settings as 'any place in which people who have been labelled as having disability are isolated, segregated and/or compelled to live together'. Congregated settings have been described slightly differently as a living arrangement where more than ten people share a living space and live-in dormitory-like settings or jointly share housing arrangements provided and/or administered by an organisation or local authority (Health Service Executive 2011). Mansell (2006) suggested that congregated settings differ from institutional settings because they are smaller in size, house fewer people and emerged from efforts to close large institutional settings.

Berger and Luckmann (1966) argue that institutions are human inventions designed to fulfil specific social and cultural needs, and earlier in this chapter, the shift in emphasis from being educational settings to medical places of control was discussed. However, due to growing public outrage at evidence that institutional care arrangements deprive disabled people of their right to decent life, major enquiries were launched across 28 European nations. These found that the majority of those institutionalised are disabled people, living in substandard conditions and robbed of their rights to equal opportunities (Mansell et al. 2007). Whilst there are many historical examples of poor and abusive care, unfortunately current occurrences continue to be exposed, for example, the cruel and inhuman treatment of residents in Winterbourne View hospital, a specialised care settings for adults with intellectual disabilities and autism (Flynn 2012). More recently, an undercover investigation at Áras Attracta, a public funded care facility for intellectually disabled people in Ireland, found systematic abuse of residents (Murphy and Bantry-White 2021). This development, and many more across Europe, has led to a renewed focus on deinstitutionalisation.

Despite the radical shift in policy, public objections to the discriminatory practices of institutionalisation and the deinstitutionalisation movement (Morin et al. 2013), authors continue to find evidence of negative social attitudes and a eugenic legacy of institutional care. Socio-attitudinal factors such as the historical oppression of institutionalisation continue to influence present-day service 'provision' and 'regulations' for persons with intellectual disabilities in the UK (Lafferty et al. 2012:31). Nonetheless, it is argued that this issue emanates from inappropriate and loose application of the concept of deinstitutionalisation as solely referring to support provision in the community (instead of a long-stay hospital), regardless of where and how many people they now share a living space with—for example, 'nursing homes' (McCarron et al. 2018:13).

Changing Philosophies

Several core philosophical ideas have emerged over the years regarding the conceptualisation of persons labelled as intellectually disabled. Chief amongst these are the traditional models of disability, which provide the lenses for understanding and explaining how others relate to the concept of disability (Ferndale et al. 2016).

There are concerns that the philosophical drive behind the traditional medical and social models of disability are founded on stigmatised assumptions concerning the identity of disabled persons and disability. The medical model portrays disability as inherent in the person rather than the social environment (Taub and Foster 2020). The implication is that support for disabled individuals is then medically driven (Taub and Foster 2020) and is focused on 'curing' or 'fixing' the individual. However, the assumption that the cause of disability lies within the person has been challenged arguing that the medical model itself is considered disabling (Taub and Foster 2020) and fails to support disabled individuals' human rights (Joint Committee on Human Rights 2008).

Challenges to the medical model led to acknowledgement of the social dimensions of disability and ushered in the social model of disability (Reed 2000), which sees disability as a socially constructed term that significantly influences perceptions of individuals so labelled (Taub and Foster 2020). This ideological shift also attributes disabled persons' negative everyday experiences at the doorstep of society (Oliver 1984). The philosophical assumptions underpinning the social model portray disability as arising from societal barriers that prevent full participation in society.

The social model of disability has, however, had limited impact on support for people with intellectual disability. Instead, it was the principle of normalisation (Wolfensberger 1972) and subsequently social role valorisation that shaped the development of services and support. The philosophy of normalisation originated in Scandinavia (Nirje 1972) and focused on strengthening disabled persons' rights to inclusion and normal patterns of everyday living (Emerson 1992). It prioritised the promotion of disabled people's rights as accepted and valued members of their society (Summers and Jones 2004). For Wolfensberger (1983), however, the development of valued social roles for people with intellectual disabilities and others at risk of social devaluation would enhance their acceptance by society.

This subsequent development by Wolfensberger to focus on the creation of socially valued roles to enhance 'social acceptance' has been criticised for its failure to value individual difference, a perceived lack of a person-centred approach and the requirement for disabled individuals rather than society, to change to enhance social acceptance (Summers and Jones 2004). Wolfensberger (1983) argued this was a misinterpretation by others and suggested 'social role valorisation' (SRV) as the new name suggesting it aimed to promote socially valued roles for socially devalued individuals in society. However, the new name was never generally accepted (Emerson 1992) and was rejected by the disability movement for seeking to pressure disabled people to change to 'fit in' rather than seeking to change society to accept and include (Summers and Jones 2004). Mindful of these concerns, others warned that society must learn from the past and thoroughly scrutinise approaches to disabled persons to avoid blind adherence to a philosophy with a conflicting and damaging effect to the one intended (Bruininkis et al. 1981).

Development of Inclusive, Community-Based Supports

An agreed definition of inclusion is elusive (Nes et al. 2018). Nevertheless, most authors agreed that it involves acceptance, belonging and having an active and equitable role in the community (Taub and Foster 2020). This reflects the guiding principle of the United Nations' Convention on the Rights of Persons with Disabilities, namely, that disabled individuals have the right to full inclusion and participation in society (United Nations 2006: para. 1).

Community-based accommodation exists in a variety of forms ranging from group homes housing no more than eight people with 24-h support provided by staff subject to individual needs, to individualised accommodation in which the person lives and receives personalised support in their own home (McConkey et al. 2016). Such arrangements have been described as representing an ideological shift in service planning and provision arising from the normalisation and inclusion movements (Felce 1997). Community support arrangements have been credited with improving the quality of life, social inclusion, satisfaction, access to commonly shared space and health and social care services for disabled people (Ginneá 2019). In addition to their compliance with international standards on equal rights amongst citizens (UN 2006), they are perceived as cost effective (Mansell et al. 2007) and have been well received by the civil rights movement (Miller et al. 2008).

In order to promote inclusion (Scior and Furnharm 2011), the wider move across the UK to include people with intellectual disabilities in community life gave rise to the need for greater consideration of the right to live independently in a place of their own choosing (McCarron et al. 2018). This was further strengthened with the adoption of the personal care budgets (Spicker 2013) and a person-centred community-focused approach where individuals are central to decisions about their own lives (Adams 2007).

However, despite the persuasive arguments for community-based support, it has not been without challenge. Some families felt that moving their relatives with intellectual disabilities from institutional to community-based settings violated the right to self-determination amongst individuals who may not be willing to live in community settings (Ginneá 2019). Similarly, due to variations in the definition of inclusion (Taub and Foster 2020), the emergence, rate of acceptance and development of a community-based support differ across time and country (Mansell and Beadle-Brown 2010). In addition, despite claims that a community-based service is cost effective (Mansell et al. 2007), other research would suggest they are more expensive (Braddock 2002).

Currently, there is a focus on the provision of person-centred support/practice in many countries. Whilst this has been defined in many ways, one helpful example is that offered by McCormack et al. (2020: 20), which states that such practice is 'underpinned by the core values of respect for personhood, authenticity, shared autonomy, respect, mutuality, therapeutic caring and healthfulness'. It can be seen that adoption of such an approach promotes a reciprocal relationship between those who provide services and those who are supported and recognises the importance of respect for the person and their autonomy. If this is translated into services and supports that reflect and respond to individual need, there is the potential to address some of the concerns highlighted in this chapter and to change societal perceptions to regard individuals with intellectual disabilities as valued citizens.

Changes Across the Lifespan

Models of care and support can also vary according to the age of individuals with intellectual disability. Intellectual disability is a lifelong condition and, as with their non-disabled peers, the support and care needs of people with intellectual disabilities vary across the lifespan. A person-centred approach to care and support (advocated above) requires that such changing needs are responded to in a person-centred manner. However, this can give rise to challenges regarding what is the most appropriate model of support and who should provide this.

When a child is identified as having an intellectual disability advice, information and support should be provided for them and their family. An important principle in relation to children with intellectual disabilities is that they are 'children first' and have the same needs and wishes as all other children (Dearing and Pallisera 2022). This means that, in relation to models of support, in many countries the focus is on including children with intellectual disabilities in generic children's services, be they health, social care or education (rather than providing support via specialist intellectual disability services). However, the complexity of some children's needs means they may require additional support or for services to be delivered in a different way.

The age at which a child is identified as having an intellectual disability will vary. Some will be identified at birth, whilst for others it may be a longer process that is only initiated as usual developmental milestones are delayed or missed. A formal diagnosis is usually provided by a paediatrician (Dearing and Pallisera 2022), and this should provide a basis for additional support where required. It will also usually mean that the child will continue to be monitored by children's health services until they reach adulthood. In relation to educational provision, then varying options may be available dependent on local provision, parental preference and the child's needs. These include mainstream education, mainstream education with additional support, a special unit within a mainstream school, special school provision or a mixed model approach with time spent in different settings (see Chap. 7).

Service systems, however, tend to be organised based on age groups and reference has been made to 'separate and compartmentalised' child and adult health services (Brown et al. 2018). Hence when young people reach the late teenage years, the transition to adult services needs to be negotiated by them and their families. This will include adult health (organised very differently to children's services) and social services as well as decisions being made as to future options for day-time occupation. Outside of service provision, it is also a time when young people need to negotiate new identities and relationships, and hence it can be challenging.

The transition to adult services has often been reported as being a negative experience (Brown et al. 2018), with families having to assume an advocacy role but with limited information (Brown et al. 2018) leaving them feeling unsupported (Codd and Hewitt 2020). Young people themselves also report that they lack information regarding their future options (Scanlon and Doyle 2021) (see Chap. 16).

As noted earlier in this chapter, the recorded prevalence of intellectual disabilities reduces during early adulthood (Hatton et al. 2016) since many do not make the transition to adult services. The reasons given above provide some insight into why this may be the case and why this can be a difficult period for both the young people and their families to negotiate. Calls have therefore been made for a more coordinated and collaborative approach to the provision of support (Brown et al. 2018; Codd and Hewitt 2020).

There are likely to be many transitions during the lifespan of people with intellectual disabilities, but to date, much of the research has focused on the post-school transition (Strnadova et al. 2021). However, another key transition that raises challenges concerning appropriate models of service provision is the transition to older adulthood.

Defining older adulthood amongst people with intellectual disabilities can be a difficult process since some of the social conventions that often mark this (such as retirement from employment) are often missing for this group of people. Another approach to defining this is what might be referred to as biological ageing (Northway et al. 2022), whereby the physiological and psychological deterioration that often accompanies the ageing process is used to identify 'old age'. People with intellectual disabilities (as with the non-disabled peers) will vary in terms of the age at which this occurs due to a range of physical, genetic, social and environmental factors. However, there is evidence that the ageing process often occurs earlier amongst people with intellectual disabilities with consensus that age-related health problems often occur during their 50s (Hermans and Evenhuis 2014).

The onset of age-related health problems often brings with it increased support needs such as adapted environments and additional personal care needs, which sometimes cannot be met within the individual's current place of residence. This then gives rise to discussions as to whether additional support can be provided in situ to enable 'ageing in place'. Where this is not possible, then decisions need to be made as to whether the most appropriate alternative provision should be a service for people with intellectual disabilities with higher support needs or general services for older adults (such as nursing homes). Both may have their challenges with intellectual disability services having limited knowledge of supporting older, frail individuals, whilst services for older people may have limited understanding of intellectual disabilities.

Conclusions

As can be seen from the discussion above, whilst key criteria have been agreed by which the presence of intellectual disabilities may be identified, how it is understood and perceived by others has changed over time and continues to vary within and between cultures. Indeed, at a given point in time, varying understandings may be present within a community. This can impact negatively on the lives of people with intellectual disabilities where, for example, they are subjected to discrimination and abuse. Indeed, at certain times attitudes and beliefs that perhaps were felt to be consigned to the past remerge, and hence there is a need to remain vigilant.

This then leads to consideration of what the future might hold. Whilst it is not possible to predict with certainty, we do know that the population of people with intellectual disabilities is likely to continue to grow as the survival of those with complex needs into adulthood increases and overall life expectancy extends. This will mean new challenges in terms of the support required, and these will occur in the context of global economic constraints that mean financial resources available are likely to be limited. This could be viewed as a very difficult future. However, if we look to the past, it will be seen that views can and do change and that increasingly people with intellectual disabilities and their allies are having a positive and significant impact. This provides hope for future, positive developments.

Key Concepts Discussed

- Understandings and concepts of intellectual disability across history and cultures
- Historical models of care
- Differing models of care across the lifespan
- Implications for future developments

References

Adams R (2007) Foundation of Health and Social Care. Palgrave Macmillan, Basingstoke

Ajuwon PM, Brown I (2012) Family quality of life in Nigeria. J Intellect Disabil Res 56(1):61–70. https://doi.org/10.1111/j.1365-2788.2011.01487.x

Aniek van Herwaarden E, Rommes WM, Peters-Scheffer NC (2021) Cultural competence in lifelong care and support for individuals with intellectual disabilities. Ethn Health 26(6):922–935. https://doi.org/10.1080/1 3557858.2019.1591348

BBC News On-Line (2021) 'Woman with Down's syndrome loses abortion law fight'. BBC news. https://www.bbc.com/news/uk-england-coventry-warwickshire-58662846. Accessed 20 Aug 2022

Berger PL, Luckmann T (1966) The social construction of reality: A treatise in the sociology of knowledge. Doubleday Anchor Books, Garden City, NY

Bjornsdottir K, Traustadottir R (2010) Stuck in the land of disability? The intersection of learning difficulties, class, gender and religion. Disabil Soc 25(1): 49–62

Braddock DL (2002) Public financial support for disability at the dawn of the 21st century. Am J Ment Retard 107:478–489

Brown M, Macarthur J, Higgins A, Chouliara Z (2018) Transitions from child to adult health care for young people with intellectual disabilities: A systematic review. J Adv Nurs 75:2418–2434

Bruininkis RH, Hauber FA, Hill BK, Lakin KC, Sigford BB, Wieck CA (1981) Summary findings of the 1978-1979 In-depth National Interview Survey of public and community residential facilities for mentally retarded persons. Minneapolis, Minnesota: University of Minnesota, Department of Psychoeducation Studies. Brief No. 5, 3(1): 1–20. Retrieved from the University of Minnesota Digital Conservancy. https://hdl.handle.net/11299/203362

Capri C, Abrahams L, McKenzie J, Coetzee O, Mkabile S, Saptouw M et al (2018) Intellectual disability rights and inclusive citizenship in South Africa: what can a scoping review tell us? Afr J Disabil 7:1–17. https://doi.org/10.4102/ajod.v7i0.396

Codd J, Hewitt O (2020) Having a son or daughter with an intellectual disability transition to adulthood: a parental perspective. Br J Learn Disabil 49:39–51

D'Andre R (1995) The development of cognitive anthropology. Cambridge University Press, Cambridge

Dearing M, Pallisera M (2022) Childhood. In: Atherton H, Crickmore D (eds) Intellectual disabilities towards inclusion. 7th edn. Elsevier, Scotland, pp 363–379

Emerson E (1992) What is normalisation? In: Brown H, Smith H (eds) Normalisation: A reader for the nineties. Routledge, London, pp 1–18

European Coalition for Community Living—ENIL (2013) Briefing on structural funds Investments for People with disabilities: achieving the transition from institutional care to community living. http://www.enil.eu/wp-content/uploads/2013/11/Structural-Fund-Briefing-final-WEB.pdf. Accessed 16 Sept 2022

Felce D (1997) Defining and applying the concept of quality of life. J Intellect Disabil Res 41:126–135

Ferndale D, Munro L, Watson B (2016) A discourse of "abnormality": exploring discussions of people living in Australia with deafness or hearing loss. J Am Ann Deaf 160(5):483–495

Flynn M (2012) Winterbourne view hospital: A serious case review. South Gloucestershire Council, Gloucestershire

Ginneá RN (2019) An exploratory study of the impact of a proposed move to dispersed housing on the perceptions and attitudes of family members of people with intellectual disabilities. Master's thesis. Limerick Institute of Technology, Ireland

Hatton C, Glover G, Emerson E, Brown I (2016) People with Learning Disabilities in England 2015: Main Report. https://assets.publishing.service.gov.uk/government/uploads/system/uploads/attachment_data/file/613182/PWLDIE_2015_main_report_NB090517.pdf. Accessed 08 Dec 2021

Health Service Executive (2011) Time to Move on from Congregated Settings: A Strategy for Community Inclusion. https://www.hse.ie/eng/services/list/4/disability/congregatedsettings. Accessed 6 Apr 2018

Hermans H, Evenhuis HM (2014) Multimorbidity in older adults with intellectual disabilities. Res Dev Disabil 35:776–783

Jarrett S, Tilley L (2022) The history of the history of learning disability. Br J Learn Disabil 50:132–142

Joint Committee on Human Rights (2008) A life like any other? Human rights of adults with learning disabilities. The Stationery Office, London

Keogh BK, Gallimore R, Weisner T (1997) A sociocultural perspective on learning and learning disabilities. Learn Disabil Res Pract 12(2):07–113

Kevles DJ (1999) Eugenics and human rights. Br Med J 319:435–438

Lafferty A, McConkey R, Simpson A (2012) Reducing the barriers to relationships and sexuality education for persons with intellectual disabilities. J Intellect Disabil 16(1):27–41

Mansell J (2006) Deinstitutionalisation and community living: Progress, problems and priorities. J Intellect Dev Disabil 31(2):65–76

Mansell JM, Knapp J, Beadle-Brown J, Beecham J (2007) Deinstitutionalisation and community living—outcomes and costs: report of a European study. Volume 2: Main Report. Tizard Centre, University of Kent, Canterbury

Mansell J, Beadle-Brown J, with members of the Special Interest Research Group on Comparative Policy and Practice (2010) Deinstitutionalisation and community living: position statement of the comparative policy and practice special interest research Group of the International Association for the scientific study of intellectual disabilities. J Intellect Disabil Res 54(2):104–112

McCarron M, Lombard-Vance R, Murphy E, O'Donovan M, Webb N, Sheaf G, McCallion P, Stancliffe R, Normand C, Smith V, May P (2018) Quality of life outcomes and costs associated with moving from congregated settings to community living arrangements for people with intellectual disability: an evidence review. Health Research Board, Dublin

McConkey R, Keogh F, Bunting B, Iriarte EG, Watson SF (2016) Relocating people with intellectual disability to new accommodation and support settings: contrasts between personalized arrangements and group home placements. J Intellect Disabil 20(2):109–120

McCormack B, McCance C, Martin S (2020) What is person centredness? In: McCormack B, McCance T, Bulley C, Brown D, McMillan A, Martin S (eds) Fundamentals of person-centred healthcare practice. Wiley Blackwell, Oxford, pp 13–22

Miller E, Cooper SA, Cook A, Petch A (2008) Outcomes important to people with intellectual disabilities. J Policy Pract Intellect Disabil 5:150–158

Morin D, Rivard M, Crocker AG, Boursier CP, Caron J (2013) Public attitudes towards intellectual disability: a multidimensional perspective. J Intellect Disabil Res 57(3):279–292

Murphy K, Bantry-White E (2021) Behind closed doors: human rights in residential care for people with an intellectual disability in Ireland. Disabil Soc 36(5):750–771. https://doi.org/10.1080/09687599.2020.1768052

Nes K, Demo H, Ianes D (2018) Inclusion at risk? Push- and pull-out phenomena in inclusive school systems: the Italian and Norwegian experiences. Int J Incl Educ 22:111–129. https://doi.org/10.1080/13603116.2017.1362045

Nirje B (1972) The right to self-determination. In: Wolfensberger W (ed) Normalization: the principle of normalization. National Institute on Mental Retardation, Toronto, ON, pp 176–200

Northway R, Wilson N, Rees S (2022) Growing older. In: Atherton H, Crickmore D (eds) Intellectual disabilities towards inclusion, 7th edn. Elsevier, London, pp 467–481

Oliver M (1984) The politics of disability. J Crit Soc Policy 4(11):21–32

Opoku MP, Elhoweris H, Jiya AN, Ngoh NA, Nketsia W, Kumi EO, Torgbenu EL (2021) Cross-national study of communal attitudes toward individuals with intellectual disabilities in sub-Saharan Africa: Cameroon vs. Ghana. PLoS One 16(9):e0257482. https://doi.org/10.1371/journal.pone.0257482

Reed J (2000) Monstrous knowledge: representing the national body in eighteenth-century Ireland. In: Deutsch H, Nussbaum F (eds) "Defects": engendering the modern body. University of Michigan Press, Ann Arbor, MI, pp 154–176

Ryan J, Thomas F (1987) The politics of mental handicap. Free Association Press, London

Scanlon G, Doyle A (2021) Transition stories: voices of school leavers with intellectual disabilities. Br J Learn Disabil 49:456–466

Schalock RL, Brown I, Brown R, Cummins RA, Felce D, Matikka L, Keith KD, Parmenter T (2002) Conceptualization, measurement, and application of quality of life for persons with intellectual disabilities: report of an international panel of experts. J Mental Retard 40(6):456–470

Scior K, Furnharm A (2011) Development and validation of the intellectual disability literacy scale for assessment of knowledge, beliefs and attitudes to intellectual disability. J Res Dev Disabil 32(5):1530–1541

Shakespeare T (1998) Choices and rights; Eugenics, genetics, and disability equality. Disabil Soc 13(5):665–681

Spicker P (2013) Personalisation falls short. Br J Soc Work 43:1259–1275

Starke M, Rosqvist HB, Kuosmanen J (2016) Eternal children? Professionals' constructions of women with an intellectual disability who are victims of sexual crime. J Sexual Disabil 34(3):315–328

Strnadova I, Loblinzk J, Wehmeyer M (2021) Transitions in the lives of people with intellectual disabilities. Br J Learn Disabil 49:263–270

Summers SJ, Jones J (2004) Cross-cultural working in community learning disabilities services: clinical issues, dilemmas and tensions. J Intellect Disabil Res 48(7):687–694

Taub D, Foster M (2020) Inclusion and intellectual disabilities: A cross cultural review of descriptions. Int Electron J Element Educ 12(3):275–281. https://doi.org/10.26822/iejee.2020358221

Thompson D, Fisher KR, Purcal C, Deeming C, Sawrikar P (2011) Community attitudes to people with disability: scoping project. Australian Government Department of Families, Community Services and Indigenous Affairs. Canberra, Australia. http://library.bsl.org.au/jspui/bitstream/1/2962/1/Community_attitudes_to_disability_accessible.pdf. Accessed 26 Oct 2022

Trent JW (1994) Inventing the feeble mind. A history of mental retardation in the United States. University of California Press, Berkeley, CA

United Nations (1975) United Nations declaration on the rights of disabled persons. United Nations, New York

United Nations (2006) The United Nations convention on the rights of people with disabilities. https://treaties.un.org/doc/Publication/CTC/Ch_IV_15.pdf. Accessed 26 Oct 2022

Venkatesan A (2017) Analysis of attributes in the official definitions for learning disability. Int J Indian Psychol 4(2):2349–3429

Wolfensberger W (1972) Normalization. The principle of normalization in human services. National Institute on Mental Retardation, Toronto, ON

Wolfensberger W (1983) Social role valorization: a proposed new term for the principle of normalization. J Mental Retard 21(6):234–239

Communication as a Basis for Person-Centred Support

Anne-Marie Martin and Victoria Jones

Chapter Topics

At the end of this chapter, the reader should:

- Understand that good quality, person-centred support occurs through effective communication.
- Recognise the importance of a rights-based approach in their communication and be able to consider the impact of the environment, culture and values on their practice.
- Be able to support the voice and choices of individuals with intellectual disabilities.
- Be aware of their responsibility as practitioners to promote self-advocacy and active listening.
- Be able to appreciate the importance of self-awareness, demonstrating respect, allowing time for communication processes and active listening.

Introduction

Communication is fundamental to humanity (McLeod 2018), an essential human need and a basic human right (Sen 2015). It is essential

A.-M. Martin (✉)
University College Cork, Cork, Ireland
e-mail: a.martin@ucc.ie

V. Jones
Aderdare, Wales, UK

to our expression, self-determination, sense of belonging and inclusion and in acknowledging the value of ourselves and others (McEwin and Santow 2018). Communication skills underpin positive social relationships and successful community inclusion along with education, employment and civic participation (Mulcair et al. 2018). Interpersonal communication has long been recognised as an essential component of person-centred care (Lund and Light 2007; Calculator 2009; McCormack and McCance 2010; Schwind et al. 2016). It is necessary for learning, forming relationships, social participation (Money et al. 2016) and expression of preferences and choices (Waters and Buchanan 2017).

Sharma et al. (2015) identified communication as one of the six common components of person-centred care: establishing a therapeutic relationship, shared power and responsibility, getting to know the person, empowering the person and trust and respect being the remainder. Effective person-centred practice is demonstrated through skilled interpersonal interactions that are focussed on understanding the person's needs, perceptions and motivations (Brown et al. 2016). Arguably, this places communication as a meta component of person-centred care because the other components occur through communication.

At the end of this chapter, the reader is invited to pause and reflect upon their communication. The questions can initially be considered

© The Author(s), under exclusive license to Springer Nature Switzerland AG 2023
F. Sheerin, C. Doyle (eds.), *Intellectual Disabilities: Health and Social Care Across the Lifespan*,
https://doi.org/10.1007/978-3-031-27496-1_2

regarding a person with whom the reader considers they have a strong relationship that is founded in good communication. A reader seeking more challenging opportunities for introspection and reflective practice would also benefit from considering the same questions regarding a different person with intellectual disability with whom their communication is less effective or the relationship less established.

The Right to Communicate

Communication as a fundamental right was first stated at international level in Article 19 of the Universal Declaration of Human Rights (1948):

> Everyone has the right to freedom of opinion and expression; this right includes freedom to hold opinions without interference and to seek, receive and impart information and ideas through any media and regardless of frontiers.—United Nations (UN) (1948)

Article 19 is a powerful statement in that it clearly states that all people, everyone, *'without distinction of any kind'* (UN 1948 Article 2), have the right to communicate. The right to freedom of opinion and expression is repeated in the *International Covenant on Civil and Political Rights* (UN 1966), the *Convention on the Rights of the Child* (UN 1989) and the *Convention on the Rights of Persons with Disabilities* (UN 2006).

People with intellectual disability can experience difficulties exercising their right to communicate due to communication difficulties and social or environmental barriers (Mulcair et al. 2018). The *Convention on the Rights of Persons with Disabilities (UNCRPD)* (UN 2006) came about in recognition of this and to effect change in attitudes and approaches towards this group. The UNCRPD reaffirms that people with disability must enjoy all human rights and fundamental freedoms that promote respect for their inherent dignity (UN 2006). It is built on principles of inclusion, equality, respect and non-discrimination. Article 21 (UN 2006) specifically focusses on communication rights.

Freedom of expression and opinion and access to information

> States Parties shall take all appropriate measures to ensure that persons with disabilities can exercise the right to freedom of expression and opinion, including the freedom to seek, receive and impart information and ideas on an equal basis with others and through all forms of communication of their choice, as defined in article 2 of the present Convention… (UN 2006)

There is a strong mandate for the European Union and its member states to improve the lives of persons with disabilities, and it is everyone's responsibility to take the necessary steps to do so. Person-centred practice based in optimal communication practices offers a clear pathway to facilitate these rights.

From an intellectual disability and health perspective, The European Declaration on the Health of Children and Young People with Intellectual Disabilities and their Families (WHO Regional Office for Europe 2010) sets out ten priorities for action to uphold the rights of this group. Priority no. 7 is particularly pertinent in relation to communication, decision-making and person-centred care. It states…

> Empower children and young people with intellectual disabilities to contribute to decision-making about their lives.
>
> Children and young people with intellectual disabilities can and will make their needs and wishes known and contribute to their community, given appropriate support and a receptive environment. Family members and advocates also need encouragement and support to make themselves heard.— (WHO Regional Office for Europe 2010)

It is unanimous, clear and unquestionable that people with intellectual disability have an internationally established right to communication and social inclusion. The right to understand what is communicated, express one's own thoughts, desires and needs and being able to relate to others is undisputed (Tabacaru 2016). Fulfilment of this right for people with intellectual disability requires skilled communication partners who communicate in a person-centred way and who recognise, respect and promote their partners rights, autonomy, individuality and culture.

Communication, Culture and Person Centredness

All human communication occurs in a cultural context. This requires an ethical practitioner to consider the culture they themselves bring. This is in addition to attending to the culture of the people and families they seek to be person centred with and the systems in which they practice. Each person has a cultural identity that has been influenced by a wealth of factors including their community, food, spirituality, language, religion, rites of passage throughout life and family heritage, amongst many others (Purnell 2012). In order to engage with an individual, and their family, in ways that are person centred, it is vital to be thoughtful about how culture can, and does, impact and influence what is done, with whom and how. Each person's (both the 'helped' and the 'helper's') cultural background shapes and creates concepts of norms and establishes their expectations of others. These norms and expectations, in turn, shape and influence what we can make possible, through communication, in our practice.

Person-centred communication begins before we meet a person, for example, the information that is developed to promote services, including the images and languages within it; referral systems and assessment tools and how accessible they are; the design of buildings and whether they communicate 'you are welcome here', 'you are valued' and 'this is a place for you'; the smile that greets someone to a service for the first or tenth time; or the way that professionals describe the interventions that they offer.

Inclusive communication is an approach that seeks to promote equality through addressing the communication culture and environment in communities and services. It recognises that professionals must make shifts in their attitudes and approach to communication to ensure that every person has the best opportunities to communicate and be heard. As communication partners it is our role to create an optimal environment for a person's views and wishes to be sought, expressed, truly heard and responded to effectively. This requires us to value every possible mode of communication as equal, for example, not to prioritise speech over other modes of communication such as signing, symbols, photographs, gestures, objects, eye gaze, expressions, routines, behaviour or technologies and to ensure that we align our communication with the abilities and needs of the individual (Money et al. 2016).

A significant proportion of human interaction also occurs in language. In the diverse communities of the twenty-first century, person-centred communication practice must also attend to considerations of language. People encode and construct their sense of the world and their memories, emotions and identities in the languages in which they experienced them (Costa 2021). For a person who does not use speech, it may be easier for them to connect with these aspects of themselves in the language they grew up with. Thus, if we are not to silence a person's sense of self and deskill them, person-centred communication may also require us to become familiar with the language a person knows best or work with others who are.

Interpersonal Communication for Person-Centred Care

Interactions with people with intellectual disability have been found to be influenced by the approach of people supporting them (Bradley et al. 2020). People with intellectual disability often make decisions with other people, and therefore, it is important to have a supporter who recognises a person's individuality, who listens to them and who supports the translation of this information into specific and concrete steps towards realising their goals and living a fulfilled life. Williams and Porter (2017) demonstrated that people with intellectual disability identified the important role of a support person facilitating individuals to not only express their choices but build their confidence to decide.

Skilled and Reflexive Advocates Facilitating Person-Centred Care

Listening to the person with intellectual disability is foundational and fundamental to planning person-centred care. Responding to and enacting these preferences is foundational and fundamental to realising it. Listening and responding are essential communication skills. An effective listener and responder is reflexive, respectful and patient, taking the time to actively listen and observe the person with intellectual disability in order to support, plan and facilitate their person-centred care.

Reflexivity/Self-Awareness

Self-awareness is an important component of an interpersonal relationship that influences how a person uses their own insight and presence to communicate in an original and authentic way (Turan 2018). A skilled communicator needs to be aware of their own characteristics, behaviours, reactions and attitudes (Rasheed and Parveen 2015) and how these influence those they communicate with. It requires introspection to bring these from the subconscious to the conscious to develop the skills, behaviours and attitudes necessary to communicate openness and willingness to listen, understand and respect the perspective and individuality of the person with intellectual disability. Much emphasis is placed on reflexivity and reflective practice as a means of becoming self-aware (Phelvin 2013). Reflection is a process of stepping back, observing an incident or encounter and understanding and evaluating it as a means of developing insight and understanding for future encounters (Bennett-Levy et al. 2001). Todd (2005) uses the idea of an internal supervisor as a metaphor to explain the dialogue that takes place within a person's consciousness whilst engaged in reflective practice, such as questioning personal bias and subjectivity to gain a more objective perspective. Reflection enables recognition and exploration of the key aspects of effective communication in an encounter to become more aware of how verbal and non-verbal communication can affect an encounter (Tregoning 2015).

Another technique used to enhance person-centred communication involves taking time to reflect upon how we form relationships and the ways in which we communicate with each other. This is called relational reflexivity and refers to the efforts made by two people to nurture and sustain a relationship that has therapeutic potential. It relates to every step of the ways in which we come together to discover and learn about how we can best relate with each other (Burnham 2005). In other words, our collaborative and coproduced person-centred practice should begin with, and be sustained by, continuous efforts to create a framework for how we will communicate together.

For example, how does this person like to communicate? When is the best time of the day to see them? What sort of space is likely to enable them to feel the most able to engage? Asking, 'whilst we are together what word would you (or the people who support you) like to use for this?' When you look like that I wonder if you are feeling sad about it? Or noticing that when I lower the tone of my voice this person seems to be more able to show me what they want. Finally, after spending time with a person, relational reflexivity invites us to reflect on what we have learned about what works and does not work in our communication together and share this information for the benefit of the individual and the whole system around them. Relationally reflexive processes such as these are especially important when we are in a therapeutic relationship with a person whose voice may not have been heard or attended to previously as is so often the case for many people with intellectual impairments (Jones 2019).

Respect

Respect is a value and a guiding principle of person-centred care. Tondora et al. (2020) repeatedly emphasise the importance of respect in terms of the way we engage with a person, respecting the communication preferences of the person and respecting their priorities and preferences for their lives. In a study by Petner-Arrey and Copeland (2015), people with intellectual disability and their support workers discussed the importance of respect in interactions. These participants asserted that respect and person-centred care are demonstrated through communication; communicating respect, listening for and attending to what is important to the person with intellectual disability and taking action to realise those aspirations (Petner-Arrey and Copeland 2015).

In a similar vein, participants in a study by Cummins et al. (2020) called for those supporting them to recognise and respect their communication preferences. They asserted that verbal communication may not always be possible or that supports such as clarification or repetition may be required (Cummins et al. 2020).

Failing to respect the person's communication preferences can contribute to several problems such as the risk of misguided tokenism (Thurman et al. 2005). Further, Hare et al. (2011) discuss how everyday communication between staff and people with intellectual disabilities can involve power and reciprocity imbalances that result in the person not being listened to. People with intellectual disability have expressed their concerns in this regard including feeling vulnerable or disempowered to be assertive (Cummins et al. 2020), their voices and preferences not being listened to or their rights to dignity and to make choices not being respected (Petner-Arrey and Copeland 2015).

Therefore, truly person-centred care is respectful of the person, their means and methods of communicating and their expressed preferences. That respect is demonstrated through communication and interactions.

Patience and Time

Patience and time are needed to actively listen and hear the person's choices and preferences to provide truly person-centred care. The importance of taking time to get to know the person

with intellectual disability and to establish and maintain a therapeutic relationship is well recognised (Jaques et al. 2018).

Spending time with a person is important to building a relationship, understanding their perspective and learning about their preferences and goals. Interactions with people with intellectual disability can take time due to difficulties with expression and comprehension experienced by both parties to the interaction. The availability and use of time, therefore, require careful and conscious consideration. The importance of time is not an issue to be dismissed or discounted as an obvious consideration. Research has shown that the influence of time on interactions may be recognised by interaction partners but does not translate easily into practice (Stans et al. 2018). Consequently, this seemingly obvious consideration continues to be an important priority for effective person-centred support.

Active Listening

Active listening refers to a person's willingness and ability to attend to all aspects and levels of communication including the verbal and non-verbal elements, perceiving explicit and implied messages (Van Servellen 2009). It challenges the notion that listening is a passive process and rather is an active process that involves attending to and noticing the plethora of expressive communication methods, reflecting on and showing genuine interest in what this conveys and making every attempt to understand the person's perspective (Bottomley and Pryjmachuk 2019). As interactions with people with intellectual disability often rely on non-verbal methods of communicating, the need for skilled communicators who recognise, attend to and understand their expressions is critical and has been identified as a key factor influencing quality of life (García et al. 2020). As previously mentioned, person-centred care cannot occur without active listening as it is how the choices, preferences and perspectives of the person with intellectual disability become known.

Advocacy

Advocacy is the process of standing alongside a person to ensure that they have voice, choice and, as much as possible, control in the decisions that affect their lives. In this context, voice refers to the myriad ways in which a person might communicate their views and wishes, for example, through vocalising, behaviour or inaction. Advocacy promotes, protects and defends the human rights of people with intellectual disabilities (Australian Government 2018). It is inherently intertwined with McCormack et al. (2020) values of person-centred practice, as both incorporate respect for personhood, shared autonomy, respect and mutuality. Advocacy and person-centred practice reinforce and enhance each other. It is not possible for practice to be person centred without attending to assuring relationships and service environments where advocacy can flourish. These relational processes all occur through communication.

The goal of advocacy is to support an individual to advocate for themselves as much as possible. This is known as self-advocacy. Supporting self-advocacy might involve augmenting the decision-making process, working with an individual to enhance their understanding of the elements of an issue from their perspective, helping a person to prepare for an important meeting, enabling them to weigh up the pros and cons of any given decision that may affect them or having a better understanding of their rights. For a group of people who are likely to need longer to process and consider a decision, such skills may need developing daily from childhood, throughout adulthood and into older age. Effective person-centred practice ensures that people are supported to make the same choices as their similarly aged peers, for example, by engaging people's views in choosing what to wear, how they will spend their day, whether to have coffee/juice or which piece of fruit to have from the fruit bowl. Such daily practices of communicating choice (involving active listening on the part of those around the individual) create possibilities for bigger decisions, such as where to live, who to date or how to spend income, to be made *with* a person rather than *for* them.

The entire process of advocacy is embedded in effective and inclusive communication. Often people with intellectual disabilities are very skilled at communicating, for example, that they do not like something, are really happy in a particular place or thrive when they are with a special person, but the professionals and services around that person are not responsive to their communication. No amount of support to build communication skills and decision-making by a person with intellectual disability will be effective if the people in power around that person do not know how to listen to them. It is unethical to support a person to have a voice, or make a choice, if their communication is going to be ignored. Indeed, this could be the most effective way to ensure that they give up trying to communicate altogether. Thus, effective person-centred practice necessarily demands that practitioners address enhancing the communication and advocacy environment around an individual by ensuring that the people in their wider system know how to 'listen' to their preferred methods of communication and then to actively respond.

There are also occasions when the role of an advocate may be to speak on behalf of an individual. Professionals who work with a group of people who are frequently marginalised and whose voice may be diminished, as is so often the case for women and men with intellectual disability, are often invited to assume the role of advocate. Whilst it is the responsibility of every person-centred practitioner to consider how they support the voices and choice-making skills of the people they support, it is equally necessary to recognise that, despite their best endeavours, supporters are often compromised when it comes to advocating effectively. For example, this might be because they know the competing needs of other people who use the service or because it is difficult to argue against the wishes of a manager or employer. These conflicts of interest can be avoided by referring the person being supported to an independent advocate who is 'structurally, financially, and psychologically free from interests such as being a provider of services, a gatekeeper of services, a funder of services, a statutory body or family and friends' (Scottish Independent Advocacy Alliance 2019:16).

Many nations have independent advocacy services that citizens are legally entitled to access. In a systematic review of the evidence supporting independent advocacy, Townsley et al. (2009) highlighted the need for further research regarding its impact on outcomes. However, they found good-quality evidence to suggest that independent advocacy, based upon a rapport built over time, can enable severely disabled young people to 'direct' an advocate to represent them effectively (Sounds Good Project 2006). Additionally, they found that independent advocacy has the potential to alter patterns of communication; improve communication between a person, their family and professionals; and empower young people and disabled parents to feel engaged (Townsley et al. 2009). Being an effective, person-centred communicator involves knowing both when and how to seek out independent advocacy alongside, or on behalf of, a person with intellectual disabilities. Indeed, consistently promoting a person-centred service culture and ethos may well be the best advocacy many professionals can provide.

Conclusion

It is clear that to communicate in truly person-centred ways we must consider the cultural backgrounds of each person who participates in a given communication interaction, the cultural environment in which the interaction occurs and the culture of communication in our practice, our services and our communities. As professional communication partners, it is the responsibility of practitioners to adapt their skills and expertise to enhance the communication culture of the people whom they serve. This benefits everyone.

Key Concepts Discussed
- Person-centred support occurs through communication. This places communication processes as the foundation or 'meta-component' of effective person-centred care.
- Skilled, person-centred practitioners will apply a rights-based approach in their communication, exploring the impact of the environment, culture and values on their practice.

- The duty to support the voice and choices of individuals with intellectual disabilities includes the responsibility of practitioners to promote self-advocacy and active listening.
- The essential skills of self-awareness, demonstrating respect, allowing time for communication processes and active listening must be considered.
- Good communication is everybody's responsibility and fundamental to the good life that person-centred support seeks to assure.

Questions to Promote Reflective Person-Centred Communication Support
Thinking about a person you support and know well, consider…

1. What do I bring to our communication?
   - What aspects of my cultural heritage are different from theirs or their family? How might this affect our communication? What assumptions do I make about this person or their family? What do I need to learn or discover about them and myself to be culturally relevant in my support?
   - What languages/dialects/vocabulary do they use at home? What is the best language for this person to feel safe, contained and understood? What vocabulary do I need to learn? Do we need to work with a translator?
2. Active listening…
   - How do I know when they like, dislike, want or do not want something?
   - How do I adapt my communication to assist them to communicate more effectively?
   - When was the last time I really listened to them through attending to their vocalisations, gestures, eye

gaze, breathing rate, body movement, smile, etc.?

- In what circumstances with this person can my communication sometimes become less effective, respectful or patient? Do I always allow enough time for us to communicate effectively? How might I address this?

3. The communication environment...
   - How do I show this person that I value their communication?
   - How do I share what I know about this person's communication and find out what others have learned about them?
   - How do I ensure that the people spending time with this person can read their communication? How and where is this knowledge recorded, e.g. through descriptions, photos, videos, etc.?
   - In what ways does our service show the public that we value all forms of communication?
   - How does my service show all of our community that they are welcome?

4. Advocacy...
   - How do I help this person to make choices in their daily life?
   - How often have I prioritised someone else's needs or wishes (mine, another client, another staff member, their relatives, the service managers) over what I thought this person might choose for themselves?
   - What structural, financial or psychological factors might create a conflict of interest for me in supporting this person's communications? For which issues may this be especially relevant?
   - If I wanted to refer this person to an independent advocate, how would I do so?

- In what ways might this person's communication benefit from the specialist assessment and intervention that a speech and language specialist could provide? How might we consult such a professional?

We invite you to repeat this exercise whilst thinking about a person with whom you are less confident communicating.

References

Australian Government (2018) Disability advocacy what is disability advocacy and why is it important? https://www.dss.gov.au/sites/default/files/documents/12_2018/disability-advocacy-fact-sheet.pdf. Accessed 2 Apr 2022

Bennett-Levy J, Turner F, Beaty T, Smith M, Paterson B, Farmer S (2001) The value of self-practice of cognitive therapy techniques and self-reflection in the training of cognitive therapists. Behav Cogn Psychother 29:203–220

Bottomley J, Pryjmachuk S (2019) Communication skills for your nursing degree. Critical Publishing, St. Albans

Bradley S, Crawford H, Nozedar H (2020) Communication. In: Heslop P, Hebron C (eds) Promoting the health and Well-being of people with learning disabilities. Springer, Cham

Brown M, Chouliara Z, MacArthur J, McKechanie A, Mack S, Hayes M, Fletcher J (2016) The perspectives of stakeholders of intellectual disability liaison nurses: A model of compassionate, person-centred care. J Clin Nurs 25(7–8):972–982. https://doi.org/10.1111/jocn.13142

Burnham J (2005) Relational reflexivity: A tool for socially constructing therapeutic relationships. In: Flaskas C, Mason B, Perlesz A (eds) The space between: experience, context, and process in the therapeutic relationship. Karnac Books, London, pp 1–17

Calculator SN (2009) Augmentative and alternative communication (AAC) and inclusive education for students with the most severe disabilities. Int J Incl Educ 13(1):93–113. https://doi.org/10.1080/13603110701284656

Costa B (2021) Psychological therapies in a multilingual world: building the confidence of psychological therapists to work across languages. In: de Medeiros A, Kelly D (eds) Language debates. Theory and reality in language learning, teaching and research. John Murray Learning/Hodder and Stoughton, London, pp 209–220

Cummins C, Pellicano E, Crane L (2020) Autistic adults' views of their communication skills and needs. Int

J Lang Commun Disord 55:678–689. https://doi.org/10.1111/1460-6984.12552

García JC, Díez E, Wojcik DZ, Santamaría M (2020) Communication support needs in adults with intellectual disabilities and its relation to quality of life. Int J Environ Res Public Health 17(20):7370. https://doi.org/10.3390/ijerph17207370

Hare DJ, Searson R, Knowles R (2011) Real listening—using personal construct assessment with people with intellectual disabilities: two case studies. Br J Learn Disabil 39:190–197. https://doi.org/10.1111/j.1468-3156.2010.00650.x

Jaques H, Lewis P, O'Reilly K, Wiese M, Wilson NJ (2018) Understanding the contemporary role of the intellectual disability nurse: A review of the literature. J Clin Nurs 27(21–22):3858–3871. https://doi.org/10.1111/jocn.14555

Jones V (2019) Relational reflexivity: talking about how we do talking and being together. In: Jones V, Haydon-Laurelut M (eds) Working with people with learning disabilities: systemic approaches. Red Globe, London, pp 290–294

Lund SK, Light J (2007) Long-term outcomes for individuals who use augmentative and alternative communication: part III-contributing factors. Augment Altern Commun 23(4):323–335. https://doi.org/10.1080/07434610600720442

McCormack B, McCance TV (2010) Person-centred nursing: theory and practice. Wiley-Blackwell, Chichester. https://doi.org/10.1002/9781444390506

McCormack B, McCance C, Martin S (2020) What is person centredness? In: McCormack B, McCance T, Bulley C, Brown D, McMillan A, Martin S (eds) Fundamentals of person-centred healthcare practice. Wiley Blackwell, Oxford, pp 13–22

McEwin A, Santow E (2018) The importance of the human right to communication. Int J Speech Lang Pathol 20(1):1–2

McLeod S (2018) Communication rights: fundamental human rights for all. Int J Speech Lang Pathol 20(1):3–11

Money D, Hartley K, McAnespie L, Crocker A, Mander C, Elliot A, Burnett CA, Hazel G, Bayliss R, Beazley S, Tucker S (2016) Inclusive communication and the role of speech and language therapy. Royal College of Speech and Language Therapists Position Paper, RCSLT, London. www.rcslt.org

Mulcair G, Pietranton AA, Williams C (2018) The international communication project: raising global awareness of communication as a human right. Int J Speech Lang Pathol 20(1):34–38

Petner-Arrey J, Copeland SR (2015) 'You have to care.' perceptions of promoting autonomy in support settings for adults with intellectual disability. Br J Learn Disabil 43:38–48. https://doi.org/10.1111/bld.12084

Phelvin A (2013) Getting the message: intuition and reflexivity in professional interpretations of non-verbal behaviours in people with profound learning disabilities. Br J Learn Disabil 41:31–37. https://doi.org/10.1111/j.1468-3156.2011.00719.x

Purnell LD (2012) The Purnell model for cultural competence. In: Purnell L (ed) Transcultural health care: A culturally competent approach. FA Davis, Philadelphia PA, pp 15–44

Rasheed SP, Parveen S (2015) Self-awareness as a therapeutic tool for nurse/client relationship. Int J Caring Sci 8(1):211–216

Schwind JK, McCay E, Metersky K, Martin J (2016) Development and implementation of an advanced therapeutic communication course: an interprofessional collaboration. J Nurs Educ 55(10):592–597. https://doi.org/10.3928/01484834-20160914-11

Scottish Independent Advocacy Alliance (2019) Independent Advocacy Principles, Standards & Code of Best Practice. Edinburgh. https://www.siaa.org.uk/wp-content/uploads/2021/02/SIAA-Principles-Final-2nd-print-run-with-ISBN.pdf. Accessed 2 Apr 2022

Sen AF (2015) Communication and human rights. Procedia Soc Behav Sci 174:2813–2817

Sharma T, Bamford M, Dodman D (2015) Person-centred care: an overview of reviews. Contemp Nurse 51(2):107–120. https://doi.org/10.1080/10376178.2016.1150192

Sounds Good Project (2006) Growing up, speaking out. A guide to advocacy for young learning disabled people at transition (14–25 years). Advocacy Resource Exchange, Southampton

Stans SEA, Dalemans RJP, Roentgen UR, Smeets HWH, Anna JHMB (2018) Who said dialogue conversations are easy? The communication between communication vulnerable people and health-care professionals: A qualitative study. Health Expect 21(5):848–857. https://doi.org/10.1111/hex.12679

Tabacaru CD (2016) Verbal and nonverbal communication of students with severe and profound disabilities. Res Pedagogy 6(2):111–119

Thurman S, Jones J, Tarleton B (2005) Without words meaningful information for people with high individual communication needs. Br J Learn Disabil 33(2):83–89. https://doi.org/10.1111/j.1468-3156.2005.00342.x

Todd G (2005) Reflective practice and Socratic dialogue. In: Johns C, Freshwater D (eds) Transforming nursing through reflective practice. Chapter 4, 2nd edn. Blackwell, London

Tondora J, Croft B, Kardell Y, Camacho-Gonsalves T, Kwak M (2020) Five competency domains for staff who facilitate person-centered planning. National Center on Advancing Person-Centered Practices and Systems, Cambridge, MA

Townsley R, Marriott A, Ward L (2009) Access to independent advocacy: an evidence review. Office for Disability Issues, Bristol

Tregoning C (2015) Communication skills and enhancing clinical practice through reflective learning: A case study. Br J Healthcare Assistants 9(2):66–69. https://doi.org/10.12968/bjha.2015.9.2.66

Turan N (2018) Chapter 31: self-awareness in the nurse-patient relationship. In: Alexandrova E, Shapekova NL, Ak B, Ozcanaslan F (eds) Health sciences research in the globalizing world. St. Kliment Ohridski University Press, Sofia, pp 270–278

United Nations (1948) Universal declaration of human rights. http://www.un.org/en/universal-declaration-human-rights/. Accessed 14 Feb 2022

United Nations (1966) International Covenant on Civil and Political Rights. https://www.ohchr.org/en/professionalinterest/pages/ccpr.aspx. Accessed 14 Feb 2022

United Nations (1989) Convention on the Rights of the Child. https://www.ohchr.org/en/professionalinterest/pages/crc.aspx. Accessed 14 Feb 2022

United Nations (2006) Convention on the Rights of Persons with Disabilities. https://www.un.org/development/desa/disabilities/convention-on-the-rights-of-persons-with-disabilities.html. Accessed 14 Feb 2022

Van Servellen G (2009) Communication skills for the health care professional: concepts, practice, and evidence. Jones and Bartlett Publishers, Sudbury, MA

Waters RA, Buchanan A (2017) An exploration of person-centred concepts in human services: A thematic analysis of the literature. Health Policy (Amsterdam) 121(10):1031–1039. https://doi.org/10.1016/j.healthpol.2017.09.003

Williams V, Porter S (2017) The meaning of 'choice and control' for people with intellectual disabilities who are planning their social care and support. J Appl Res Intellect Disabil 30:97–108. https://doi.org/10.1111/jar.12222

World Health Organization Regional Office for Europe (2010) European declaration on the health of children and young people with intellectual disabilities and their families. Better Health, Better Lives https://apps.who.int/iris/handle/10665/108010. Accessed 14 Feb 2022

Care and Support in a Multi/Interdisciplinary Context

3

Aud Elisabeth Witsø and Mary-Ann O'Donovan

Chapter Topics

After reading this chapter, the reader should have knowledge about:

- The differences between multi- and interdisciplinary ways of working
- The importance of interdisciplinary services for people with intellectual disability
- The translation and comparison of collaborative policy and practice in two cases—Norway and Australia (NSW)
- Recommendations for future multi- and interdisciplinary care models for people with intellectual disability

Approaches to including people with intellectual disability as key members of the healthcare team.

A. E. Witsø (✉)
Norwegian University of Science and Technology, Department of Mental Health, The National Institute on Intellectual Disability and Community (NAKU), Trondheim, Norway
e-mail: aud.e.witso@ntnu.no

M.-A. O'Donovan
Centre for Disability Studies, Affiliate of the University of Sydney, Sydney, Australia
e-mail: mary-ann.odonovan@sydney.edu.au

Introduction

Public health and social services for people with intellectual disability face multiple challenges to effective collaboration and coordination. Professional knowledge within services has become increasingly specialised and coherence is difficult to handle. To have professionals from different disciplines working together in service provision for people with disability is regarded as the most effective approach to promote holistic development across life domains (Rapport et al. 2004). However, collaboration does not happen automatically, and guidance is needed to facilitate effective interdisciplinary care, as well as a cultural shift within healthcare institutions.

It is also naïve to assume that health professionals have access to appropriate training and skill development to work specifically with the population of people with intellectual disability. The work of Trollor et al. (2016, 2018) highlighted inadequate intellectual disability content at a tertiary level and within recognised professional development across medical and nursing qualifications in Australia.

In addition to promoting and guiding health practitioners in how to work in an interdisciplinary way, and ensuring curriculum adequately addresses the specific health and communication needs of people with intellectual disability, the authors argue that core to interdisciplinary

© The Author(s), under exclusive license to Springer Nature Switzerland AG 2023
F. Sheerin, C. Doyle (eds.), *Intellectual Disabilities: Health and Social Care Across the Lifespan*,
https://doi.org/10.1007/978-3-031-27496-1_3

working is the inclusion of the voice and perspective of the person with intellectual disability.

In this chapter, we will explore current discrepancies and misunderstandings with key terminology guiding collaborative working in the health setting, outline why multi- and interdisciplinary working is important to meet the needs of people with intellectual disability and propose some ways to include people with intellectual disability as key members of these teams. Descriptive case studies of two settings, Norway and Australia (specifically NSW), are presented with the intention of exploring the translation of collaborative policy in practice in two settings and comparing similarities and differences across these jurisdictions. Recommendations for future multi- and interdisciplinary care models for people with intellectual disability will be made.

What Is and What Is the Purpose of Multi- and Interdisciplinarity?

There are many terms used to describe collaborative working arrangements between professionals (Xyrichis and Lowton 2008). Frequently mentioned forms of collaboration between disciplines in the literature are multi- and interprofessional teams and multi-, inter- and transdisciplinarity (Collin 2009). These terms are often used interchangeably in the literature to refer to different types of teams and different processes within them (Nancarrow et al. 2013). Multidisciplinary processes are characterised by different groups of professionals working independently to illuminate a problem and within their own disciplinary boundaries. Bell et al. (2010) define multidisciplinary approaches as typical medical model-based teams, with limited communication between involved professionals. Multidisciplinary collaboration can be suitable when a person with intellectual disability has problems that are delineated and can be considered effectively isolated from each other. This is often rare in people with intellectual disability, particularly as people age and complexity increases.

Multidisciplinarity can be regarded as a condition for interdisciplinarity. However,

interdisciplinary approaches differ from multidisciplinarity and are characterised by bridge-building amongst professionals from different disciplines (Collin 2009) working together in interactive ways to achieve a coordinated and coherent whole (Rapport et al. 2004). Interdisciplinary approaches are considered suitable when problems are complex and intertwined. A transdisciplinary approach occurs when professionals collaborate from the beginning to develop a holistic intervention plan based on the individual's needs, rather than on the professional expertise (Bell et al. 2010). The three concepts do not involve user involvement per se, but including the person and their supporters at the centre of planning and service provision is both a right (UN 2006) and a prerequisite for successful goal setting and attainment in service provision (Doherty et al. 2020).

There are several purposes of inter- and transdisciplinary collaboration. One purpose is to illuminate problems and situations from different angles to see interactions and coherence. The aim with these approaches is not to find simple solutions to problems or to ascribe results to single therapy forms or singular actions (Bredland et al. 2011). Inter- and transdisciplinary collaboration processes aim to coordinate effort and secure consensus. There is a strong emphasis on shared information so that all disciplines in the collaboration process work together to reach the goals of and best outcomes for the individual. This is the person-centred nature of inter- and transdisciplinary care. However, this does not mean that all the collaborating professionals are present at the same time with the person with intellectual disability. For instance, even though a family doctor may not have as frequent contact with a patient as other partners may have in daily service provision, it is recommended that he/she should be defined as part of the interdisciplinary team and communication flow. This is also applicable for other professionals that provide less frequent services but where actions are important for achieving the person's goals, such as physiotherapists and pharmacists (The Norwegian Health Directorate 2017).

Competence is an important subject related to multi- and interdisciplinarity. Multiple professionals with education at bachelor and higher levels are relevant in multi- and interdisciplinary collaboration in services for persons with intellectual disability, from health professionals like intellectual disability nurses, occupational therapists, physiotherapists and clinical nutritionists, community pharmacists and family doctors to professionals within social work and special education (Bobbette et al. 2020). A fundamental problem seems however to be low levels of curriculum content that focus on intellectual disability.

Only a few European countries provide specialist education and training options for working with people with intellectual or other cognitive disabilities. According to Jaques et al. (2018), the United Kingdom and Ireland are the only twenty-first-century jurisdictions to have a specialist preregistration programme for intellectual disability nursing. There is also the Norwegian social educator programme, which is comparable to the intellectual disability nursing programme, a certified health professional bachelor-level education with people with intellectual disability

and complex needs as the key focus population (Grung 2016). In Australia, many nurses work in services for people with intellectual disability but without specialisation within intellectual disability (Jaques et al. 2018). Social workers are also recognised as core in working with adults with intellectual and developmental disability in system navigation roles and case management of complex health and social issues (Bobbette et al. 2021). No single profession can fill the roles and competence needed in quality health and social care for people with intellectual disability. However, one may argue that specialised professions in intellectual disability have important roles to recognise, initialise and contribute to multi- and interdisciplinary collaboration (Fig. 3.1).

Teamworking is often used in conjunction with the concepts of multi- and interdisciplinarity (Nancarrow et al. 2013). Although there is no single way to provide or accomplish multi- and interdisciplinary collaboration, there are some general recommendations to be found in the literature.

Fig. 3.1
Recommendations for interdisciplinary teamwork (source: adapted from Nancarrow et al. (2013) and The Norwegian Health Directorate (2021))

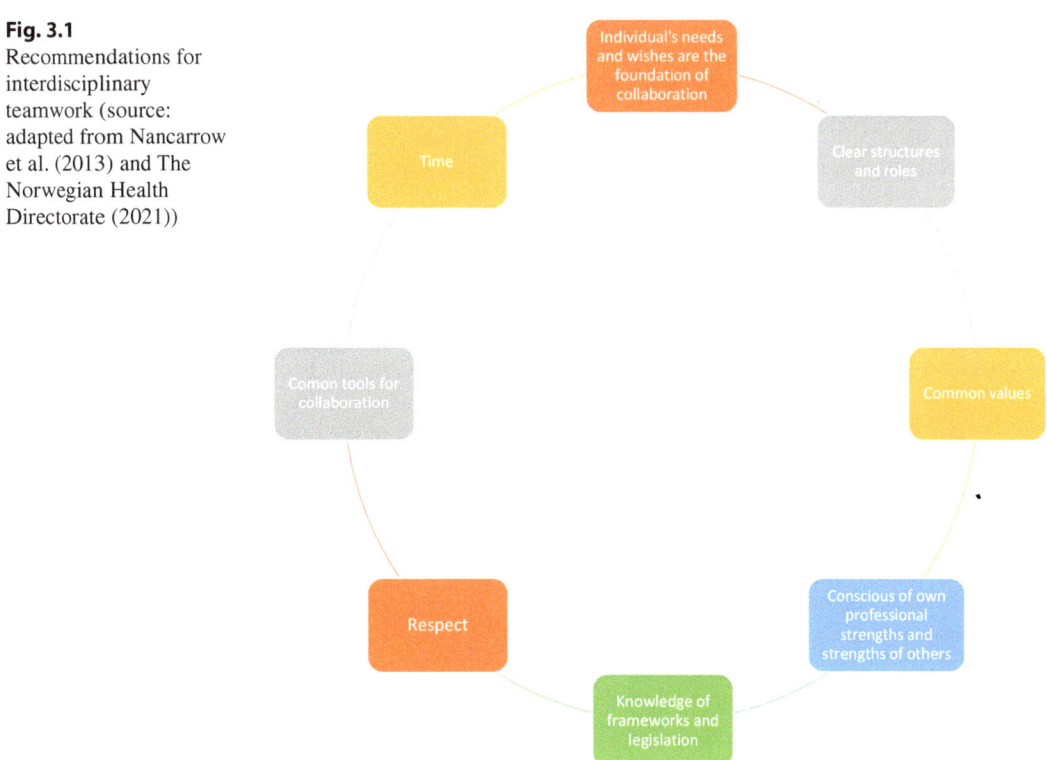

Why Should Service Provision for People with Intellectual Disability Be Interdisciplinary?

People with intellectual disability experience higher rates of multi-morbidity, when compared with the general population (McCarron et al. 2011, 2017). Multi-morbidity refers to the presence of two or more chronic conditions. In the Netherlands, 47% of the population of people with intellectual disability were found to have four or more chronic conditions (Hermans and Evenhuis 2014). In addition to greater morbidity, people with intellectual disability are at higher risk of mortality (Trollor et al. 2017; Reppermund et al. 2019), and due to persistent health inequities that exist at a system, access and utilisation level, people with intellectual disability are at greater risk of early mortality and death due to preventable causes (Reppermund et al. 2019).

Life expectancy has increased (Reppermund et al. 2019) and with this increased life expectancy we have had the opportunity to understand how people with intellectual disability age. People with intellectual disability are one of the most frail population groups (Ahlström et al. 2020), with earlier onset of frailty and age-related chronic conditions (Goddard et al. 2008). In tandem with exposure to earlier onset of multiple chronic conditions, people with intellectual disability are prone to greater medication use and potentially inappropriate prescribing is known to increase with age and morbidity (O'Dwyer et al. 2018).

The complexity of need exhibited by the population of people with intellectual disability requires interdisciplinary expertise and intervention to holistically, and comprehensively, address the health needs. This was mooted by Wilson et al. (2020) when they stated people with intellectual disability with complex and chronic needs often require unique models of care that can be both costly and intensive. However, health systems tend not to be organised in a manner conducive to this holistic care approach, and as Ahlström et al. (2020) report, the healthcare system has typically developed to respond to specific disease needs rather than to the needs of people with multi-morbidity. Such a singular disease-specific approach is likely to result in inefficiencies in the system if each disease is treated separately rather than through an integrated care model (Ahlström et al. 2020). For the individual, these inefficiencies could translate into neglect of healthcare needs should one condition be prioritised when a multi-pronged approach is required. The Australian healthcare system has been criticised for this very reason by Goddard et al. (2008), and they call for a greater focus on the chronic and complex need profile of people with intellectual disability and subsequent need for policy, practice and research to address this.

Australian Case

Context

It is estimated that 18% of the Australian population has a disability (AIHW 2020), with over 400,000 people with an intellectual disability (CID, IA 2019). The National Disability Insurance Scheme (NDIS) is a national funding scheme that provides individualised payments for disability-related supports. The legislation to establish the NDIS came into effect in 2013. As of June 2022, the NDIS has over 500,000 participants with 18% reporting a primary disability of intellectual disability (NDIS 2022). Thus, not every person with a disability qualifies for and can access NDIS funding.

In Australia, responsibility for different aspects of health and disability exists at federal or state level. For example, at a very basic level, primary care and ageing is the responsibility of the federal government, while hospital care and disability are the responsibility of the state governments. There are six states and two territories in Australia, with differences in legislation, policy and practice. Due to such differences across states, and territories, this case study will focus on the State of New South Wales. NSW is also of particular interest as it has been at the forefront of many health initiatives for people with intellectual disability. Within NSW, people with intellectual disability represent about 1% of the population (Srasuebkul et al. 2021).

Policy

The National Roadmap for Improving the Health of People with Intellectual Disability (AGDH 2021) was launched in 2021 and emphasises multidisciplinary and person-centred care. There is also an emphasis on trauma-informed care. A core goal is to achieve better integration within the health system (point B3) with multidisciplinary teams (where appropriate) involving GPs, nurses, midwives, allied health professionals, dentists, medical specialists and pharmacists. A second goal is for better coordination across sectors, including collaboration of health with disability and education sectors (point B4).

Case conferences are one approach recommended to facilitate multidisciplinary teams working together to support the care of people with intellectual disability, with a noted role for technology to enable this. The roadmap states that people with intellectual disability should be central to the multidisciplinary team and involved in decisions and case conferences. However, there is the caveat 'where appropriate' and no indication of how and who would make this judgement? Active engagement of the person with intellectual disability in their healthcare decision-making is not a minimum expectation in this document.

In addition, there is no specific guidance on how a multidisciplinary team is established and how it operates in practice. Given the complexity of need and subsequent diversity in disciplines and interventions that will be required, coordinating responsibility would be desirable.

Models of Integrated Care

One example to examine in this space is the specific model of integrated care—Specialist Team for Intellectual Disability Sydney (STriDeS), which has been established in Sydney and is referenced within the Roadmap. At present there are six teams located in six of the local health districts (LHDs). The teams have a specific remit around building capacity in understanding and working with people with intellectual disability within the mainstream health system, as well as providing health assessments with people with intellectual disability of all ages. No evaluation of these teams has taken place and some local health districts do not have a team in place and people with intellectual disability in those areas can access outreach services. People with intellectual disability are referred to one of the teams, if there is a persistent health problem that requires further investigation and diagnosis. The teams provide a health assessment and referral to appropriate services and then discharge the individual. It is not an ongoing service and there is no mechanism for annual health assessments for people with intellectual disability (which has been noted as best practice). In addition, the health outcomes and experiences in navigating the system with and without these intellectual disability specialist teams have not been undertaken. It is therefore unclear if current challenges in navigating the health system as a person with chronic and complex needs will be overcome or if a cycle of repeated 'one-off' assessments will ensue. Indeed, based on longitudinal studies on ageing and intellectual disability internationally, we can be sure that challenges will arise for people with more complex chronic conditions and as they age, who are at higher risk of preventable hospitalisation (Balogh et al. 2010). Some people with intellectual disability will need ongoing investigation, review and monitoring. The capacity within primary care and amongst GPs is known to be limited and also hampered by limited experience and skills in working with people with intellectual disability. In NSW, future funding for the only specialist intellectual disability clinic in Sydney, which operates with a multidisciplinary team to provide comprehensive annual assessments, is uncertain.

In some countries, specialist intellectual disability nurses and community pharmacists play an important role in the care of people with intellectual disability, and though the roadmap mentions nurses and pharmacists as members of multidisciplinary teams for people with intellectual disability, some current challenges for these disciplines in working with people with intellectual disability presently in NSW should be noted.

Education and Curriculum

In Australia there is no formal accreditation of the intellectual disability nurse available. However, the Professional Association of Nurses in Developmental Disability Australia (PANDDA) has developed practice guidelines for nurses working with people with intellectual and developmental disability (PANDDA 2020). NSW was the first state in Australia to establish specific nursing roles of clinical nurse consultant and educator within community-based allied health professional teams that work with the intellectual disability population (Wilkes et al. 2015).

Pharmacists are another discipline who can play an important role in a multidisciplinary team supporting the care of people with intellectual disability. However, there is no legislative or policy guidance in NSW on the administration and management of medication to people with intellectual disability, and much medication management falls to non-health professionals such as disability support workers, who have no requirement to have training in medications (Duckworth and Wilson 2022).

These are just some examples of the challenges for some disciplines in having a role in an integrated multidisciplinary model of care.

Funding

Another challenge to multi- and interdisciplinary care is the funding mechanism for people with disability. As noted above, the NDIS is the mechanism for individual payments for disability supports. However, there is a distinction, and some would say a false one, made between disability supports and health needs. Essentially health is not funded under the NDIS and is under the remit of NSW Health (or the relevant state). NDIS have as their remit to provide funding for supports related to disability, and supports to live one's life, but not health-related supports. For example, if an individual has an accident or is injured, the funding for rehabilitation is not provided under the NDIS; this is referred to the health services. The distinction more recently has been made with disability-related health supports that are defined by the NDIS (2022, no page number) as 'a support you may need to help you manage a health condition directly because of your disability. Or, to help you to manage your health or health condition if your disability means you can't do this on your own'.

Disability-related health supports include supports for dysphagia, respiratory, nutrition, diabetes management, continence, epilepsy, podiatry, wound and pressure care. Thus, the interaction of health and disability is not fully acknowledged, and this demarcation is another fictional one, like the demarcation between responsibility for disability and ageing. Current systems and policy treat the individual as someone with a disability *or* someone who is ageing *or* someone with a health condition, as if there is no comorbidity or correlation between them. This presents challenges not only from a funding perspective but also from the perspective of holistic, multidisciplinary and interdisciplinary care and subsequently impacts on health outcomes.

Norwegian Case

Context

Approximately 25,000 persons are registered with intellectual disability in Norway. However, the systems for diagnosing and reporting intellectual disability have limitations and inaccuracies with focus by the authorities on the importance of improving and clarifying responsibilities and systems (The Norwegian Health Directorate 2019a).

In 2017, it was estimated that the 356 municipalities in Norway each had approximately 50 service recipients with intellectual disability. However, the smallest municipalities have none or only a few, while the capital city Oslo has approximately 1700 citizens with intellectual disability. The age distribution of persons with intellectual disability receiving services in 2015 was as follows: under 18 years, 12.1%; 18–49 years, 57.1%; 50–66 years, 21.6%; 67–79 years, 7.4%; and 80+ years, 1.4%. Of all service recipients with intellectual disability receiving services, 58% were registered with complex comprehensive needs (The Norwegian Health Directorate 2017).

Funding

The Norwegian welfare system is based on the Nordic model that is characterised by a public social policy of high contribution rates, with comprehensive systems and services covering most situations of citizens' welfare across the lifespan. Public services are prioritised, and each municipality plays a central role (Sandvin et al. 2020). Another characteristic of the model is universal social rights for all citizens independent of income. Further, there is a strong orientation towards work/employment, which means that welfare systems are organised to support as many people as possible in employment. This includes free education, strong worker protection rules, financial security systems when unemployed and ill, support to return to work and good financial security for people retiring from work because of age or disability. Until 2015 the diagnosis of severe and profound intellectual disability was a prerequisite to receiving disability insurance without consideration of capacity to work. This was the case, for example, for people with multiple disabilities or persons with severe autism. Then the term 'severe' was removed from legislative text. Having the diagnosis of intellectual disability regardless of level of severity is now sufficient to be fast-tracked to disability insurance and onward referral to municipal health and care services. Thus, and despite some specific and interesting work to improve inclusive practice, there are very few pathways for people with intellectual disability into employment in Norway. Persons with intellectual disability in work are usually in adapted municipal day centres or different kinds of supported employment (Wendelborg and Tøssebro 2018).

The responsibility for providing health and social care services in Norway exists at both municipal/local government level and at state/national level. The municipalities are obliged to provide health and care services, which are established by the Health and Care Services Act (Ministry of Health and Care Services 2011a) aiming to ensure the quality of the services and to provide equal service provision. Another objective is to prevent, treat and accommodate for coping with illness, damage, suffering and reduced functioning (The Norwegian Health Directorate 2017).

Policy

In 2021 the national guide 'Good health and care services for persons with intellectual disability' was published by The Norwegian Health Directorate (2021). The background for this national guide is, in short, research and several published reports on setbacks after the deinstitutionalisation period, serious violation of human rights during the past 10–15 years and increased focus on the CRPD in Norway, for example, the Official Norwegian Report 2016:17 (The Ministry of Children and Families 2016). This guide uses the wording shall/must, can or should. The wording 'shall and must' denotes that claims are fixed by law or statute or are so deeply professionally rooted that it would be difficult not to align with the guide. The wording 'should' is a strong recommendation from the Health Directorate. If the municipality decides to utilise other solutions than recommended by the Health Directorate, it is recommended to document a professional reason for this. The wording 'can' is applied for example or recommended suggestions for how to comply with legal claims or a strong recommendation. The following main themes are included in the national guide, collaboration and competence, person-centred and individualised services, life phases and transitions, habilitation and daily life support, healthcare, collaboration with family, relatives and guardians and documentation and professional secrecy (The Norwegian Health Directorate 2021). The national guide has considerable potential to influence the development and realisation of the rights to quality health and social services by people with intellectual disability. However, it is too early to decide if and how the municipalities and professionals embrace it, and at present there is little knowledge about how to evaluate the municipalities' use of the guide.

Models of Integrated Care

Areas that specifically require interdisciplinary collaboration are habilitation, rehabilitation, coordination of services and individual planning. These areas are captured in the Habilitation, Rehabilitation and Coordinator Act (Ministry of Health and Care Services 2011b) and in the Individual Planning for the Provision of Welfare Services Act (Ministry of Children and Families 2022). Interaction, interdisciplinarity and competence in healthcare services in the municipalities are mentioned in the Health and Care Services Act §3–4 (Ministry of Health and Care Services 2011a, b). The municipality is, for example, obliged to arrange for collaboration and to work with the county authorities and the state in questions regarding health (Health and Care Services Act).

One effort to promote interdisciplinary collaboration and improve and coordinate services has been the use of individual plans. If one needs prolonged and coordinated health and care services, which is the case for many people with intellectual disability, one has the right to an individual plan (IP) under the Patient and User Rights Act, § 2–5 (The Ministry of Health and Care Services 1999). It is also a right to participate in the development of one's own individual plan, that should be adjusted for, and family should be included to the extent the user or the family wish to do so (Patient and User Rights Act, § 3–1). Both municipal and specialist healthcare levels are responsible for providing these areas. In addition, the municipality is responsible for having coordinating units that have the general responsibility for dealing with individual plans and for designating, training and counselling of coordinators. However, how municipalities organise this and to what extent the unit is visible and active in the municipal services varies greatly. In 2015, 41% of service users with intellectual disability were registered with an IP, 52% did not have an IP,

and 3% did not want to have one (The Norwegian Health Directorate 2017). Another example to mention is the use of case management teams that has been widespread in Norway, especially when it has come to preparation of individual plans; there is little research or evaluation on their use. In the new national guide (The Norwegian Health Directorate 2021), case management teams are just barely mentioned, while a model of structured interdisciplinary follow-up teams is referred to.

The national guide points out that municipalities and medical doctors should adapt for yearly health assessments for persons with intellectual disability. There are checklists for yearly health assessments available (The Norwegian Health Directorate 2021). A report by The Norwegian Health Directorate (2020) showed that in 2018 family doctors participated in one or more interdisciplinary meetings regarding 20% of their patients with intellectual disability and had communication with family members regarding 15% of their patients with intellectual disability. The same report points to the county authorities that have responsibility for public dental services and are decreed by law to provide regular and outreaching service to persons with intellectual disability, independent of age (The Norwegian Health Directorate 2020). In 2015, it was estimated that 80% of persons with intellectual disability over 18 years were being examined or treated by dental services. However, there were significant differences between the municipalities (The Norwegian Health Directorate 2017).

Education and Curriculum

The Norwegian authorities expect the municipalities to have an overview of the competence and training requirements in relation to service recipients' needs for services and associated service delivery. The previously mentioned health profession 'social educator' (vernepleier) programme has people with intellectual disability and complex needs as the key target population. Typically, the social educator works in different aspects of services for people with intellectual disabilities, home-based municipal care services, but also in respite care homes, care homes for older people, other municipal health and social services as well as in specialist healthcare like habilitation services and in psychiatry. The social educator's contribution in meeting the care needs of people with intellectual and other disabilities is defined as important for identifying the need for and contributing to multi- and interdisciplinary services. Social education includes broad knowledge of intellectual disability, milieu therapy, habilitation, rehabilitation, health promotion and healthcare as described in the Guideline for Social Education Act (Ministry of Education and Research 2019). However, a report by the Norwegian Union of Social Educators and Social Workers (FO) and The Norwegian National Institute on Intellectual Disability and Community (NAKU) (FO and NAKU 2020) shows that there is a deficit of 20,000 social educators in services for people with intellectual disability. The Official Norwegian Report 'On Equal Terms' (Ministry of Children and Families 2016:17) concluded that lacking competence is a continuous challenge in services for people with intellectual disability in Norway. Both municipalities and specialist healthcare lack necessary knowledge about intellectual disability and their human rights, challenges and needs. Knowledge of methods, treatment, accommodations and statutory obligations are insufficient as well as consciousness about self-determination, the right to participate and being included in society.

Case Comparison of Collaborative Working in Two Jurisdictions

The two cases illustrate that the terms multi- and interdisciplinary care are used interchangeably in policy documents, guidelines and practice. In the Australian case, the term multidisciplinary seems to be more commonly used than interdisciplinary, while the opposite is true of the Norwegian case.

Multi- and interdisciplinarity and coordination of services are emphasised and recommended across cases in political documents and in guidelines within the field of intellectual disability.

However, documentation in terms of how it works in practice is more difficult to identify.

Multidisciplinarity receives focus in the Australian roadmap, but greater focus on interdisciplinarity is required. There are limited specialist roles in health with specific responsibility for people with intellectual disability in NSW, with no accredited pathway for intellectual disability nursing. A focus on multidisciplinary rather than inter- and transdisciplinary care risks retaining a medical model of care, which does not value the individual voice and has limited collaboration in practice, with singular focus on condition specific care, rather than the holistic care of the individual with intellectual disability.

Both cases provide examples of how multi- or interdisciplinary collaboration is organised in the two countries. However, it seems that models of collaboration to provide multi- and/or interdisciplinarity are inconsistent and evaluation of models is insufficient. If the terms are not fully understood or continue to be used interchangeably in policy and strategy documents, there is a risk that incorrect/inconsistent team models will persist in practice.

The main responsibility for disability service provision lies with states and municipalities in Australia and Norway. Thus, large variability in this service provision for people with intellectual disability exists across municipalities and states. In both jurisdictions there is a continuation to demarcate 'older people' from 'people with disability' at a policy, funding and system level with people with disability who are ageing at risk of exclusion from age-related services.

How disability and health services are funded is likely hampering the health needs of people with intellectual disability being met. There is a lack of clarity and agreement on what is a health need, what is a disability-related health need and what is disability focus, with the categorisation linked to different funding sources. For example, in Australia, the National Disability Insurance Scheme has a strong focus on funding disability supports but not health needs.

Another topic illuminated in both cases is the role of qualified health personnel in identifying the need for interdisciplinary collaboration as well as being a collaboration partner and link between different professionals. Both cases have identified the need for strengthening recruitment and competence in intellectual disability in all parts of the service organisation. One fundamental way to address the unmet needs of people with intellectual disability is to focus on improving the education of students within health and social education regarding intellectual disability.

Involvement of the Voices of People with Intellectual Disability in Service Planning and Development

There have been many differing iterations related to how disciplines work together and how these can be truly inclusive of the voices of those whose care and support are being planned and provided.

The aim of involving users in development of their own services is to increase their control, choice, influence and the quality of services. However, the involvement of people with intellectual disability in service development has often been unjustly treated (Gjermestad et al. 2019). Consequently, in Norway, the national guide 'Good health and care services for persons with intellectual disability' (The Norwegian Health Directorate 2021) stated that services *must* be designed in collaboration with the person and his/her family. It is also stated that involvement includes planning, designing, accomplishing and evaluating services and actions. It is fundamental to recognise individuals' right to make own choices to be included as an equal participant in society (Fiala-Butora 2016). A question is how to involve persons' needs and wishes, and this has been subject to a variety of projects and research.

There is an increased focus on the right to choose and autonomy and a move away from guardianship models of care towards the development of supported decision-making tools and mechanisms to include the voice of all people with intellectual disability regardless of level of ability, across all aspects of their life. Though often people with intellectual disability are absent

from decisions regarding their health, there are mechanisms by which this involvement can be made possible.

'Peer-led' and 'peer-involved' approaches to managing the burden of chronic health conditions amongst people with intellectual disability were mooted in the report by the National Disability Services on 'Chronic Illness and People with Intellectual Disability Prevalence, Prevention and Management' (Banks 2016). Active support, collaboration based on the principles of person-centred supports that holds the person at the centre of decision-making and planning, has grown in prominence in disability services (Bigby et al. 2020), with some application evident in healthcare settings (Banks 2016). 'Expert-patient' programmes (EPP) are one application within chronic disease setting, by and for persons with chronic disease and an emphasis on empowerment and self-management. An adaptation of this model for people with intellectual disability has been trialled by Wilson and Goodman (2011). Supported decision-making is another mechanism to ensure that the individual demonstrates autonomy and control, with the appropriate supports as required. The role of the supporter in these 'peer-involved' and 'supported decision-making' approaches is essential to success. Carney et al. (2021) highlight that the will, preferences and rights of persons with intellectual disability may better be realised through training of supporters designed to enable greater participation by persons being supported and greater reflection and deliberation on wise and effective ways of providing such support by supporters.

Thus, competence and cultures that contribute to and adjust for active involvement must be developed and strengthened. This in turn requires respect, openness and sensitivity of individuals' wishes and needs, confidence building, accessible information about alternatives, advantages and disadvantages outlined and communication, including *alternative* and *augmentative* means of *communication*. Adapted inclusive contexts for collaboration about treatment and services should be developed, where the person, and his/her family members if suitable, should be invited. Examples could be case management team meetings, meetings in structured follow-up teams, the use of individual plans and meetings to develop long-term and short-term goals and actions (The Norwegian Health Directorate 2019b). Other examples are dialogue meetings (Gjermestad et al. 2019) together with relevant participants (depending on the challenges or goals) like the family doctor, intellectual disability nurse, physiotherapist, specialist healthcare professionals and teacher.

A contact person close to the person with intellectual disability (could be a family member or other supporter) should be present at the meetings if necessary to mediate the person's expressions when challenges with communication are experienced. If the person doesn't wish to be involved, this should be respected, but ways to communicate the person's wishes, experiences and needs should still be prioritised. Openness, good communication, respect for and shared competence and clarifying different alternatives are prerequisites for active participation and involvement. Defining the responsibility for coordination is also fundamental for succeeding with involvement and collaboration (The Norwegian Health Directorate 2017).

Conclusion

People with intellectual disability are more likely to experience multi-morbidity compared with the general population. Therefore, in the field of intellectual disability, it is of great importance to recognise the need of multi-, inter- and transdisciplinarity in policy, practice and teaching. The differences and understanding of the concepts should also be recognised. In this chapter it is argued that a singular disease-specific approach represents a medical model viewpoint, which draws similarity with the multidisciplinary approach. Thus, it is recommended to enhance focus on inter- and transdisciplinary teams and collaboration to provide coherent healthcare. No single profession can fill the roles and competence needed in quality healthcare for people with intellectual disability, but one may argue that specialised professions in intellectual disability have

important roles to recognise, initialise and contribute to multi- and interdisciplinary collaboration. Core to this collaboration is the inclusion of the voice and perspective of the person with intellectual disability.

Key Concepts Discussed

- Multi- and interdisciplinarity require different ways of team working and collaboration.
- Multidisciplinary working may be viewed as like the medical model due to its restricted focus and lack of holistic care.
- People with intellectual disability have complex care needs that require input from multiple health professionals; thus emphasis should be placed on inter- and transdisciplinary ways of working.
- The false separation of health and disability in policy, funding and health system structures requires revision to contribute to better health outcomes for people with intellectual disability.
- People with intellectual disability should be central to their healthcare and involved in all health-related decisions.

References

Ahlström G, Hansson J, Kristensson J, Runesson I, Persson M, Bökberg C (2020) Collaboration and guidelines for the coordination of health care for frail older persons with intellectual disability: a national survey of nurses working in municipal care. Nurs Open 8(3):1369–1379. https://doi.org/10.1002/nop2.753

Australian Government Department of Health (AGDH) (2021) National Roadmap for Improving the Health of People with Intellectual Disability. https://www.health.gov.au/resources/publications/national-roadmap-for-improving-the-health-of-people-with-intellectual-disability. Accessed 8 Dec 2021

Australian Institute of Health and Welfare (AIHW) (2020) People with disability in Australia. Australia, AIHW

Balogh R, Brownell M, Ouellette-Kuntz H, Colantonio A (2010) Hospitalisation rates for ambulatory care sensitive conditions for persons with and without an intellectual disability-a population perspective. J Intellect Disabil Res 54(9):820–832. https://doi.org/10.1111/j.1365-2788.2010.01311.x

Banks S (2016) Chronic illness and people with intellectual disability: prevalence, prevention and management. National Disability Services. Australia. https://

www.nds.org.au/images/LearnNDevelop/Chronic-Illness-and-People-with-Intellectual-Disability.PDF. Accessed 20 Aug 2022

Bell A, Corfield M, Davies J, Richardson N (2010) Collaborative transdisciplinary intervention in early years–putting theory into practice child: care. Health Dev 36(1):142–148. https://doi.org/10.1111/j.1365--2214.2009.01027.x

Bigby C, Bould E, Iacono T, Kavanagh S, Beadle-Brown J (2020) Factors that predict good active support in services for people with intellectual disability: a multilevel model. J Appl Res Intellect Disabil 33(3):334–344. https://doi.org/10.1111/jar.12675

Bobbette N, Ouellette-Kuntz H, Tranmer J, Lysaght R, Ufholz L-A, Donnelly C (2020) Adults with intellectual and developmental disabilities and interprofessional, team-based primary health care: a scoping review. JBI Evid Synth 18(7):1470–1514. https://doi.org/10.11124/jbisrir-d-19-00200

Bobbette N, Lysaght R, Ouellette-Kuntz H, Tranmer J, Donnelly C (2021) Organizational attributes of interprofessional primary care for adults with intellectual and developmental disabilities in Ontario, Canada: a multiple case study. BMC Fam Pract 22:157. https://doi.org/10.1186/s12875-021-01502-z

Bredland E, Linge O, Vik K (2011) Det handler om verdighet og deltakelse. Verdigrunnlag og praksis i rehabiliteringsarbeid (It's about dignity and participation. Values and practice in rehabilitation). Gyldendal Akademisk, Oslo

Carney T, Bigby C, Then S-N, Smith E, Wiesel I, Douglas J (2021) Paternalism to empowerment: all in the eye of the beholder? Disabil Soc. https://doi.org/10.1080/09687599.2021.1941781

Collin A (2009) Multidisciplinary, interdisciplinary, and transdisciplinary collaboration: implications for vocational psychology. Int J Educ Vocat Guid 9(2):101–110. https://doi.org/10.1007/s10775-009-9155-2

Council for Intellectual Disability (CID), Inclusion Australia (IA) (2019) The Health of People with Intellectual Disability: Budget and Federal election 2019 Commitments sought from Australian political parties. https://cidorgau/wp-content/uploads/2019/06/Intellectual_disability_health_bid_200219pdf Accessed 21 Aug 2022

Doherty AJ, Atherton H, Boland P et al (2020) Barriers and facilitators to primary health care for people with intellectual disabilities and/or autism: an integrative review. BJGP Open. https://doi.org/10.3399/bjgpopen20x101030

Duckworth NJ, Wilson NJ (2022) Medication oversight, governance, and administration in intellectual disability services: legislative limbo. Res Pract Intellect Dev Disabil 9(1):73–83. https://doi.org/10.1080/23297018.2021.2015424

Fellesorganisasjonen (FO) and Nasjonalt kompetansemiljø om utviklingshemmede (NAKU) (2020) Ingen tid å miste. En kartlegging av kompetansesituasjonen i tjenester til personer med utviklingshemming. (No time to lose. A mapping of competence situation in services

to people with intellectual disability). https://www.fo.no/getfile.php/1330661-1599214029/Filer/Rapport%20om%20kompetanse%20i%20tjenester%20til%20utviklingshemmede%20-%20nettversjon.pdf. Accessed 21 Aug 2022

Fiala-Butora J (2016) Reconstructing personhood: legal capacity of persons with disabilities. Ph.D. thesis. Harvard Law School, USA

Gjermestad A, Luteberget L, Midjo T, Witsø AE (2019) Preparing a dialogue conference together with persons with intellectual disability. Nordic Soc Work Res 10(4):343–355. https://doi.org/10.1080/2156857X.2019.1602558

Goddard L, Davidson P, Daly J, Mackey S (2008) People with an intellectual disability in the discourse of chronic and complex conditions: an invisible group? Aust Health Rev 32(3):405–414. https://doi.org/10.1071/AH080405

Grung RM (2016) The role of the Norwegian social educator. Learn Disabil Pract 19(10):24–26

Hermans H, Evenhuis HM (2014) Multimorbidity in older adults with intellectual disability. Res Dev Disabil 35(4):776–783. DOU: 10.1016/j.ridd.2014.01.022

Jaques H, Lewis P, O'Reilly K et al (2018) Understanding the contemporary role of the intellectual disability nurse: a review of the literature. J Clin Nurs 27(21-22):3858–3871. https://doi.org/10.1111/jocn.14555

McCarron M, Swinburne J, Burke E et al (2011) Growing older with an intellectual disability in Ireland 2011: first results from the intellectual disability supplement to the Irish longitudinal study on ageing (IDS-TILDA). School of Nursing and Midwifery, Trinity College Dublin, Dublin

McCarron M, Cleary E, McCallion P (2017) Health and health-care utilization of the older population of Ireland: comparing the intellectual disability population and the general population. Res Aging 39(6):693–718[a]. https://doi.org/10.1177/0164027516684172

Ministry of Children and Families (2016) On Equal Terms—Eight Steps to Realise Rights for People with Intellectual Disability. https://www.regjeringen.no/no/dokumenter/nou-2016-17/id2513222/. Accessed 20 Aug 2022

Ministry of Children and Families (2022) Individual Planning for the Provision of Welfare Services. https://lovdatano/dokument/SF/forskrift/2022-06-22-1110?q=individuell%20plan. Accessed 13 Sept 2022

Ministry of Education and Research (2019) The Guideline for Social Education Act. https://lovdata.no/dokument/SF/forskrift/2019-03-15-411. Accessed 20 Aug 2022

Ministry of Health and Care Services (1999) Patient and User Rights. https://lovdata.no/dokument/NL/lov/1999-07-02-63?q=pasient%20og%20brukerrettighetsloven. Accessed 20 Aug 2022

Ministry of Health and Care Services (2011a) Health and Care Services Act. . https://lovdata.no/dokument/NL/lov/2011-06-24-30. Accessed 20 Aug 2022

Ministry of Health and Care Services (2011b) Habilitation, Rehabilitation, Individual Plan, and Coordination

Act. https://lovdata.no/dokument/SF/forskrift/2011-12-16-1256/KAPITTEL_3#%C2%A75. Accessed 20 Aug 2022

Nancarrow SA, Booth A, Ariss S et al (2013) Ten principles of good interdisciplinary teamwork. Hum Resour Health 11:19. https://doi.org/10.1186/1478-4491-11-19

National Disability Insurance Scheme (2022) What so We Mean by Disability-Related Health Supports? https://ourguidelines.ndis.gov.au/supports-you-can-access-menu/disability-related-health-supports/what-do-we-mean-disability-related-health-supports. Accessed 20 Aug 2022

O'Dwyer M, McCallion P, McCarron M, Henman., M. (2018) Medication use and potentially inappropriate prescribing in older adults with intellectual disability: a neglected area of research. Therap Adv Drug Safety 9(9):535–557. https://doi.org/10.1177/2042098618782785

Professional Association of Nurses in Developmental Disability Australia Inc. (PANDDA) (2020) Standards for nursing practice. 2nd edition. http://www.pandda.net/files/PANDDA-2020-Standards.pdf. Accessed 8th Dec 2021

Rapport MJK, McWilliam RA, Smith BJ (2004) Practices across disciplines in early intervention: the research base. Infants Young Child 17(1):32–44

Reppermund S, Srasuebkul P, Dean K, Trollor JN (2019) Factors associated with death in people with intellectual disability. J Appl Res Intellect Disabil 33(3):420–429. https://doi.org/10.1111/jar.12684

Sandvin J, Vike H, Anvik C (2020) Tjenester til personer med utviklingshemming—i spennet mellom ny og gammel omsorgsideologi (Services for people with intellectual disability, between new and old ideology of care). In: Høj Anvik C, Sandvin JT, Paulsen Breimo JI, Henriksen Ø (eds) (ebook) Velferdstjenestenes vilkår. Nasjonal politikk og lokale erfaringer (The conditions for welfare services. National policy and local experienes). Universitetsforlaget, Oslo. https://www.idunn.no/doi/pdf/10.18261/9788215034713-2020. Accessed 15 Sept 2022

Srasuebkul P, Cvejic R, Heintze T, Reppermund S, Trollor JN (2021) Public mental health service use by people with intellectual disability in New South Wales and its costs. Med J Aust 215(7):325–331. https://doi.org/10.5694/mja2.51166

The Norwegian Health Directorate (2017) Tverrfaglig samarbeid som grunnleggende metodikk i oppfølging av personer med behov for omfattende tjenester [nettdokument]. (Interdisciplinary collaboration as basic method in follow-up of people with complex service-needs) Oslo: Helsedirektoratet. https://www.helsedirektoratet.no/veiledere/oppfolging-av-personer-med-store-og-sammensatte-behov/strukturert-oppfolging-gjennom-tverrfaglige-team/tverrfaglig-samarbeid-som-grunnleggende-metodikk-i-oppfolging-av-personer-med-behov-for-omfattende-tjenester. Accessed 21 Aug 2022

The Norwegian Health Directorate (2019a) Pilot for strukturert tverrfaglig oppfølgingsteam. Oslo: Helsedirektoratet. https://www.helsedirektoratet.no/om-oss/forsoksordninger-og-prosjekter/pilot-for-strukturert-tverrfaglig-oppfolgingsteam. Accessed 21 Aug 2022

The Norwegian Health Directorate. (2019b) Utredning og diagnostisering av utviklingshemming. Rapport til Helse- og omsorgsdepartementet (Medical examination and diagnostication of intellectual disability. Report to the Department of Health and Human Services). Oslo: Helsedirektoratet. https://www.helsedirektoratet.no/rapporter/utredning-og-diagnostisering-av-utviklingshemming/Rapport%20om%20utredning%20og%20diagnostisering%20av%20psykisk%20utviklingshemming.pdf/_/attachment/inline/f6c8ed73-c1d0-4819-9f83-b69bfbe17f38:bd58feb11efd678f91da43e173453bcef93ffb97/Rapport%20om%20utredning%20og%20diagnostisering%20av%20psykisk%20utviklingshemming.pdf. Accessed 21 Aug 2022

The Norwegian Health Directorate (2020) Fastlegers oppfølging av sine hjemmeboende pasienter med utviklingshemming. Basert på data fra Kommunalt pasient og brukerregister (KPR). (Family doctors' follow-up of their patients with intellectual disability living at home) Report: IS-2883. https://www.helsedirektoratet.no/rapporter/fastlegers-oppfolging-av-sine-hjemmeboende-pasienter-med-utviklingshemming/Fastlegers%20oppf%C3%B8lging%20av%20sine%20hjemmeboende%20pasienter%20med%20utviklingshemming.pdf/_/attachment/inline/236c1b80-edce-4600-8b85-fcf1d199f226:d13b4c855f866f6c9ce335eb3b6364c7fa467855/Fastlegers%20oppf%C3%B8lging%20av%20sine%20hjemmeboende%20pasienter%20med%20utviklingshemming.pdf. Accessed 21 Aug 2022

The Norwegian Health Directorate (2021) Gode helse- og omsorgstjenester til personer med utviklingshemming (good health and welfare services for people with intellectual disability). Helsedirektoratet, Oslo. https://www.helsedirektoratet.no/veiledere/gode-helse-og-omsorgstjenester-til-personer-med-utviklingshemming. Accessed 21 Aug 2022

Trollor JN, Eagleson C, Turner B et al (2016) Intellectual disability health content within nursing curriculum: an audit of what our future nurses are taught. Nurse Educ Today 45:72–79. https://doi.org/10.1016/j.nedt.2016.06.011

Trollor J, Srasuebkul P, Xu H, Howlett S (2017) Cause of death and potentially avoidable deaths in Australian adults with intellectual disability using retrospective linked data. BMJ Open 7(2). https://doi.org/10.1136/bmjopen-2016-013489

Trollor JN, Eagleson C, Turner B et al (2018) Intellectual disability content within tertiary medical curriculum: how is it taught and by whom? BMC Med Educ 18:182. https://doi.org/10.1186/s12909-018-1286-z

United Nations (2006) Convention on the rights of persons with disabilities (CRPD). WHO, Geneva

Wendelborg C, Tøssebro J (2018) Personer med utviklingshemming og arbeid—arbeidslinje eller fasttrack til kommunal omsorg (people with intellectual disability and work, pathways to work or fasttrack to municipal care)? Fontene Forskning 11(2):58–71

Wilkes L, Luck L, O'Baugh J (2015) The role of a clinical nurse consultant in an Australian Health District: a quantitative survey. BMC Nurs 14:25. https://doi.org/10.1186/s12912-015-0075-9

Wilson PM, Goodman C (2011) Evaluation of a modified chronic disease self-management programme for people with intellectual disability. J Nurs Healthc Chronic Illn 3(3):310–318. https://doi.org/10.1111/j.1752-9824.2011.01105.x

Wilson N, Riches V, Riches T, Durvasula S, Rodrigues R, Pinto S (2020) Complex support needs profile of an adult cohort with intellectual disability transitioning from state-based service provision to NDIS-funded residential support. J Intellect Dev Disabil 45(4):355–364. https://doi.org/10.3109/13668250.2020.1717069

Xyrichis A, Lowton K (2008) What fosters or prevents interprofessional teamworking in primary or community care? A literature review. J Nurs Stud 45:140–143. https://doi.org/10.1016/j.ijnurstu.2007.01.015

Attachment, Cognitive Dissonance and Reciprocation in Intellectual Disability Care Provision

Jan de Vries and Eimear McGlinchey

Chapter Topics

- This chapter will introduce three psychological mechanisms and their implications for people with an intellectual disability and those that support and care for them. The three mechanisms are attachment, cognitive dissonance and reciprocity.
- Attachment is the vehicle whereby infants learn and develop and may be compromised in children with an intellectual disability. Intellectual disability care and support workers need to be aware of this and find ways of generating attachment through sensitive interactions.
- Cognitive dissonance occurs when inconsistencies are encountered in information, cognition or behaviours. It generates tension and discomfort that motivates effort to reduce it. As such it represents a regulating mechanism to maintain consistency in all humans. People with an intellectual disability may require assistance in managing dissonance discomfort and maintaining peace of mind.
- Reciprocity is at the core of how communities function. The issue for people with an intellectual disability is that they often do not contribute to communities but are limited to receiving care and support. This confirms stigma and exclusion.

- The chapter clarifies each of the mechanisms and suggests ways in which intellectual disability workers can assist the people they support in navigating the issues involved. Four activities provide practical applications of the principles discussed.

Introduction

While psychology forms part of the curriculum for most healthcare professionals, the depth in the way in which it is applied tends to be limited. As a result, the potential of what psychology has to offer to inform the care and support for people with an intellectual disability tends to be underestimated. This chapter is intended to challenge this and offer a practical perspective on three core psychological mechanisms that have considerable implications for the understanding of thinking and behaviour in the person with an intellectual disability and consequently for the care and support that can be provided. Of course, in what way psychology might be useful depends on the care or support setting, the severity of the intellectual disability of the persons to be supported, level of independence, living and working circumstances and communicative abilities. However, the principles addressed here apply regardless.

The three mechanisms are attachment, cognitive dissonance and reciprocity. Each of these is

J. de Vries (✉) · E. McGlinchey
Trinity College Dublin, Dublin, Ireland
e-mail: devriej@tcd.ie; mcgline@tcd.ie

© The Author(s), under exclusive license to Springer Nature Switzerland AG 2023
F. Sheerin, C. Doyle (eds.), *Intellectual Disabilities: Health and Social Care Across the Lifespan*,
https://doi.org/10.1007/978-3-031-27496-1_4

based on demonstrated neurological processes, and research suggest that the facility to process information related to each has neurological correlates and is most likely hardwired in the brain (Escobar et al. 2013; de Vries et al. 2015; Tooby and Cosmides 2008). Considering that these are fundamental mechanisms, we may assume that they function in people with an intellectual disability in similar ways as in the general population. They may not operate at the same level of cognitive sophistication, but the neurological basis is most likely the same, unless it is demonstrated that neural functioning is considerably disrupted and makes it impossible.

In regard to *attachment*, it is not too farfetched to think that children with an intellectual disability have the same need for attachment and benefit from it largely in the same way in terms of emotional stability, mental health and learning. We discuss the premise of attachment theory and its application and considerations for intellectual disability and caregiver response.

The application of *cognitive dissonance theory* is of particular relevance and provides a lens through which a care worker can address issues of ambivalence and inner conflict with the person with an intellectual disability. All humans seek to maintain *cognitive consistency*, to avoid chaos in our thinking and maintain peace of mind. The recognition and effective processing of inconsistency or dissonance is essential for people with an intellectual disability as much as it is in the general population. We posit that while the mechanisms may operate in the same fashion as in the general population, the ability to effectively reduce complex inconsistencies may be reduced. Care and support workers may be able to provide assistance with managing these processes.

Finally, we apply the principle of *reciprocity* as a cornerstone of social cognition and community interaction. While this is not new by any means, the suggestion of a hardwired evolutionary adaptation (Tooby and Cosmides 2008; Buss 2019) puts it in a new light and suggests the urgent need for creative applications in providing intellectual disability support. Our suggestion is that people with an intellectual disability need to be given more opportunities to contribute to their communities rather than be limited to receiving support.

Attachment: Emotional Connection and Learning

Psychological evidence shows that the bonds and relationships we develop early in our lives are the foundation for the development of adult neuro-affective functioning and behaviour (Hart 2011). Positive relationships in infancy contribute to mental health, and negative relationships can lead to emotional distress, which may extend into adulthood. In particular, early attachments to caregivers have a lasting impact on well-being (Andrews and Hicks 2017) but also learning (Bosmans et al. 2020) and social cognition (Nolte et al. 2013).

As we strive to understand the underlying processes, ethologists have looked to the animal kingdom. Lorenz's (1935) observations of baby geese revolutionised the understanding of attachment, also in humans. Lorenz observed that a gosling would follow the first moving object it saw upon hatching and become attached to this. There is a critical period in which what he called 'imprinting' takes place (for goslings this appears to be 12–17 h after hatching), after which it appears to be irreversible, and the gosling will remain attached to this person or object from then on (Hess 1958). This adaptive mechanism would normally ensure that the gosling will receive the protection of the mother and through observing the mother's behaviour will learn everything it needs to learn to survive. The same principle applies to many other birds. Lorenz's (1935) work showed that an innate mechanism that does not require reinforcement is the start of all learning and without this process learning and development will be limited. Parallels between imprinting in geese and attachment in mammals have been established.

Through experiments with primates, we have learned that attachment, while not developing as quickly as imprinting in goslings, also follows innate patterns. Harlow and Zimmermann (1959) conducted experiments with rhesus monkeys in which the monkeys were separated from their mothers and placed with one of two inanimate surrogate mothers: one made of wire that provided milk and the other made of soft material, but did not provide milk. The baby monkeys seemed to be pre-programmed to favour the soft comforting 'surrogate mother' and spent most of their time literally attaching itself to it, even though it didn't provide any food. In nature we see the same pattern and even when the infant primate starts exploring the world, it continuously returns to the mother for comfort, thus availing of protection and learning opportunities just like the goslings. Because the early development of human infants is highly similar to that of primates, the same mechanisms have been assumed and investigated (Suomi 1997).

Attachment Theory in humans

Building on these animal studies, attachment theory in humans was developed in the 1960s by John Bowlby (1958, 1969) and Mary Ainsworth (1978) to highlight the importance of early physical and emotional relationships between children and their primary caregivers, both in terms of later relationships and in developing learning and a sense of self (Ainsworth and Bowlby 1991).

Bowlby observed that a human infant will display attachment behaviours such as grasping, searching and crying in order to increase proximity to the primary caregiver. These behaviours are part of what Bowlby called the child's 'attachment behavioural system'. For a secure attachment relationship to develop, the primary caregiver must respond to these behaviours with their own 'caregiving behavioural system' (Bowlby 1979; Bretherton 1992). These two systems must work in harmony to develop secure attachment. Turn-taking, mirroring emotions, dispelling fears and providing physical warmth and support are essential. In particular, touch is considered essential (Stack and Muir 1990). The so-called 'still face' studies have demonstrated that if

the primary caregiver does not respond effectively to the infant's attachment behaviour, infants get upset and attempt to regain attention. If this fails consistently, the emotional tie may be damaged, which may reduce the infants' ability to connect fully with the caregiver and become a precursor for difficulties forming emotional relationship in adulthood (Adamson and Frick 2003). To compensate, the infant will develop alternative strategies to try to remain close to their caregiver and avoid rejection—these alternative strategies are known as insecure strategies (BPS 2017). These patterns become internalised and generalised, and consequently the child may see itself as being valued and accepted (secure) or as being incompetent and unacceptable (insecure). These internal working models of interaction and self, whether positive or negative, can endure beyond the early need for proximity to primary caregivers and may be internalised as templates for relationships in adulthood. Ainsworth (1978) conducted laboratory experiments with infants and their primary caregivers to test these attachment theories. Her studies involved leaving the child for 3 min and observing its response when the caregiver leaves, during their absence and when reunited. From their behaviour the attachment relationship was inferred. This experiment was called 'The Strange Situation', and from it, Ainsworth (1978) wrote about four attachment styles and the caregiver style that was associated with them.

A 'secure' attachment style was considered to be shown whenever children were happy when the carer was present, upset when they left, but easily settled again when the caregiver returned. It was thought that secure attachment was generated if caregivers were generally available to meet the emotional needs of the child. When the child was seen to avoid the caregiver on return or to show little emotion, they were labelled as having developed an 'insecure-avoidant' attachment. In this case caregivers may have lacked closeness to the child. If the child showed high levels of distress when the caregiver left and could not to be comforted by the caregiver when they returned, they were considered to display an 'insecure ambivalent' attachment style. It was thought that this may be the result of the caregiver responding inconsistently to the child. The final style noted was referred to as 'disorganised' attachment, which included unexpected behaviours such as rocking, freezing and alternating between approach and avoidance of the caregiver. It was believed that this could show that the caregiver may be both a source of comfort and distress and could even indicate abuse (Ainsworth 1978).

Application of Attachment Theory in Intellectual Disability

It is evident that disruption in the interactions around attachment can prevent the attachment process from fully developing. Research has shown that infants with an intellectual disability and their caregivers are at increased risk of this (Hamadi and Fletcher 2021). An infant with intellectual disability may not display attachment behaviours such as proximity seeking, contact maintenance or distance interactions (Ganiban et al. 2000), which generally trigger attachment processes in the caregiver. Instead, the child may display compensatory behaviours, such as rocking, challenging or withdrawal, which may be misinterpreted or go unnoticed. Infants with Down syndrome have been described as less emotionally reactive than other infants and show higher rates of insecure attachment (Ganiban et al. 2000). Children with Down syndrome also have high rates of neuromotor impairment such as hypotonia and ataxia, which may disrupt attachment-related behaviours (Ganiban et al. 2000). Research on dual diagnosis of intellectual disability and autism spectrum disorder (ASD) suggest that the intellectual disability, rather than ASD, was the biggest risk factor for attachment disorganisation (Rutgers et al. 2004).

In addition, parents may lack expertise or motivation or have difficulty accepting an intellectual disability diagnosis. If this interferes with their interaction with the child, this can disrupt the development of secure attachment. An early diagnosis is advantageous because it allows parents to come to terms with the matter and acquire expertise and support early on. Children with Down syndrome are at an advantage because they are often diagnosed antenatally, whereas autism is diagnosed at an average of 3.5 years (van't Hof et al. 2021).

In the general population, as children grow older, the need for physical proximity lessens as attachment becomes more verbally expressed. At this point the attachment need is replaced by internal working models of attachment and a theory of mind. Furthermore, during adolescence attachment needs and abilities are transferred from the primary caregivers to other meaningful relationships. In older children with an intellectual disability, obstacles to this natural development may have the result that attachment expressions remain at a primary level. In this case ongoing physical proximity may be needed to generate safety and security (Fletcher and Gallichan 2016).

An issue of relevance in residential or group home settings is that high workload and frequent changes in staff can lead to inconsistent response to attachment behaviour, with subtle cues being missed (Schuengel et al. 2010). Since the quality of caregiving is based on the interpersonal relationship between caregiver and person with intellectual disability, a constant turnover in staff will impede the development and expectation of secure relationships and ultimately relationship skills in the person with an intellectual disability. The occurrence of challenging behaviours, rocking, avoidance and absence of emotional expression, as noted by Ainsworth (1978), may need to be examined and considered as evidence of possible attachment problems. In summary, attachment styles developed in early childhood are linked to learning and developing relationships and bonds throughout adult life. Obstacles to secure attachment put a person at an increased risk of psychological distress later in life, including paranoia, depression, obsessive compulsive disorder and other psychiatric problems (BPS 2017).

Implications for the Intellectual Disability Support Worker

Given what we know about attachment and how attachment is formed, there is a need to examine how services can best support *secure attachment*, as this promotes learning, and the development of relationships from early childhood through to late adulthood in the person with an intellectual disability. It is essential that, especially early supports should not be transitory in nature, and as the research in children in general shows, awareness of the 'caregiving behavioural system' as outlined by Bowlby (1958, 1969, 1979) is required. This means emphasis on responsiveness, physical contact and turn-taking.

A greater understanding of the signs and implications of insecure attachment will be beneficial to intellectual disability care and support workers. A more accurate interpretation of attachment behaviours such as crying, clinging or searching and responding sensitively in light of this interpretation is crucial (Skelly 2016). From Harlow's work, we know of the importance of physical contact and comfort in developing a sense of security, so there is a need to consider how services can respond to this need. Implementing care and support while interpreting behaviour through an attachment lens can complement other more common interventions such as applied behaviour analysis and positive behaviour support through understanding the cause of the behaviour and focussing on relationship building and development of emotional bonds, rather than on symptomatic change, such as reduction in frequency of certain behaviours (Skelly 2016). It is likely that reinforcement of desired behaviours without attachment between person and caregiver may not be fully effective. Thus, moving from a purely behavioural approach to an attachment-led approach may be beneficial. The exercise in Activity 4.1 provides an opportunity to apply these ideas to a scenario.

Activity 4.1   Attachment principles and their application in intellectual disability

Narrative

Jack (22) has Down syndrome, a moderate level of intellectual disability and difficulties with language production but a good level of understanding. Hypotonia and poor mobility are other challenges he is facing. Jack's parents struggled in early years but ensured that Jack had access to supports available from services. In his adolescence, Jack started visiting a day centre. This transition was successful. He became close to a key worker, Susan, who worked closely with Jack and coordinated his care. As well as providing support for Jack, Susan provided education and support to Jack's parents, allowing them to better support Jack. This meant that Susan and Jack's parents were working in harmony and reacting consistently to Jack's non-verbal cues. All were sensitive to facial expressions, noises, eye contact and touch. Alternative methods of communication were found that worked best for Jack and allowed him to express himself. Jack felt valued and accepted. Unfortunately, Susan moved out of the service and while a successor was appointed, the new care relationship did not work out as well. Soon after the transition, Jack was found reluctant to return to the day centre and when he went there showed challenging behaviour, withdrew from interactions, ignored staff and was sometimes found rocking himself

Discuss the following:

Can you interpret the scenario in terms of attachment development?	Can you suggest how the situation can be improved with reference to attachment aspects?

Consistency/Dissonance Processing: Cognitive Dissonance Theory

One of the principles that allows the human system to operate as a unit is that it strives towards consistency (Festinger 1957). We discriminate between consistent and inconsistent information, and we recognise when our actions or thoughts are consistent or inconsistent with our goals (Harmon-Jones et al. 2009), principles or beliefs (Aronson 1969). Whenever we become aware of inconsistencies, our brain produces an alarm signal, a small one for small incongruencies and a big one for more significant ones. We tend to respond to the discomfort of the alarm by setting in motion efforts to reduce the discrepancy or find other ways of silencing it (de Vries and Timmins 2016). This is a regulatory system that helps us avoid chaos in our thinking and ensures that actions remain goal directed (Harmon-Jones et al. 2009). This principle affects all humans and there is no reason to think that it would be different for a person with an intellectual disability.

Cognitive Dissonance Theory

While psychology has yielded many theories that address this aspect of our functioning, cognitive dissonance theory (Festinger 1957) is perhaps of most interest here because of the abundance of empirical research, theoretical scrutiny and broad application (Gawronski 2012). When Festinger developed the model, he defined cognitive dissonance as arising from a psychological inconsistency between two (or more) notions, which generate a tension that is experienced as discomfort and serves as a drive to engage in efforts to reduce the inconsistency. The motivational aspect added a core element to cognitive theory. It gave it an engine! (Gerard 1992). Later research highlighted that it may not be necessary to reduce the inconsistency itself to diminish the discomfort. Seeking distraction, for instance, may also reduce the discomfort (McGrath 2017). A variety of revisions of the theory have highlighted that self-related dissonance (Aronson 1969) may have the highest intensity, while the most recent innovations emphasise the importance of dissonance as a signal to regulate our actions (Harmon-Jones et al. 2009). If our actions are inconsistent with the goals we try to achieve, dissonance discomfort alerts us to this problem, and motivates adjusting the action, until it is consistent with the goals again. It follows that it is important to discriminate between dissonance induction and reduction (Tryon and Misurell 2008) and the contrasting states they bring about in humans: inner conflict or peace of mind.

Application of Dissonance Theory in Intellectual Disabilities

Looking at the life of a person with intellectual disability through the lens of dissonance theory may provide a new clarity and has significant implications for understanding how support can be optimised, hence its inclusion here. We will look at its application at different levels of functioning.

At its most basic, the processing of consistency/inconsistency takes place at the physiological level. Coordination of muscle groups, joints, endocrine and cardiovascular activity relies on it. Normally an intellectual disability would not interfere with the core mechanisms involved, although a person affected by multiple physical and intellectual disabilities may experience problems with proprioception and muscle coordination. While this would not necessarily be experienced at the level of cognitive awareness, the frustration at not being able to satisfy a need or achieve a valued basic goal such as feeding oneself may well bring about persistent dissonance felt as frustration, which affects the life satisfaction of the person. Caregivers would most likely be aware of this and through attentive care and support minimise this source of dissonance discomfort.

At a cognitive level, processing of consistency and inconsistency may still occur without conscious awareness. Essential knowledge of what is good and bad requires limited awareness and even awareness of an implicit expectation may not require complex cognitive processing. More cognitive complexity is involved in identifying whether a rule is violated or whether behaviour or thinking is inconsistent with an important principle, belief or standard (see Activity 4.2).

It is situations like this that may create a conundrum that people with an intellectual disability may find hard to address. The initial dissonance can apparently rather easily be resolved by undoing the violation of the rule; however the sudden risk of public shaming leads to momentary averting of more intense dissonance

Activity 4.2   Cognitive dissonance roleplay

Scenario

Jeni (16) has just dropped her chewing gum on the floor. She did it on purpose, although she is well aware that chewing gum should go in the bin. She feels bad about it and is just getting ready to pick it up, when it is noticed by another resident. 'Who threw their chewing gum on the floor?' he yells. Jeni says 'It wasn't me' and walks away. Now she feels worse. Not only has she violated the chewing gum rule, but now she has lied, and she likes to think of herself as an honest person. Jeni is in a bad mood during the rest of the day, unable to resolve her dissonance. In the evening a support worker starts a conversation with Jeni ....

Dissonance analysis

Initial dissonance:
I have dropped my chewing gum on the floor <> chewing gum should go in the bin

Subsequent dissonance:
I have lied <> I am an honest person

Roleplay: Read the scenario and the underlying dissonance analysis. Make use of the dissonance reduction and exacerbation elements below to roleplay with a colleague how you will talk (and not talk) with Jeni to address her bad mood.

Possible dissonance reduction:

- Changing behaviour: (I will always put my gum in the bin from now on)
- Adapting cognitions (it is a stupid rule)
- Adding cognitions (I always clean up after myself)
- Seeking justifications (if he had not yelled, I would have picked up the gum)
- Diversion of responsibility (there should be more bins around)
- Trivialisation (who cares, it is not important)
- Shifting attention (I am going to enjoy my dinner)
- Finding distraction (if I watch television, I won't think about it)
- Denial (I dropped the gum by accident, I did not throw it)

Possible ways in which dissonance may be exacerbated:

- Highlighting the importance of the gum-in-the-bin rule
- Highlighting how unhygienic gum on the floor is
- Accusing someone else
- Making a big deal out of it
- Emphasising the importance of honesty
- Emphasising that lying is a sin

(*I have been caught*) through a response that unfortunately leads to added dissonance (*now I have lied*). Resolving the dissonance in this situation requires courage, mental flexibility and perhaps social skills and creative thinking. This may be hard for people with an intellectual disability.

Research on the reduction of cognitive dissonance makes it clear that whenever an action to reduce dissonance is not possible or blocked, other approaches are used. Typically, we would see efforts to reconcile the incongruity by adapting cognitions, adding positive cognitions, seeking justifications, diversion of responsibility, but also trivialisation, shifting attention, finding distraction and even denial (McGrath 2017). Each of these efforts may be successful, but sometimes only to a point. In which case, the person may have to continue to look for other ways of reducing the dissonance. In such situations dissonance may become a continuous presence and the efforts to reduce it may become a major distraction from other things in life. Being unable to resolve dissonance generates great upset and unhappiness.

A common source of prolonged dissonance is the incongruence people with an intellectual disability may experience around their personal identity as deviating from the norm. One of the most relevant revisions of cognitive dissonance theory suggests that the most intense dissonance discomfort is generally experienced when the inconsistency is with aspects of the self. Aronson (1969) suggested that whenever we do something or experience something that is dissonant with the belief that we are good, right, smart, etc., we feel intense discomfort. This perspective has specific relevance to the person with an intellectual disability who may question the core of their identity. They may, for instance, experience dissonance such as illustrated in Activity 4.3. In such situations the support worker is in a prime position to provide existential support by helping the person develop an acceptable and stable perspective on their identity and a repertoire of dissonance reduction strategies.

Activity 4.3 Cognitive dissonance roleplay (continued)

Scenario	Underlying dissonance analysis
Jeni (16) expresses being unhappy with the fact that she is different from other people. You have noticed periods of low mood and withdrawal in which she seemed to be ruminating. When a support worker approaches her to talk, she tells you of the reason for her unhappiness ……	**Source of dissonance** I have an intellectual disability and am therefore not worthy <> I am a good person

Roleplay: Read the scenario and the underlying dissonance analysis. Make use of the dissonance reduction and exacerbation elements below to roleplay with a colleague how you will talk (and not talk) with Jeni to address this fundamental issue.

Possible ways of dissonance reduction	Possible ways in which dissonance may be exacerbated:
• Changing behaviour (I will do my best and do things just like everyone else) • Adapting cognitions (an intellectual disability does not mean I am worthless) • Adding cognitions (while I have an intellectual disability, I am also kind and friendly) • Seeking justifications (it must be something that I got from my parents) • Diversion of responsibility (I can't help it) • Trivialisation (I am who I am, it is not important) • Shifting attention (I am going to enjoy my life) • Finding distraction (if I do things I like, I won't think about it) • Denial (I am as smart as anyone)	• Highlighting how important it is to be smart • Seeing others be successful in unattainable ways • Emphasising evidence of diminished capabilities • Demonstrating how the person with an intellectual disability cannot function at a high intellectual level • Highlighting disappointing experiences related to the intellectual disability • Allowing humiliations to take place

Implications for the Intellectual Disability Support Worker

Because dissonance may not be explicitly revealed by the person with an intellectual disability, a support worker will need to learn to read the signals and be prepared to investigate them. Preoccupation with dissonance tends to show as tension, upset, frustration, absent-mindedness, fretting or typical dissonance emotions such as shame, embarrassment, regret and self-directed anger. When dissonance emotions linger, they can lead to excessive worry and rumination. Worry should be seen as efforts to cognitively resolve dissonance, but when it slides into rumination, the cyclical repeat of the same thoughts yields no new solutions, and the process loses its aim. Rumination may lead to difficulties concentrating, loss of sleep, irritability and low mood, which can become a health and mental health risk (Lyubomirsky et al. 2003). When someone seems perturbed without an obvious reason, we ask 'What is wrong?'. We should expect that there is an aspect of dissonance involved in the answer. When people say they don't want to talk about it, it is generally because they have been trying to divert their attention away from it, and by naming it, the dissonance discomfort is felt again.

It is important to assist the person with an intellectual disability in reducing or managing this discomfort. For starters, they can be assisted to effectively navigate common sources of dissonance, such as displayed in the roleplay scenario (Activity 4.2), providing support to reduce dissonance and help disqualifying approaches that make it worse. This should be part of day-to-day coping skills. In addition, the support worker can help the person to come to terms with possible long-term sources of dissonance such as outlined in the continuation of the roleplay (Activity 4.3). This may require conversations with the person to discover which dissonance reduction approaches may lead to long-term improvements in peace of mind. This should go beyond showing empathy. For instance, when addressing a person's struggle to come to terms with a mild intellectual disability and the limitations this brings, it is not enough to say, 'I know how important this is for you'. While this shows empathy, it may only increase the dissonance discomfort. Furthermore, it is not enough to help identify the core of the dissonance, such as in 'So you want a boyfriend/girlfriend, but it is not possible because you have an intellectual disability. Is this the problem?' It needs to be followed by finding ways of reducing the dissonance. Support workers need to be cautious in this respect because the person may not have capacity to face the issue in a fundamental fashion and may need to resort to shifts in attention, trivialisation or even denial. It is essential for the care worker to check the impact of any cognitive-behavioural interventions. If we look at it through the dissonance lens, it is dissonance reduction that should be the outcome. Feeling relief through reduction of dissonance is the litmus test!

In short, applying the cognitive dissonance perspective to problems encountered by people with an intellectual disability will be useful for the support worker. It explains the origin of inner turmoil, resulting in preoccupations, and helps us recognise efforts to reduce the discomfort and the emotions. Our conclusion is that an effective intellectual disability support worker needs to: (a) be aware of the dissonance mechanism and understand how it can arise in the lives of the people they support; (b) recognise signs of dissonance, particularly when it is prolonged; and (c) assist the person with an intellectual disability in reducing dissonance discomfort to enhance their peace of mind.

Reciprocity: No Community Without Reciprocity

One of the authors once attended a remarkable theatre play. The story of Tristan and Isolde was performed by a large cast, with singing and music by actors with varying levels of intellectual disability. Some actors were vocal, while others were not. It was a riveting show in which a narrator told the story from the top of a medieval tower high above the action. She performed her role in unforgettable fashion moving the audience and drawing laughter. Her bright light and exceptional talent were a source of real entertainment. The show received a standing ovation at the end. Her parents were in tears of joy only a few seats away from the author.

Talking with them afterwards, it became clear that the reason why they were so moved was not just because she was doing so well but that she had been in a position to 'give' joy to the community. With all the care and support she had received over the years, she had now given something to be remembered in return.

Many people with an intellectual disability are commonly at the receiving end of care and support and not usually in a position to provide a service in return. This is a problem because it places the person outside of the community. With all our efforts to integrate people with an intellectual disability into education and society, this is something that requires more attention. There is no community without reciprocity. So, if people with an intellectual disability cannot contribute to a community, are they really a part of it? Sociologists and anthropologists have pointed out that doing favours and receiving them is essential to the social fabric and cohesion in families and communities (Bell 1991). This exchange is the engine of social interaction, as social psychologists (Cialdini et al. 1987) have pointed out. The spark that keeps this engine going has been understood in a new way by evolutionary psychologists Tooby and Cosmides (2008).

Reciprocity and Cheater Detection

When someone does us a favour, we experience pleasure, but at the same time, we feel an obligation to return the favour. This is like a mental itch. We feel uncomfortable if we can't return the favour (Cialdini et al. 1987). Moreover, we keep track of who we owe a favour to and who owes us a favour. In addition, in a broader sense, we generalise a favour done to us, by becoming more prone to do favours to others in general after having received a favour. This goes by the name 'indirect reciprocity' (Panchanathan and Boyd 2004). Being magnanimous may have its origin in feeling that one has been treated well by others. Tooby and Cosmides (2008) have suggested that this is motivated by signals from the brain that are triggered by receiving something from others. Pro-social behaviour is promoted and maintained in this way. The opposite is also the case. If we fail to receive a return for a favour, we may feel hard done by, perhaps insulted, and trust might be reduced. We may tell ourselves to exclude the person. Because this brings to a halt the free flow of favour and counter favour, the basis of community living, it is essential to prevent this.

Tooby and Cosmides (2008) have argued that this is the reason we are so sensitive on this front. In their research they asked participants to solve problems and found that if the problem contained an element of identifying a cheater, they were more effective at solving the problem. In their studies, the experimental group received information that a cheater needed to be identified, while a control group received the same problem, but without this element (Cosmides and Tooby 2005). The research was conducted in numerous variations but with the same outcome. The researchers concluded that humans must be particularly sharp and motivated to address cheating. They proposed a 'cheater detection' module in the brain and argued for it as an evolutionary adaptation. Neuroscience has provided some support for this notion (Krill et al. 2007; Cosmides and Tooby 2004, 2005). But even without this, the idea that we are subject to a cognitive mechanism that keeps track of checks and balances is not too far-fetched. And therefore, it is unsurprising that we feel better when we are 'contributing' instead of 'receiving', or not 'in the red', so to speak. Our self-esteem and well-being are affected by this, as research on volunteer work shows (Wilson 2000; Brown et al. 2012).

well focussed (Fulton et al. 2021). The problem for people with an intellectual disability is that their opportunities to contribute to society are limited. A minority of people with an intellectual disability are gainfully employed or work in a voluntary capacity (Garrels and Sigstad 2019; McCausland et al. 2020; Meltzer et al. 2020). Moreover, they tend to receive care and support by self-effacing parents and care providers who may not have educated them to be on the giving end of social and economic relationships. In short, they are often systematically 'in the red'. There is evidence that this has a negative impact on their health and quality of life (Dean et al. 2018).

In a broader sense, applying the reciprocity principle sheds a new light on the stigma people with an intellectual disability experience. While often described with indignation as socially constructed (Scior and Werner 2016), it could also be seen as an evolutionary adaptation to avoid people who will not or cannot contribute in an economic or social sense to the tribes in which the human race lived in its hunter-gatherer days. This perspective shifts the focus, and the implication is that if we want to successfully integrate people with an intellectual disability in society, our efforts to reduce stigma through enlightening society may not be as essential as the need to ensure that people with an intellectual disability can contribute in one way or another. Of course, this is easier said than done. The obstacles to social integration are similar to those for economic integration. Nonetheless, this perspective offers an alternative focus with practical implications that can be applied in all support and care settings.

Application of the Reciprocity Principle in Intellectual Disability

The importance of reciprocity for people with an intellectual disability has been recognised as essential in generating social inclusion and belonging; however the research within the context of intellectual disability is sparse and not

Implications for the Intellectual Disability Support Worker

While the intellectual disability support worker may not be able to affect the reciprocity balance in people with an intellectual disability in general, there are obvious opportunities to address this within the lives of people with an intellectual dis-

Activity 4.4 Reciprocity balance—support workers can complete this grid with people they support

Activity 4:Reciprocity balance-Support workers can complete this grid with people they support		
What I do for others	What I do for myself	What others do for me

ability they support. Key is to look for opportunities to bring the person with an intellectual disability into situations in which they can contribute. Shared living accommodation generally provides excellent opportunities for this. Often the emphasis is on promotion of self-support. Research on older adults in nursing homes has emphasised the benefits of this within care settings (Langer and Rodin 1976). However, it follows from the argument made here that doing something for others is perhaps even more important.

The support worker is in a prime position to provide education and identify opportunities to put this principle in practice. In congregated care settings, the focus may be on reinforcing turn-taking and reciprocation in all interactions and where possible promoting opportunities to contribute. For those with moderate and mild intellectual disability who venture into the community, this includes assisting in finding fitting paid or voluntary work. Also, in most staffed housing, a system of reciprocity around cleaning, shopping and other household chores can be set up. The care worker can help with this and be involved as a referee in ensuring fairness. To motivate the person with an intellectual disability, awareness can be created by discussing a system of checks and balances (see Activity 4.4).

In addition to awareness of the balance or imbalance, filling in such a diagram may generate ideas as to where improvements can be made. For instance, if someone is really good at doing something for him-or herself, this could then be considered to be done for others. Furthermore, once the practice of doing things for others and the personal pleasure derived

from it has become clear, the thought of contributing could become part of a person's routine. More than anything this often involves a change in mindset. Initially it may be easier to do things *for* the person with an intellectual disability rather than supporting them to do things themselves, let alone *for others*, but the long-term benefits are likely to prevail. The reciprocity principle can also be applied in rethinking the relationship people with an intellectual disability who live within the community have with that community. Very often the interactions are minimal (Sheerin et al. 2015). The exploration and implementation of activities that people with an intellectual disability can be involved in to visibly contribute to the people in the community may be crucial to changing this!

Conclusion

In this chapter we have endeavoured to provide a perspective on three core aspects of cognitive and behavioural functioning that have implications for people with an intellectual disability and subsequently for those who care and provide support for them. These principles are attachment formation, consistency and dissonance processing and reciprocity and contribution to community. Understanding the principles and the psychological mechanisms involved provide a lens through which intellectual disability care and support workers can not only develop a better understanding of core issues but also improve care and support. This has been summarised below.

Summary of conclusions

	Core issues in intellectual disabilities	Implications for intellectual disability care/support
Attachment formation	1. Development of attachments with primary caregivers is based on the successful interaction of a child's 'attachment behavioural system' and the 'caregiver behavioural system' 2. Limitations in these interactions in early infancy may have interfered with the development of *secure attachments* 3. Compensatory behaviours (rocking, avoidance) may have developed and learning may have been hampered 4. Current attachment relationship may be limited by staff turnover and time available for care and support relationships	1. To support and educate the person, the caregiver needs to ensure that an attachment relationship is generated 2. Early childhood attachment needs, such as physical contact, may still dominate, if early attachment was compromised 3. Rocking and avoidance of social contact may need to be understood as insecure attachment 4. Consistency in care and support relationships is important, especially for those who have not developed 'secure attachments'
Consistency and dissonance processing	1. Just like in the general population, the person with an intellectual disability needs to come to terms with inconsistency in information, actions and personal identity 2. Inconsistency is experienced as discomfort and motivates efforts to reduce it. This self-regulatory system helps maintain peace of mind 3. Proficiency to reduce dissonance may be lower in people with an intellectual disability 4. Inability to reduce salient self-related dissonance in people with intellectual disability may lead to frustration, stress and mental health problems	1. The caregiver/support worker needs to be alert to potential inconsistencies for the person in their care 2. The caregiver/support worker needs to be alert that signs of distress could be the result of dissonance 3. When the person with an intellectual disability seems unable to reduce dissonance, assistance may need to be provided 4. Self-related dissonance may need to be addressed so that the person with an intellectual disability can come to terms with being different
Reciprocity and contribution to community	1. Reciprocity is at the basis of the formation of personal relationships and community 2. We are hard-wired to be sensitive to who we owe and who owes us. This principle is also at work in people with intellectual disability 3. Self-esteem is higher when people owe us, rather than the other way around 4. People with an intellectual disability are more likely to thrive when they can contribute to community and society (do things for others)	1. Formation of relationships with the person with an intellectual disability should involve reciprocal activities 2. A person with an intellectual disability may not be entirely happy when only on the receiving end of care and support 3. People with an intellectual disability should be given opportunities to do things for others and be noted for this. This is often absent and therefore limits relationships within the community 4. To ensure long-term thriving in people with an intellectual disability, integration within community and society needs to be based on reciprocation in any way possible

Key Concepts Discussed

• Attachment formation: The bonds and relationships we form contribute to our well-being and also influence learning processes and social cognition. Understanding of the attachment process for those caring for people with an intellectual disability can support the development of secure attachment.

• Dissonance and inconsistency: As humans, we strive for consistency. When our thoughts or actions are inconsistent with our goals, beliefs or principles, this can lead to feelings of discomfort and inner turmoil. Through awareness and understanding of the dissonance mechanism, support workers can support people with intellectual disability to reduce discomfort when dissonance occurs.

- The importance of reciprocal activities in relationship formation: Reciprocity is key for the formation of relationships, self-esteem and community integration. Relationships with the person with intellectual disability should involve promoting contributing to their community and practicing reciprocity.

References

Adamson LB, Frick JE (2003) The still face: A history of a shared experimental paradigm. Infancy 4(4):451–473

Ainsworth MDS (1978) The Bowlby-Ainsworth attachment theory. Behav Brain Sci 1(3):436–438

Ainsworth MS, Bowlby J (1991) An ethological approach to personality development. Am Psychol 46(4):333

Andrews EE, Hicks RE (2017) Dealing with anxiety: relationships among interpersonal attachment style, psychological wellbeing and trait anxiety. Int J Psychol Stud 9(4):53–64

Aronson E (1969) The theory of cognitive dissonance: a current perspective. Adv Exp Soc Psychol 4:2–34. https://doi.org/10.1016/S0065-2601(08)60075-1

Bell D (1991) Reciprocity as a generating process in social relations. J Quantit Anthropol 3(3):251–260

Bosmans G, Bakermans-Kranenburg MJ, Vervliet B, Verhees MW, van IJzendoorn, M. H. (2020) A learning theory of attachment: unraveling the black box of attachment development. Neurosci Biobehav Rev 113:287–298

Bowlby J (1958) The nature of the child's tie to his mother. Int J Psychoanal 39:350–373

Bowlby J (1969) Attachment and loss: Vol. 1 Attachment. Basic Books, New York

Bowlby J (1979) The Bowlby-Ainsworth attachment theory. Behav Brain Sci 2(4):637–638

Bretherton I (1992) The origins of attachment theory: John Bowlby and Mary Ainsworth. Dev Psychol 28(5):759

British Psychological Society (2017) Incorporating attachment theory into practice: clinical practice guideline for clinical psychologists working with people who have intellectual disabilities. Leicester UK, BPS

Brown KM, Hoye R, Nicholson M (2012) Self-esteem, self-efficacy, and social connectedness as mediators of the relationship between volunteering and Well-being. J Soc Serv Res 38(4):468–483

Buss DM (2019) Evolutionary psychology: the new science of the mind, 6th edn. Routledge, New York

Cialdini RB, Schaller M, Houlihan D, Arps K, Fultz J (1987) Empathy-based helping: is it selflessly or selfishly motivated? J Pers Soc Psychol 52(4):749–758. https://doi.org/10.1037/0022-3514.52.4.749.   PMID 3572736

Cosmides L, Tooby J (2004) Social exchange: the evolutionary design of a neurocognitive system. In: Gazzaniga MS (ed) The cognitive neurosciences. Boston Review, Boston, MA, pp 1295–1308

Cosmides L, Tooby J (2005) Neurocognitive adaptations designed for social exchange. In: Buss DM (ed) Handbook of evolutionary psychology. Wiley, Hoboken, NJ, pp 584–627

de Vries JMA, Timmins F (2016) Care erosion in hospitals: problems in reflective nursing practice and the role of cognitive dissonance. Nurse Educ Today 38:5–8

de Vries J, Byrne M, Kehoe E (2015) Cognitive dissonance induction in everyday life: an fMRI study. Soc Neurosci 10(3):268–281

Dean EE, Shogren KA, Hagiwara M, Wehmeyer ML (2018) How does employment influence health outcomes? A systematic review of the intellectual disability literature. J Vocat Rehabil 49(1):1–13

Escobar MJ, Rivera-Rei A, Decety J, Huepe D, Cardona JF, Canales-Johnson A et al (2013) Attachment patterns trigger differential neural signature of emotional processing in adolescents. PLoS One 8(8):e70247

Festinger L (1957) A theory of cognitive dissonance, vol 2. Stanford University Press, Stanford, CA

Fletcher HK, Gallichan DJ (2016) An overview of attachment theory: Bowlby and beyond. Attach Intellect Dev Disabil:8–32

Fulton L, Kinnear D, Jahoda A (2021) Belonging and reciprocity amongst people with intellectual disabilities: A systematic methodological review. J Appl Res Intellect Disabil 34(4):1008–1025

Ganiban J, Barnett D, Cicchetti D (2000) Negative reactivity and attachment: down syndrome's contribution to the attachment–temperament debate. Dev Psychopathol 12(1):1–21

Garrels V, Sigstad HMH (2019) Motivation for employment in Norwegian adults with mild intellectual disability: the role of competence, autonomy, and relatedness. Scand J Disabil Res 21(1):250–261

Gawronski B (2012) Back to the future of dissonance theory: cognitive consistency as a core motive. Soc Cogn 30(6):652

Gerard HB (1992) Dissonance theory: A cognitive psychology with an engine. Psychol Inq 3(4):323–327

Hamadi L, Fletcher HK (2021) Are people with an intellectual disability at increased risk of attachment difficulties? A critical review. J Intellect Disabil 25(1):114–130

Harlow HF, Zimmermann RR (1959) Affectional response in the infant monkey: orphaned baby monkeys develop a strong and persistent attachment to inanimate surrogate mothers. Science 130(3373):421–432

Harmon-Jones E, Amodio DM, Harmon-Jones C (2009) Action-based model of dissonance: A review, integration, and expansion of conceptions of cognitive conflict. Adv Exp Soc Psychol 41:119–166

Hart S (2011) The impact of attachment: developmental neuroaffective psychology. W.W. Norton & Co., New York

Hess EH (1958) "Imprinting" in animals. Sci Am 198(3):81–93

Krill AL, Platek SM, Goetz AT, Shackelford TK (2007) Where evolutionary psychology meets cognitive neuroscience: A précis to evolutionary cognitive neuroscience. Evol Psychol 5(1):147470490700500114

Langer EJ, Rodin J (1976) The effects of choice and enhanced personal responsibility for the aged: a field experiment in an institutional setting. J Pers Soc Psychol 34(2):191

Lorenz K (1935) Der Kumpan in der Umwelt des Vogels. Der Artgenosse als auslösendes Moment sozialer Verhaltungsweisen. J Ornithol Beiblatt (Leipzig)

Lyubomirsky S, Kasri F, Zehm K (2003) Dysphoric rumination impairs concentration on academic tasks. Cogn Ther Res 27(3):309–330

McCausland D, McCallion P, Brennan D, McCarron M (2020) In pursuit of meaningful occupation: employment and occupational outcomes for older Irish adults with an intellectual disability. J Appl Res Intellect Disabil 33(3):386–397

McGrath A (2017) Dealing with dissonance: A review of cognitive dissonance reduction. Social Personal Psychol Compass 11(12):e12362. https://doi.org/10.1111/spc3.12362

Meltzer A, Robinson S, Fisher KR (2020) Barriers to finding and maintaining open employment for people with intellectual disability in Australia. Soc Policy Adm 54(1):88–101

Nolte T, Bolling DZ, Hudac CM, Fonagy P, Mayes L, Pelphrey KA (2013) Brain mechanisms underlying the impact of attachment-related stress on social cognition. Front Hum Neurosci 7:816

Panchanathan K, Boyd R (2004) Indirect reciprocity can stabilize cooperation without the second-order free rider problem. Nature 432(7016):499–502

Rutgers AH, Bakermans-Kranenburg MJ, van Ijzendoorn MH, van Berckelaer-Onnes IA (2004) Autism and attachment: a meta-analytic review. J Child Psychol Psychiatry 45(6):1123–1134

Schuengel C, Kef S, Damen S, Worm M (2010) 'People who need people': attachment and professional caregiving. J Intellect Disabil Res 54:38–47

Scior K, Werner S (2016) Intellectual disability and stigma. Palgrave Macmillan, Basingstoke

Sheerin F, Griffiths C, de Vries J, Keenan P (2015) An evaluation of a community living initiative in Ireland. J Intellect Disabil 19(3):266–281

Skelly A (2016) Maintaining the bond: working with people who are described as showing challenging behaviour using a framework based on attachment theory. Attachment in intellectual and developmental disability: A clinician's guide to practice and research. John Wiley & Sons, Chichester, West Sussex, pp 104–129

Stack DM, Muir DW (1990) Tactile stimulation as a component of social interchange: new interpretations for the still-face effect. Br J Dev Psychol 8(2):131–145

Suomi SJ (1997) Early determinants of behaviour: evidence from primate studies. Br Med Bull 53(1):170–184

Tooby J, Cosmides L (2008) The evolutionary psychology of the emotions and their relationship to internal regulatory variables. In: Lewis M, Haviland-Jones JM, Barrett LF (eds) Handbook of emotions. The Guilford Press, New York, pp 114–137

Tryon WW, Misurell JR (2008) Dissonance induction and reduction: A possible principle and connectionist mechanism for why therapies are effective. Clin Psychol Rev 28(8):1297–1309

van't Hof M, Tisseur C, van Berckelear-Onnes I, van Nieuwenhuyzen A, Daniels AM, Deen M et al (2021) Age at autism spectrum disorder diagnosis: A systematic review and meta-analysis from 2012 to 2019. Autism 25(4):862–873

Wilson J (2000) Volunteering. Annu Rev Sociol 26(1):215–240

Part II

From Birth to Adolescence

Nature of Intellectual Disability

5

Lynne Marsh and Paul McAleer

Chapter Topics

At the end of this chapter, readers should be able to:

- Gain a better understanding of the prevalence of intellectual disabilities.
- Identify the common prenatal, perinatal, postnatal and genetic causes of intellectual disabilities.
- Recognise the modifiable risk factors associated with intellectual disabilities and an increased awareness of the importance of focused public health campaigns.
- Appreciate the complexities of receiving a diagnosis of an intellectual disability.
- Recognise the role of healthcare professionals in supporting the person with intellectual disabilities and their families beyond the initial disclosure.

Overview of the Prevalence of Intellectual Disabilities

Life expectancy of individuals with intellectual disabilities, a lifelong condition (Kishore et al. 2019), has increased at two ends of the age continuum (Dolan et al. 2021). This changing trend in life expectancy has been attributed in part to the survival of premature babies with multiple and complex disabilities coupled with significant advances in medical care and treatment options, advancements in earlier assessment and diagnosis of intellectual disabilities and a deeper understanding of genetics and associated healthcare needs. There have also been medical, social and economic advances that have improved the quality of life (QoL) considerably for individuals with intellectual disabilities and their families. However, it is important to say that even with all these advancements, individuals with intellectual disabilities still to this day die on average, 19 years earlier than their peers in the general population (McCarron et al. 2015; Glover et al. 2017). This changing landscape has resulted in a global increase in the survival of children and adults with intellectual disabilities into older age, a welcome trend for this population group (McKenzie et al. 2016; McBride et al. 2021). There could potentially be an explosion of individuals with intellectual disabilities at both ends of the age continuum requiring additional support that will lead to increasing prevalence rates over the coming years.

Nevertheless, the prevalence rates of children and adults with intellectual disabilities across studies are quite variable and are dependent on variations in data collection methods, how intellectual disabilities is defined, the use of combined

L. Marsh (✉) · P. McAleer
Queen's University, Belfast, Northern Ireland, UK
e-mail: l.marsh@qub.ac.uk; p.mcaleer@qub.ac.uk

© The Author(s), under exclusive license to Springer Nature Switzerland AG 2023
F. Sheerin, C. Doyle (eds.), *Intellectual Disabilities: Health and Social Care Across the Lifespan*,
https://doi.org/10.1007/978-3-031-27496-1_5

terms such as learning difficulties with intellectual disabilities and the recent increase in autism spectrum disorder (ASD) diagnoses and its relationship to intellectual disabilities (Friedman et al. 2018; Anderson et al. 2019). However, in an effort to extend and understand more broadly the definition of intellectual disabilities, there has been a welcome shift in the focus of this diagnosis from one that was based primarily on intelligence quotient (IQ) to one that recognises that intellectual disabilities may manifest at different ages, under different circumstances, and can be informed by significant difficulties with activities of daily living such as communication as well as an impairment in an individual's level of adaptive functioning (McKenzie et al. 2016). This change in position has invariably led to a reconsideration of both incidence and prevalence of this lifelong condition and has allowed for a broader understanding of the nature and construct of intellectual disabilities.

Prevalence rates, irrespective of the lack of standardisation of definitions used, are still drawn globally from data collection methods such as general population census data (McBride et al. 2021), national household surveys (Maenner et al. 2016; McKenzie et al. 2016; McGuire et al. 2019) and national intellectual disability databases (Hourigan et al. 2018). Within such data collections, there is high variability in the estimates of prevalence rates of intellectual disabilities. As a consequence, these prevalence rates must be viewed with caution, as there may be some individuals with intellectual disabilities within society who have not been assessed as having an intellectual disability. There may also be some individuals who may not have availed or accessed intellectual disabilities services yet. Ultimately, as the population of individuals with intellectual disabilities and family carers age, there may be an increase in the number of older adults with intellectual disabilities surviving into old age (Heller 2019). Often, it is in the event of a family carer becoming sick and unwell or dying that some individuals, primarily older adults, come to the attention of services at a later stage in their life and may

require additional support (Forrester-Jones 2021). In summary, while prevalence rates can often be underestimated, they are a useful measure in estimating and predicting the current and future needs of individuals with intellectual disabilities, there is an inevitably of prevalence rates being underestimated and must be viewed with caution.

A meta-analysis by McKenzie et al. (2016) of 20 studies from Canada, the United States (USA), Taiwan, Denmark, India, Australia and Norway published between 1980 and 2009 suggested that the best estimate of prevalence for that time period was 1%. This estimation is much lower than Hourigan et al. (2018) findings of a prevalence rate of 5.96 per 1000 population in the Republic of Ireland. As they were able to draw from an Irish National Intellectual Disability Database (NIDD), they were also able to identify that 10,032 children between birth and 19 years of age were registered with an intellectual disability out of a total population of 28,388 people (Hourigan et al. 2018). Similar estimations by McBride et al. (2021) in Northern Ireland indicated a prevalence rate of 2% for the overall population, of which there was a prevalence rate of 3.8% for children aged between birth and 15 years of age. It is important to determine prevalence rates of the number of individuals who have an intellectual disability, as this key information will help to inform and plan future healthcare planning and interventions, educational needs and social care requirements for each and every individual with intellectual disabilities across the lifespan.

In summary, current practice in estimating the number of individuals with intellectual disabilities demonstrates an over-reliance on household surveys and census data and, whilst helpful, is not always reliable or accurate, and future prevalence rates need to be viewed with caution. What is clear, however, is that there is an increased life expectancy for individuals with intellectual disabilities at both ends of the continuum. As they age, they may require additional age-related health and social care services as their peers in the general population.

Prenatal, Perinatal and Postnatal Diagnosis of an Intellectual Disability

With significant advances in diagnostic screening measures such as amniocentesis, chorionic villus sampling, nuchal translucency and foetal anomaly imaging and genetic testing, many syndromes and conditions associated with intellectual disabilities are diagnosed prenatally, perinatally and postnatally. A diagnosis of an intellectual disability is primarily based on a prenatal, perinatal or postnatal diagnosis and is largely informed by a clinical history, family history, genetic history and the child's presentation of other associated health-related conditions (Patel et al. 2020).

Conditions such as spina bifida and hydrocephaly (Vasudevan and Suri 2017; Vogel et al. 2019) can be diagnosed prenatally, whilst perinatal causes of intellectual disabilities may be associated with maternal infections such as rubella and cytomegalovirus (Simpson et al. 2016). A postnatal diagnosis of an intellectual disability may be identified immediately at birth due to the visible features of a condition like Cri-du-chat syndrome in which the facial features are quite distinct (Su et al. 2019). Other postnatal causes may be attributed to traumatic events at birth or immediately after birth resulting in a brain injury or anoxia (Linn et al. 2019). For others, a postnatal diagnosis can occur at a later stage when a child is experiencing feeding difficulties within days or weeks of their birth or there is a concern that the child is not reaching the typical child development milestones resulting in a global developmental delay (GDD) (Vasudevan and Suri 2017).

Whilst the aetiology of some intellectual disabilities is idiopathic in nature, with the cause remaining unknown, the diagnosis of an intellectual disability may also be confirmed at birth due to an infant's low birth weight and/or smaller head circumference. These traits can be associated with syndromes like Cornelia de Lange syndrome (CdLS) (Boyle et al. 2015), which will be confirmed with further genetic investigations postnatally. For others, a genetic diagnosis may be pursued by parents due to concerns about their child demonstrating severe behavioural issues, hyperactivity or anxiety, which could later be confirmed as fragile X syndrome through genetic testing (Hagerman et al. 2017). Table 5.1 identifies some of the common prenatal, perinatal and postnatal risk factors associated with intellectual disabilities.

Reader Activity 5.1

The aetiology of some intellectual disabilities is idiopathic in nature, with many of the causes remaining unknown.

1. List three emotions that a family member may experience when they realise there may be no clear cause for their child's intellectual disability.
2. What are the key implications of not knowing the cause of a child's intellectual disability?
3. What would you consider as your key role in supporting family members at this time?

Genetic Diagnosis of an Intellectual Disability

Arguably, the growth of genetic research has been largely positive and welcomed by parents of children with intellectual disabilities, geneticist and healthcare professionals as it has led to a more accurate diagnosis of intellectual disabilities, better identification of specific care and management processes associated with the condition as well as enhanced understanding of possible physical, psychological and behavioural issues (Vasudevan and Suri 2017). Furthermore, knowing and understanding the genetic cause of an intellectual disability assists parents to identify specific

Table 5.1 Common prenatal, perinatal and postnatal risk factors associated with intellectual disabilities

Prenatal risk factors	Perinatal risk factors	Pre- and postnatal causes
Advanced maternal age	Male sex	Down syndrome
Maternal black race	Low birth weight	Fragile X syndrome
Low maternal education	Preterm birth	Klinefelter's syndrome
Third or more parity		Cornelia de Lange syndrome (CdLS)
Non-modifiable risk factors		
Health-related risk factors	**Traumatic events during labour and at birth**	**Neurodevelopmental disabilities**
Maternal infections (i.e. rubella, cytomegalovirus, syphilis, toxoplasmosis)	Birth trauma	Foetal alcohol spectrum disorder (FASD)
Maternal hypertension	Head trauma	Autism spectrum disorder (ASD)
Maternal diabetes	Prolonged delivery	
Maternal epilepsy	Anoxia (oxygen deprivation)	
Maternal asthma		
Maternal nutrition		

This is not an exhaustive list

genetic risk factors for subsequent pregnancies and to plan accordingly. This growth in genetic screening and testing has inevitably changed the disability landscape for many individuals and plays an important role in identifying prenatal, perinatal and postnatal conditions genetically associated with intellectual disabilities that had traditionally been diagnosed months and even years after birth. For example, whilst Klinefelter's syndrome had long been associated with a delayed diagnosis at puberty when the child failed to develop secondary sex characteristics (Bourke et al. 2014), the advances in non-invasive diagnostic testing and screening, conditions such as Klinefelter's syndrome, can now be detected prenatally (Herlihy and McLachlan 2015; Zampini et al. 2021) and is only one of many sex chromosome anomalies that can be detected much earlier during pregnancy. With this genetic disclosure, parents can gain an enhanced understanding of the specific genetic condition their child presents with, allowing them to be better placed and prepared to appropriately support their child across their caregiving trajectory.

As highlighted, intellectual disabilities have heterogeneous causation that are influenced by multifactorial biological, genetic, environmental, social and psychological phenomena. Over the years, continuous advancement in diagnostic technologies have contributed to a more accurate identification of the causal factors of intellectual disabilities at earlier stages in an individual's life cycle and, in some cases, have altered the known prevalence of some conditions. Phenylketonuria (PKU), for example, is a genetic condition that causes an inborn error that prevents metabolism of the protein phenylalanine (Phe). Phenylalanine is commonly found in many foods and, when consumed by individuals with PKU, can lead to toxic accumulations in the blood plasma and brain, subsequently resulting in irreversible intellectual disabilities in 95% of cases (Bodamer 2010; Perez-Garcia et al. 2022). Evidence supporting the use of a Phe-restricted diet in the 1950s, and the development of a diagnostic screening tool known as the Guthrie test in the 1960s, have strongly influenced the course of this condition (van Vliet et al. 2018). Invariably, neonatal, whole population public health screening has led to the reduction in rates of intellectual disabilities, caused by PKU, from 95% to 1% (Bodamer 2010), further demonstrating the invaluable role for public health and genetic screening processes.

Notably, other disorders strongly associated with intellectual disabilities appear to be increasing in prevalence. A recent study of seven million children in UK state schools suggests that diagnosis of ASD has increased from 1 in 64 pupils in 2009 to 1 in 57 pupils in 2017 (Roman-Urrestarazu et al. 2021). Research suggests that rises in diagnosed cases of ASD can be attributed to expanded diagnostic criteria, increased knowledge and awareness of the disorder leading to earlier detection and a growing recognition that the disorder is lifelong (Matson and Kozlowski 2011). Whilst a diagnosis of ASD is currently dependent on psychometric testing, other forms of testing, such as genetic testing, have also contributed to the changing evidence base for prevalence of disorders that are linked to intellectual disabilities.

Over recent decades advances in genomics and genetic testing have led to greater accuracy in diagnosis of prenatal and postnatal conditions that cause intellectual disabilities and represents a move away from diagnosis, which is based on phenotypical observations of biological, psychological or social symptoms alone (Huang et al. 2016; Wolfe et al. 2017). In cases where the individual's presentation is suspected to be linked to a specific genetic disorder or condition, chromosomal microarray analysis can be used to identify the specific genetic deletions, duplications or translocations that have led to the impairment of neurodevelopmental functioning and subsequent intellectual disabilities.

As many of the syndromic disorders that will be discussed in this chapter share an increased risk of severe or moderate intellectual disabilities, it is apparent that without the advent of technological advances in genetic testing, diagnosis of these disorders is overly reliant on the presence and identification of phenotypical features and thus may lead to differential diagnosis or diagnostic overshadowing. Xiol et al. (2021) suggest that individuals with less well-defined or idiopathic diagnoses such as ASD, epilepsy or intellectual disabilities tend to show less successful biopsychosocial outcomes.

Overview to Genetic Screening and Genetic Testing

Wolfe et al. (2017) suggest that only 10% of individuals with intellectual disabilities will be referred for genetic testing. Yet, Reilly et al. (2017) contend that the lack of evidence of or delay in diagnosis could potentially contribute negatively to parental well-being with limited understanding of their child's specific health or behavioural needs. Therefore, accurate and early genetic testing can support precise diagnosis and support individualised clinical management, treatment plans or care pathways that may help to avoid a 'one size fits all' approach to treatment and intervention (Wolfe et al. 2017).

Arguably, whilst genetic testing is retrospective and cannot prevent the genetic mutations that give rise to syndromic disorders, through genetic counselling, information derived from testing regarding heredity can assist parents with decision-making prior to future pregnancy (Reilly et al. 2017). As genetic testing technologies continue to advance, it is predicted that future whole population screening approaches similar to the Guthrie test can be developed, which provide platforms for early interventions and improved health outcomes for individuals with intellectual disabilities and syndromic disorders (Reilly et al. 2017).

Still, whilst genetic screening has clearly played a significant role in supporting families and the child with intellectual disabilities, there have been numerous global ethical debates that have focused on 'screening out' rather than 'screening for' particular conditions associated with an intellectual disability with a focus on offering terminations (Klucznik and Slepian 2018). This has been clearly evidenced in Iceland where there are now fewer live births of babies being born with Down syndrome because of current screening practices and policies (Klucznik and Slepian 2018). Notably, Down syndrome is recognised as the most common genetic cause of intellectual disabilities, and the primary purpose of genetic screening should be to make an informed decision without any undue pressures to decide to continue or terminate a pregnancy (van Schendel et al. 2017). Yet, Icelandic practices and policies supports termination as the 'best' and almost 'preferred' option for mothers with a positive diagnosis of Down syndrome and warrants further attention and wider global debate (Klucznik and Slepian 2018).

However, whilst debating the ethics of genetic screening is beyond the scope of this chapter, it would be remiss not to recommend the importance of reading the arguments and current research evidence to gain that genetic understanding. Irrespective of a personal view of genetic screening practices and policies, the role of healthcare professionals nevertheless should be to ensure non-judgemental attitudes when in discussions with pregnant mothers or those planning a pregnancy and must remain central to the core of professional practice.

Nevertheless, whilst being cautious about the purpose and rights to genetic screening, testing and subsequent diagnosis, the evidence is clear that genetic screening and testing is often a vital first step for parents, to gain a deeper understanding of their genetic predisposition to the wide range of conditions that are associated with an intellectual disability.

Sharing of a Diagnosis of a Child's Intellectual Disability

The sharing of a diagnosis of intellectual disability has been featured across the research literature with many parents recalling the impact and implications of such a disclosure for their child and wider family. This diagnosis has been noted as a life-changing event for many, and in parents' narratives, which professionals were involved in the disclosure is recalled vividly as is the setting and what information and support, if any, was provided. This disclosure remained a central tenet of a parent's experience of being informed of their child's intellectual and is where their stories began in becoming a parent of a child with an intellectual disability (Marsh et al. 2018; Zampini et al. 2021).

In a recent study by Zampini et al. (2021), 48 Italian parents, 6 of whom were fathers, investigated parents' satisfaction to a prenatal diagnosis of Klinefelter's syndrome through the completion of an anonymous questionnaire. Overall, the findings identified that approximately half of parents (n = 24) were satisfied by the communication process in relation to the disclosure of the diagnosis. This satisfaction was attributed to the clarity and completeness of the information provided. Conversely, the lack of professionalism and sensitivity

by the person communicating the diagnosis was deemed to be unsatisfactory for almost 29% of parents. Whilst there was a range of professionals involved in sharing the diagnosis that included geneticist or gynaecologist, parents overall were most satisfied with how the geneticist shared their child's intellectual disability diagnosis. A secondary finding of this study highlighted some of the reasons parents went on to share their child's diagnosis with others. In relation to professionals such as teachers, family general practitioner (GP) or psychologist, parents shared the diagnosis as they required treatment, monitoring, advice and support. Notably, the fear of prejudices and discrimination were the primary reason for not disclosing the diagnosis to professionals.

Whilst the reasons for sharing a disclosure with relatives, close friends and co-workers were similar to professionals as advice and support was required, non-disclosure to relatives and friends was also similar and associated with fear of prejudices, discrimination and the desire not to worry others. Clearly, parents knowing the cause of a child's intellectual disability and then sharing the disclosure with others was deemed to be quite an emotive experience. Therefore, professionals should demonstrate sensitivity, work at a parent's pace and understand that additional time to accept a disability diagnosis may be required and valid and updated information is crucial to the disclosure process (Zampini et al. 2021), a finding articulated across other studies (Lingen et al. 2016; Shree and Shukla 2016).

In summary, there can be significant challenges in determining the exact cause of an intellectual disability, and the process of disclosure and confirmation can be extremely difficult (Shree and Shukla 2016). Understanding the prenatal, perinatal or postnatal predisposition for a condition supports parents to make informed decisions in relation to supporting the child across the trajectory of caring. Additionally, a parent's choice to share a disability disclosure may also be difficult and can be emotive as the fear of prejudice and discrimination is a very real concern. Notably, having access to genetic screening and testing assists parents in planning a pregnancy or planning a subsequent pregnancy (Kishore et al. 2019). Having this understanding of the specific health, emotional or behavioural supports and interventions required by their child can further ensure that the best possible quality of life outcomes for their child and family across the lifespan can be achieved.

Implications of a Diagnosis of Intellectual Disabilities and Genetic Conditions

Whilst there are variations in the definitions of intellectual disabilities as previously discussed, there are many implications for families in receiving such a disclosure. In order to support the child appropriately, parents and families need to understand the aetiology of the intellectual disability as well as recognise that the severity, cognitive abilities, adaptive function and communication ability will vary and each child will require a tailor-made plan of care and support across their lifespan (Patel et al. 2020).

Whilst the diagnostic process can be an emotional and lengthy process and fraught with many difficulties (Oswald et al. 2017), many parents just want to understand the cause and specific reason for their child's disability so that they can move forward and support their child appropriately (Karam et al. 2015). For example, whilst nine Japanese fathers had received a definitive diagnosis of Down syndrome about 1 month following the birth of their child in Takataya et al. (2016) qualitative study, they continued to question why their child had been born with this condition. This question of 'why' remains unresolved for some parents as often the cause of condition is random with the aetiology remaining unknown. This questioning of 'why' a child has been affected is evident across studies and is not specific to parents of Down syndrome (Marsh et al. 2018). Rather for many, understanding why their child has an intellectual disability allows them to move on and accept their child's disability and to ensure appropriate help and support can be available (Bourke et al. 2014).

Equally, some parents innately know there is a concern in relation to their child's development and understanding the specific cause and implications of a diagnosis supports parents to access appropriate health information associated with the condition. Likewise, a specific diagnosis allows parents to plan current care and support and predict future needs for care when parents may not be in a position to care for their child in the longer term. Parents often recall that if they do not have this definitive diagnosis, the right type of support may not be available to their child or family and could invariably impact negatively on their child's life and that of the wider family. Ultimately, obtaining a diagnosis can improve QoL (Lingen et al. 2016). This section of the chapter has considered the sharing of a diagnosis of an intellectual disability. The implications of receiving a diagnosis and the need for information to support a family member have also been discussed.

Overview of the Common Conditions Associated with Intellectual Disabilities

This section provides a brief overview of some of the common conditions associated with intellectual disabilities.

Pitt-Hopkins Syndrome

Pitt-Hopkins syndrome (PTHS) is a rare genetic disease first described by Australian physicians David Pitt and Ian Hopkins in 1978 with 500 confirmed clinical cases reported worldwide (Sparber et al. 2020). It is described as a rare, genetic, neurological disorder affecting both sexes and is caused by an abnormal expression of the transcription factor 4 (TCF4) gene, leading to deletions or mutations on the 18th chromosome. Some of the clinical features of PTHS include a narrow forehead, wide nasal bridge, cupid's bow upper lip, microcephaly and scoliosis. Global developmental delay, intellectual disabilities, impaired speech patterns, recurrent seizures, severe constipation, breathing anomalies, hypotonia and delayed gross motor development are usually apparent in the first year of life (Zollino et al. 2019; McAleer 2021).

Fragile X Syndrome (FXS)

Fragile X syndrome (FXS) is a single gene disorder and is the most commonly identifiable cause of intellectual disabilities and ASD, affecting approximately 1.4 per 10,000 males and 0.9 per 10,000 females (Borch et al. 2020; Crawford et al. 2020). FXS is caused by a mutation of the fragile X mental retardation 1 (FMR1) gene and leads to two distinct pathways, fragile X full mutation and fragile X premutation. It is estimated that approximately 1 in 300 women and 1850 men carry the fragile X premutation; however full mutation only occurs in offspring following maternal transmission (Smolich et al. 2020). Whilst full mutation of the FMR1 gene commonly leads to moderate to severe intellectual disabilities in males, symptomatology in females who carry the full mutation is less clear and can lead to variations in neurodevelopment ranging from no intellectual disabilities to moderate intellectual disabilities (Crawford et al. 2020). FXS can be identified by some physical features such as prominent ears, narrow face hypotonia and hyper-flexibility; however these features are variable and therefore not diagnostically significant. In addition to intellectual disabilities, individuals who have been diagnosed with FXS will experience a range of co-morbid health conditions that present biological, psychological and social care needs, including otitis media, ocular disorders, epilepsy, sleep disorders and mitral valve prolapse (in 50% of adults). There is a higher prevalence of ASD (71%), attention-deficit hyperactivity disorder (ADHD), social avoidance, aggression and self-injurious behaviour in individuals with FXS that benefit from early identification, diagnosis, assessment and intervention (Reilly et al. 2017).

Williams Syndrome (WS)

Like FXS, early diagnosis and intervention can lead to improved health outcomes in other prenatal genetic conditions such as Williams syndrome (WS; also known as Williams-Beuren syndrome). WS is caused by a microdeletion on the chromosome 7q11.23 and leads to a multisystem disorder, which affects the cardiovascular, central nervous, gastrointestinal and endocrine systems (Kozel et al. 2021). Knowledge of this clinical syndrome has been expanding over the past number of decades, and intellectual disabilities are now diagnosed in approximately 75% of cases (Kozel et al. 2021). Prevalence rates of WS are understood to be estimated at between 1 in 7000 and 1 in 20,000 for both males and females (Reilly et al. 2017). Individuals with WS present with a range of phenotypical physical features that are identifiable in early childhood, including a wide forehead, a smaller pointed lower jaw, periorbital fullness, flat nose and a long philtrum (Kozel et al. 2021).

Individuals with WS are at greater risk of developing cardiovascular disease, slow physical growth, joint laxity and/or contractures, visual and auditory disorders, constipation and gastroesophageal reflux, obesity in adulthood, decreased bone mineral density and sleep apnoea. The presence of psychosocial disorders such as ADHD, ASD, anxiety or depression are also indicated in addition to communication problems. Rates of co-morbid ASD vary from between 12 and 20% and caution is indicated regarding assessment, treatment and support; that is, support should be provided by practitioners who are knowledgeable of both ASD and WS (Kozel et al. 2021).

Tuberous Sclerosis Complex (TSC)

Other prenatal genetic multisystem disorders linked with intellectual disabilities are associated with equally pervasive symptomologies, for example, tuberous sclerosis complex (TSC). TSC is caused by multiple or sporadic mutations in either the TSC1 or TSC2 gene and results in overactivation of the mTOR pathway, which regulates cell growth and proliferation (Jozwiak and Curatolo 2021; Notaro and Pierce 2021). Evidence suggests that TSC is present in approximately 1 in 6000 to 1 in 10,000 births (Jozwiak and Curatolo 2021), and whilst 55% of individuals diagnosed with TSC do not experience impairments in cognitive functioning, 30% of individuals will have severe to profound and multiple intellectual disabilities (Ng et al. 2014).

Evidence suggests that dysregulation of the mTOR pathway could play a significant role in increasing the susceptibility of an individual with TSC to developing a range of significant health problems (Jozwiak and Curatolo 2021). mTOR pathway dysregulation leads to the growth of multiple types of benign tumours in the central nervous, cardiac, renal, ophthalmic, pulmonary, dermal and dental systems (Notaro and Pierce 2021). Cortical tubers and subependymal giant cell astrocytomas (SEGAs) are abnormal but benign growths in the brain that increase risk of epilepsy that occurs in 85% of TSC cases (Notaro and Pierce 2021). SEGAs may calcify or harden over time and lead to obstructive hydrocephalus; thus early diagnosis and intervention can improve long-term health outcomes for individuals with TSC (Northrup and Krueger 2013). Tuberous growths in the cardiac system can lead to dysrhythmias consistent with Wolff-Parkinson-White syndrome (Northrup and Krueger 2013). Tubers and benign growths known as angiomyolipomas are a significant cause of renal failure and premature mortality in TSC cases, second only to severe intellectual disabilities (Northrup and Krueger 2013). Angiomyolipomas are relatively slow growing and their identification at the earliest stage is essential in order to improve outcomes, thus highlighting the importance of accurate condition-specific knowledge, diagnosis, assessment and intervention.

Rett Syndrome (RTT)

Whilst some disorders are caused by a small number of genetic mutations that have multiple impacts on physiological systems, some disorders are caused by mutations across multiple genes that significantly affect sequencing of genomes and can lead to an array of overlapping phenotypes relating to a single disorder (Xiol et al. 2021). One example of this effect can be observed in the sequencing of genomes relating to

Rett syndrome (RTT), which is the second most common cause of severe intellectual disabilities in females, with a prevalence of 1 in 10,000 to 20,000 live births (Cosentino et al. 2019).

RTT is primarily caused by a mutation of the methyl-CpG-binding protein 2 (MECP2) gene. Whilst this suggests that RTT is caused by a single gene mutation, MECP2 is responsible for binding DNA during the process of gene expression, thus creating a mosaic pattern of 250 known gene mutations that give rise to a range of heterogeneous phenotypes and clinical manifestations (Ivy and Standridge 2021). These variations in clinical manifestations, discovered by emerging genetic testing technology, have led to some authors to propose that RTT should be considered as a spectrum disorder rather than a defined clinical syndrome (Xiol et al. 2021).

MECP2 is abundant in the brain and plays a significant role in development of neurological structures such as the brainstem and spinal cord (Cosentino et al. 2019). Individuals with RTT will experience neurodevelopmental delays within the first 30 months of life, which are characterised by failure to reach developmental milestones and an apparent loss of acquired movement and communicative skills (Neul 2019). RTT is also associated with conditions that co-occur alongside severe intellectual disabilities including epilepsy, gastrointestinal disorders, scoliosis, sleep disorders, breathing abnormalities such as apnoea, in addition to communication problems, limitations in motor control of the hands and impaired mobility (Strugnell et al. 2019). Due to the mosaic nature of the disorder, it is unsurprising that it presents phenotypical features that overlap with other genetic disorders and can lead to differential diagnosis with syndromic conditions such as Cornelia de Lange syndrome (Schönewolf-Greulich et al. 2017).

Cornelia de Lange Syndrome (CdLS)

Cornelia de Lange syndrome (CdLS) has an estimated prevalence of between 1 in 10,000 and 1 in 50,000 births; however exact figures are unknown as some individuals with CdLS may have a milder form of the disorder and thus remain undiagnosed (Boyle et al. 2015). CdLS phenotypically overlaps with the most common features of RTT, except for some additional central nervous system (CNS) abnormalities and dysmorphic facial features found in CdLS (Schönewolf-Greulich et al. 2017). It is easily recognised from birth due to the distinctive craniofacial appearance and growth pattern, as well as limb malformations (Kline et al. 2018). The range of intellectual disabilities is from mild to severe and as with many of these syndromes, there is a wide variation in presentation, and not all children will be affected in the same way. Some of the associated health needs include high arched palate, cardiovascular anomalies, oral problems and vertebral anomalies. They may also present with cognition and behaviour difficulties such as ASD and self-injurious behaviour (Kline et al. 2018).

Foetal Alcohol Spectrum Disorder (FASD)

Foetal alcohol spectrum disorder (FADS), first described in 1973 by Jones and Smith (May et al. 2021), has an estimated global prevalence of 7.7 per 1000 population (Lange et al. 2017). It is a lifelong condition caused from a mother's substantial alcohol exposure during pregnancy. It is often recognisable at birth due to the unusual facial features, microcephaly and lower birth weight. The diagnostic process should include a family, social and medical history as well as a complete physical examination and be informed by the mother's history of alcohol consumption during pregnancy. As the child develops, they may also present with a mild to severe intellectual disability, difficulties with learning and language, growth restrictions and behavioural impairments. Co-morbid conditions associated with FASD may affect the heart, kidneys, muscles and bones (Scottish Intercollegiate Guidelines Network (SIGN) 2019).

In summary, each child is unique and the individual presentation of the condition is different. Not all children will experience the range of comorbidities and the intellectual disability can range from mild to profound. However, whilst demonstrating traits of their condition, children are more like themselves and their families than each other with the same diagnosis.

Prevention of an Intellectual Disability

As previously discussed, they are many causes and risk factors associated with an intellectual disability, and for the most part, the prevention of an intellectual disability is not possible in many cases as there may be no known aetiology, the condition may be a random occurrence or there is a genetic predisposition to the condition. With the significant advancements in genetic screening and testing, and a clearer understanding of whole population public health screening and diagnostic measures, improvements have been made in terms of preventive and public health measures in relation to modifiable risks.

Preventive Health Measures: Maternal Infections

Some of the modifiable risk factors presented in the early section of this chapter may be reduced. For example, there are many maternal infections that can be dangerous to the baby during pregnancy such as cytomegalovirus (CMV), toxoplasmosis and rubella that can result in hearing loss, visual impairments, intellectual disabilities and epilepsy. Whilst it is not possible to completely prevent maternal infections, the risk can be significantly reduced through public health awareness, education and whole population vaccination programmes, which have been critical to the reduction of these conditions on a global scale. Focused public health awareness campaigns in relation to maternal infections advise expectant mothers to adhere to the following practices:

1. Wash hands with soap and hot water, often and regularly.
2. Do not share food or cutlery with young children.
3. Hug rather than kiss children on the face.

4. Follow general food hygiene in relation to preparation, cooking and storage of foods.
5. Avoid close contact with cats especially if they are sick.
6. Avoid emptying cat litter trays.

Preventive Health Measures: Alcohol Consumption

Globally, alcohol consumption in women of childbearing age is a common and significant public health issue. Over the last 20 years, alcohol abstention has been widely promoted as a preventative measure, yet there is a concern that rather than reducing FASD, there is an increased prevalence of this condition (Choate et al. 2019) suggesting that preventative measures need to be reviewed as a matter of urgency. Whilst many countries have developed public health campaigns to promote alcohol abstinence, the risk to the baby in utero remains a public health issue with incidences of FASD still being underestimated.

Whilst FASD is 100% preventable if a woman does not drink during pregnancy, clearly many pregnancies are not planned and often a woman does not know she is pregnant until a few weeks or months into the pregnancy where alcohol has already been consumed. Therefore, rather than just promoting abstinence, delivering health literacy education about safe drinking practices to all women of childbearing age is required as a first step as a preventive measure (WHO 2020). Once a pregnancy is confirmed, brief health literacy around alcohol consumption should be delivered to all women who use alcohol during pregnancy (Nawabi et al. 2021).

The focus of prevention should be to highlight the adverse effects of alcohol consumption on the unborn baby, to raise awareness that this lifelong condition can be prevented and to reduce the social stigma associated with having a child born with FASD. A National Clinical Guideline was developed and published in 2019 by Health Improvement Scotland in January 2019 (Scottish Intercollegiate Guidelines Network) for people at

risk of FASD, their families, allied health professionals, families and voluntary and statutory organisations and policymakers. Within this guideline, there are recommendations in relation to identifying those at risk, assessment and diagnostic measures and management and follow-up that may be beneficial across the range of families and professionals, supporting people with an FASD diagnosis.

Reader Activity 5.2
Some modifiable risk factors associated with intellectual disabilities may be reduced and healthcare professionals are well placed to support families through practice and education to improve their understanding.

1. Source and review one evidence-based research paper in relation to one of the following:
   - FASD
   - Maternal infections
2. Next, make some reflective notes on the key issues and concerns that were highlighted in this paper.
3. Make a list of what you would need to know to increase public health awareness campaigns about modifiable risk factors associated with intellectual disabilities.

Best Practice Guidance to Disclosure of a Diagnosis

Being informed of a child's intellectual disability can be an emotional event in a parent's life and needs to be completed in a sensitive and empathetic way. The range of professionals confirming a diagnosis of a child's intellection varies from geneticist, paediatricians, audiologists, educational psychologist and intellectual disability specialist. The emerging research evidence suggests that the disclosure experience is often negative, accompanied by a lack of support and inappropriate information (Goodwin et al. 2015). Therefore, there is a clear need for professionals who are involved in a disclosure to remember that the disclosure needs to be tailored, timely, informative and supportive to meet the needs of the family (National Best Practice Guidelines 2007, Douglas et al. 2017).

There have been many recommendations emerging from the literature in relation to parent's expectations of receiving a disclosure of their child's intellectual disability, yet few published guidelines exist. However, parents continue to highlight the need for valid, reliable and sensitive information, sharing a disclosure with kindness, care and understanding. Australian parents of 11 children with an intellectual disability in a qualitative study by Douglas et al. (2017) identified specifically 3 types of information they required: firstly, they wanted information on their baby's condition; secondly, the baby's specific needs; and finally, information on the available supports and services. Rather than being a one-off meeting with the relevant professional, a follow-up meeting would be preferred to allow parents to process the information and return with their questions. For many, this experience understandably is quite emotional and the information shared at the initial meeting is not retained or understood until sometime after.

The National Federation of Voluntary Bodies in Ireland in 2007 developed and published *National Best Practice Guidelines for Informing Families of their Child's Disability* and recommend that the following seven guiding principles should be applied in every case of a disclosure:

1. Family-Centred Disclosure
2. Respect for Child and Family
3. Sensitive and Empathetic Communication
4. Appropriate, Accurate Information
5. Positive, Realistic Messages and Hope
6. Team Approach and Planning
7. Focused and Supported Implementation of Best Practice

This is not an exhaustive list and needs to be considered and adapted to the individual needs of the parents and the child, irrespective of who is sharing this disclosure. This disclosure must be considerate, family-centred and delivered over time at a pace that suits the family. Given that an intellectual disability is a permanent and lifelong condition, ensuring the disclosure is completed with sensitivity is crucial. Healthcare professionals are well placed to deliver a diagnosis of a child's intellectual disability and continue to undertake professional training and development so that remain well placed to support the family beyond the initial disclosure.

Conclusion

It is clear that prevalence rates of intellectual disabilities can be complex to understand and highly variable depending on data collected. Furthermore, it is noted that life expectancy of individuals with intellectual disabilities has increased at both ends of the age continuum. There are a wide variety of common prenatal, perinatal, postnatal and genetic causes of intellectual disabilities, and these have been explored in more detail in this chapter. The sharing of a diagnosis of intellectual disability and the implications of such a disclosure for the child and family have been considered. Best practice guidelines are important and the need for information is identified as an essential part of the diagnostic process. Whilst the prevention of an intellectual disability is not possible in many cases, the significant advances made in genetic screening and testing allow for a clearer formation of a picture resulting in an improved plan of care. Furthermore, improvements made in terms of preventive and public health measures in relation to modifiable risks have been outlined.

Key Concepts Discussed
- Globally, there are more people being diagnosed with intellectual disabilities.
- Life expectancy is also increasing with many presenting with multiple and complex

disabilities across the lifespan requiring extended care.

- There are many prenatal, perinatal, postnatal and genetic causes of intellectual disabilities; however many of the causes remain unknown.
- For the most part, the prevention of an intellectual disability is not possible, but some of the modifiable risk factors can be reduced through education and focused public health awareness campaigns.
- The disclosure of an intellectual disability can be an emotional and difficult journey for the person with intellectual disabilities and their families.
- Healthcare professionals are well placed to support the person with intellectual disabilities and their families beyond the initial disclosure and positively influence change in practice, education and research.

References

Anderson LL, Larson SA, MapelLentz S, Hall-Lande J (2019) A systematic review of US studies on the prevalence of intellectual or developmental disabilities since 2000. Intellect Dev Disabil 57(5):421–438. https://meridian.allenpress.com/idd/article-abstract/57/5/421/364937/A-Systematic-Review-of-U-S-Studies-on-the

Bodamer OA (2010) Screening for phenylketonuria. Ann Nestlé (English ed.) 68(2):53–57. https://doi.org/10.1159/000312812

Borch LA, Parboosingh J, Thomas MA, Veale P (2020) Re-evaluating the first-tier status of fragile X testing in neurodevelopmental disorders. Genet Med 22(6):1036–1039. https://www.nature.com/articles/s41436-020-0773-x

Bourke E, Snow P, Herlihy A, Amor D, Metcalfe S (2014) A qualitative exploration of mothers' and fathers' experiences of having a child with Klinefelter syndrome and the process of reaching this diagnosis. Eur J Hum Genet 22(1):18–24. https://www.nature.com/articles/ejhg2013102

Boyle MI, Jespersgaard C, Brøndum-Nielsen K, Bisgaard A-M, Tümer Z (2015) Cornelia de Lange syndrome. Clin Genet 88(1):1–12. https://doi.org/10.1111/cge.12499

Choate P, Badry D, MacLaurin B, Ariyo K, Sobhani D (2019) Fetal alcohol spectrum disorder: what does public awareness tell us about prevention programming? Int J Environ Res Public Health 16(21):4229. https://www.mdpi.com/1660-4601/16/21/4229

Cosentino L, Vigli D, Franchi F, Laviola G, De Filippis B (2019) Rett syndrome before regression: a time window of overlooked opportunities for diagnosis and intervention. Neurosci Biobehav Rev 107:115–135. https://www.sciencedirect.com/science/article/abs/pii/S0149763418308443

Crawford H, Abbeduto L, Hall SS, Hardiman R, Hessl D, Roberts JE, Scerif G, Stanfield AC, Turk J, Oliver C (2020) Fragile X syndrome: an overview of cause, characteristics, assessment and management. Paediatr Child Health 30(11):400–403. https://www.sciencedirect.com/science/article/abs/pii/S1751722220301530

Dolan E, Lane J, Hillis G, Delanty N (2021) Changing trends in life expectancy in intellectual disability over time. Ir Med J 112(9):1006. http://www.imj.ie/wp-content/uploads/2019/10/Changing-Trends-in-Life-Expectancy-in-Intellectual-Disability-Over-Time.pdf

Douglas T, Redley B, Ottmann G (2017) The need to know: the information needs of parents of infants with an intellectual disability—a qualitative study. J Adv Nurs 73(11):2600–2608. https://doi.org/10.1111/jan.13321

Forrester-Jones R (2021) The experiences of older carers of people with learning disabilities: "I just carry on with it". Tizard Learn Disabil Rev 26(1):48–57. https://www.emerald.com/insight/content/doi/10.1108/TLDR-08-2020-0018/full/pdf?casa_token=ahSRwWNO0hQAAAAA:7z2tq2tEglaxkYHZVgFzFAIERoIL3xoe2t9r3B-32CchCOIs8KD_MSCSUG2IBvLbVb-KenwGZpOVj2bWKRsLteeo2fwRknU8JyVoRYN_WYiTw6gLCpwU

Friedman DJ, Gibson Parrish R, Fox MH (2018) A review of global literature on using administrative data to estimate prevalence of intellectual and developmental disabilities. J Policy Pract Intellect Disabil 15(1):43–62. https://doi.org/10.1111/jppi.12220

Glover G, Williams R, Heslop P, Oyinlola J, Grey J (2017) Mortality in people with intellectual disabilities in England. J Intellect Disabil Res 61(1):62–74. https://doi.org/10.1111/jir.12314

Goodwin J, Schoch K, Shashi V, Hooper SR, Morad O, Zalevsky M, Gothelf D, Campbell LE (2015) A tale worth telling: the impact of the diagnosis experience on disclosure of genetic disorders. J Intellect Disabil Res 59(5):474–486. https://doi.org/10.1111/jir.12151

Hagerman RJ, Berry-Kravis E, Hazlett HC, Bailey DB, Moine H, Kooy RF, Tassone F, Gantois I, Sonenberg N, Mandel JL, Hagerman PJ (2017) Fragile X syndrome. Nat Rev Dis Primers 3(1):1–19. https://www.nature.com/articles/nrdp201765

Heller T (2019) Bridging aging and intellectual/developmental disabilities in research, policy, and practice. J Policy Pract Intellect Disabil 16(1):53–57. https://doi.org/10.1111/jppi.12263

Herlihy AS, McLachlan RI (2015) Screening for Klinefelter syndrome. Curr Opin Endocrinol Diabetes Obes 22(3):224–229. https://www.ingentaconnect.com/content/wk/coedo/2015/00000022/00000003/art00013

Hourigan S, Fanagan S, Kelly C (2018) Annual Report of the National Intellectual Disability Database Committee 2017 Main Findings. https://www.hrb.ie/fileadmin/2._Plugin_related_files/Publications/2018_pubs/Disability/NIDD/NIDD_Annual_Report_2017.pdf

Huang J, Zhu T, Qu Y, Mu D (2016) Prenatal, perinatal and neonatal risk factors for intellectual disability: a systemic review and meta-analysis. PLoS One 11(4):e0153655. https://journals.plos.org/plosone/article?id=10.1371/journal.pone.0153655

Ivy AS, Standridge S (2021) Rett syndrome: a timely review from recognition to current clinical approaches and clinical study updates. Semina Pediatr Neurol 37:100881. https://www.sciencedirect.com/science/article/pii/S1071909121000097?casa_token=OECkxJFPdhwAAAAA:eJRv3GoFzhKVfq2To7AvWyqJzrVKm0q0EgUaBj45pgbczpFo_EgMVnndcmNYM-W5Rm2AUAJ05rQ

Jozwiak S, Curatolo P (2021) Editorial: tuberous sclerosis complex – diagnosis and management. Front Neurol 12:755868. https://www.frontiersin.org/articles/10.3389/fneur.2021.755868/full

Karam SM, Riegel M, Segal SL, Félix TM, Barros AJ, Santos IS, Matijasevich A, Giugliani R, Black M (2015) Genetic causes of intellectual disability in a birth cohort: a population-based study. Am J Med Genet A 167(6):1204–1214. https://doi.org/10.1002/ajmg.a.37011

Kishore MT, Udipi GA, Seshadri SP (2019) Clinical practice guidelines for assessment and management of intellectual disability. Indian J Psychiatry 61(Suppl 2):194–210. https://www.ncbi.nlm.nih.gov/pmc/articles/PMC6345136/?report=reader

Kline AD, Moss JF, Selicorni A, Bisgaard AM, Deardorff MA, Gillett PM, Ishman SL, Kerr LM, Levin AV, Mulder PA, Ramos FJ (2018) Diagnosis and management of Cornelia de Lange syndrome: first international consensus statement. Nat Rev Genet 19(10):649–666. https://www.nature.com/articles/s41576-018-0031-0

Klucznik S, Slepian H (2018) Iceland's abortion policy concerning children with down syndrome: an ethical analysis. J Healthcare Ethics Administr 4(1):45–48. http://www.jheaonline.org/pdf/7_klucznik_Slepian_jhea.10.7164.pdf

Kozel BA, Barak B, Kim CA, Mervis CB, Osborne LR, Porter M, Pober BR (2021) Williams syndrome. Nat Rev Dis Primers 7(1):1–21. https://www.proquest.com/docview/2542128407?pq-origsite=gscholar&fromopenview=true

Lange S, Probst C, Gmel G, Rehm J, Burd L, Popova S (2017) Global prevalence of fetal alcohol spectrum disorder among children and youth: a systematic review and meta-analysis. JAMA Pediatr 171(10):948–956. https://jamanetwork.com/journals/jamapediatrics/article-abstract/2649225?casa_token=0ElyK3_0d6IAAAAA:H9lsqbjb5sQfWKrt_dJZ8N-ZbxnHig7B9KjwiEUS1NJvS7BvsQgE95zVk8w-G1qv01tHkrcvYW7g

Lingen M, Albers L, Borchers M, Haass S, Gaertner J, Schroeder S, Goldbeck L, Von Kries R, Brockmann K, Zirn B (2016) Obtaining a genetic diagnosis in a child with disability: impact on parental quality of life. Clin Genet 89(2):258–266. https://doi.org/10.1111/cge.12629

Linn JG, Chuaqui J, Wilson DR, Arredondo E (2019) The global impact of intellectual disability. Int J Childbirth Educ 34(2):14–17. https://www.researchgate.net/profile/Emanuel-Arredondo/publication/332368245_The_Global_Impact_of_Intellectual_Disability_and_Other_Mental_Disorders_in_Children/links/5caff746a6fdcc1d498e1dbe/The-Global-Impact-of-Intellectual-Disability-and-Other-Mental-Disorders-in-Children.pdf

Maenner MJ, Blumberg SJ, Kogan MD, Christensen D, Yeargin-Allsopp M, Schieve LA (2016) Prevalence of cerebral palsy and intellectual disability among children identified in two U.S. National Surveys, 2011-2013. Ann Epidemiol 26(3):222e226. https://www.ncbi.nlm.nih.gov/pmc/articles/PMC5144825/

Marsh L, Warren PL, Savage E (2018) "Something was wrong": a narrative inquiry of becoming a father of a child with an intellectual disability in Ireland. Br J Learn Disabil 46(4):216–224. https://onlinelibrary.wiley.com/doi/full/10.1111/bld.12230?casa_token=PFuOZYgpFlgAAAAA%3A7HEU-NpA1GD7fxm4YFy8hF8cosnDYetYl1H9vUn0dEQKtcrZHccFsPY4Y5wOzQuWjqe-0t-GRyitrA

Matson JL, Kozlowski AM (2011) The increasing prevalence of autism spectrum disorders. Res Autism Spectr Disord 5(1):418–425. https://www.sciencedirect.com/science/article/pii/S1750946710000917?casa_token=uEm28pd2L8gAAAAA:IMQaLDlVdydglflb8FbLXWPSwq_qd6YCQye64Q78PIAlKS32oZ8_FoJZvfru-uNzzuBFLjwfy1g

May PA, Marais AS, De Vries MM, Buckley D, Kalberg WO, Hasken JM, Stegall JM, Hedrick DM, Robinson LK, Manning MA, Tabachnick BG (2021) The prevalence, child characteristics, and maternal risk factors for the continuum of fetal alcohol spectrum disorders: A sixth population-based study in the same South African community. Drug Alcohol Depend 218:108408. https://www.sciencedirect.com/science/article/pii/S0376871620305731?casa_token=DX4LIIgXkJQAAAAA:CL_oQo_8No8pQLefozkEj6K6wIuvyGQkU0b1QbKYRzmBE7CZB7bAnsXtPwXBHAnm6sFHt3YW_A

McAleer P (2021) Pitt-Hopkins syndrome. Learn Disabil Pract 24(4):15–16. https://doi.org/10.7748/ldp.24.4.15.s6

McBride O, Heslop P, Glover G, Taggart T, Hanna-Trainor L, Shevlin M, Murphy J (2021) Prevalence estimation of intellectual disability using national administrative and household survey data: the importance of survey question specificity. Int J Popul Data Sci 6(1). https://www.ncbi.nlm.nih.gov/pmc/articles/PMC8188522/

McCarron M, Carroll R, Kelly C, McCallion P (2015) Mortality rates in the general Irish population compared to those with an intellectual disability from 2003 to 2012. J Appl Res Intellect Disabil 28(5):406–413. https://doi.org/10.1111/jar.12194

McGuire DO, Tian LH, Yeargin-Allsopp M, Dowling NF, Christensen DL (2019) Prevalence of cerebral palsy, intellectual disability, hearing loss, and blindness, National Health Interview Survey, 2009–2016. Disabil Health J 12(3):443–451. https://pubmed.ncbi.nlm.nih.gov/30713095/

McKenzie K, Milton M, Smith G, Ouellette-Kuntz H (2016) Systematic review of the prevalence and incidence of intellectual disabilities: current trends and issues. Curr Dev Disord Rep 3(2):04–115. https://link.springer.com/article/10.1007/s40474-016-0085-7

National Federation of Voluntary Bodies (2007) Informing families of their child's disability— National Best Practice Guidelines. National Federation of Voluntary Bodies, Ireland. http://www.informingfamilies.ie/_fileupload/Informing_Families_Guidelines.pdf

Nawabi F, Alayli A, Krebs F, Lorenz L, Shukri A, Bau AM, Stock S (2021) Health literacy among pregnant women in a lifestyle intervention trial: protocol for an explorative study on the role of health literacy in the perinatal health service setting. BMJ Open 11(7):e047377. https://www.ncbi.nlm.nih.gov/pmc/articles/PMC8252873/

Neul JL (2019) Can Rett syndrome be diagnosed before regression? Neurosci Biobehav Rev 104:158–159. https://europepmc.org/article/med/31283955

Ng KH, Ng SM, Parker A (2014) Annual review of children with tuberous sclerosis. Arch Dis Childh Educ Pract Ed 100(3):114–121. https://ep.bmj.com/content/edpract/100/3/114.full.pdf?casa_token=mGv2_22zaE8AAAAA:Kag39yD4mx5fz1mz8scZhkP5GasTNEPPgbCyWTCPmkD91b9rI9IAPU3OJ3a-R162OmblnK3gi70

Northrup H, Krueger DA (2013) Tuberous sclerosis complex diagnostic criteria update: recommendations of the 2012 international tuberous sclerosis complex consensus conference. Pediatr Neurol 49(4):243–254. https://www.sciencedirect.com/science/article/pii/S0887899413004906

Notaro K, Pierce B (2021) Tuberous sclerosis complex. J Am Acad Phys Assist 34(3):28–33. https://journals.lww.com/jaapa/fulltext/2021/03000/tuberous_sclerosis_complex__a_multisystem_disorder.3.aspx?casa_token=CKt_baavW6QAAAAA:AuWBG1-LGxC9GhZwaTE2Z-wRl4cvdfJwWgLriuPx6koampyALDr20N8ensUMtdgvGkDE0rW3cJZuGCXEEgr9V4GSX64Z4g

Oswald DP, Haworth SM, Mackenzie BK, Willis JH (2017) Parental report of the diagnostic process and outcome: ASD compared with other developmental disabilities. Focus Autism Dev Disabil 32(2):152–160. https://journals.sagepub.com/doi/pdf/10.1177/1088357615587500?casa_token=o1cVAdSMQmMAAAAA:WEifANeCv68LG9Ur7aOdJoNV1mu0n23YJWk0Qpj4lny940OCyF3fuU6831e-qkkCNuQwUcus4DH0

Patel DR, Cabral MD, Ho A, Merrick J (2020) A clinical primer on intellectual disability. Transl Pediatr 9(Suppl 1):S23. https://www.ncbi.nlm.nih.gov/pmc/articles/PMC7082244/

Perez-Garcia CG, Diaz-Trelles R, Vega JB, Bao Y, Sablad M, Limphong P, Chikamatsu S, Yu H, Taylor W, Karmali PP, Tachikawa K, Chivukula P (2022) Development of an mRNA replacement therapy for phenylketonuria. Mol Ther Nucleic Acids 28:87–98. https://www.sciencedirect.com/science/article/pii/S2162253122000488

Reilly C, Murtagh L, Senior J (2017) Factors associated with age of diagnosis in four neurogenetic syndromes. J Policy Pract Intellect Disabil 14(3):180–186. https://doi.org/10.1111/jppi.12202

Roman-Urrestarazu A, van Kessel R, Allison C, Matthews FE, Brayne C, Baron-Cohen S (2021) Association of Race/ethnicity and social disadvantage with autism prevalence in 7 million school children in England. JAMA Pediatr 175(6):e210054. https://jamanetwork.com/journals/jamapediatrics/article-abstract/2777821

Schönewolf-Greulich B, Bisgaard A-M, Møller RS, Dunø M, Brøndum-Nielsen K, Kaur S, Van Bergen NJ, Lunke S, Eggers S, Jespersgaard C, Christodoulou J, Tümer Z (2017) Clinician's guide to genes associated with Rett-like phenotypes-investigation of a Danish cohort and review of the literature. Clin Genet 95(2):221–230. https://pubmed.ncbi.nlm.nih.gov/29023665/

Scottish Intercollegiate Guidelines Network (SIGN) (2019) Children and young people exposed prenatally to alcohol. Edinburgh: SIGN; (SIGN publication no. 156). [January 2019]. https://www.sign.ac.uk/media/1092/sign156.pdf

Shree A, Shukla PC (2016) Intellectual disability: definition, classification, causes and characteristics. Learn Commun Int J Educ Soc Dev 7(1):9. https://www.indianjournals.com/ijor.aspx?target=ijor:lco&volume=7&issue=1&article=002

Simpson N, Mizen L, Cooper SA (2016) Intellectual disabilities. Medicine 44(11):679–682. https://www.sciencedirect.com/science/article/abs/pii/S1357303916301694

Smolich L, Charen K, Sherman SL (2020) Health knowledge of women with a fragile X premutation: improving understanding with targeted educational material. J Genet Couns 29(6):983–991. https://onlinelibrary.wiley.com/doi/full/10.1002/jgc4.1222?casa_token=fFkBUjoZ7C0AAAAA%3AeHd2Y5NiTtJhBTVlReYf_S2xDlYhWMbN2Qbk1Y08rIfNsBH9F_e19tnkGUVBV3dTnxZ-S-OPQ2IEaQ

Sparber P, Filatova A, Anisimova I, Markova T, Voinova V, Chuhrova A, Tabakov V, Skoblov V (2020) Various haploinsufficiency mechanisms in Pitt-Hopkins syndrome. Eur J Med Genet 63(104088):1–4. https://www.sciencedirect.com/science/article/pii/S1769721220307989?casa_token=CQlfy4i4Wd4AAAA:8WvtPVxC2O_vAVbNSgSklyYp5qPhHUjRfFg7Qn1wUTgbaKu3ATf8rQDmFwf-hd7RTdjrQ9aczw

Strugnell A, Leonard H, Epstein A, Downs J (2019) Using directed-content analysis to identify a framework for understanding quality of life in adults with Rett syndrome. Disabil Rehabil 42(26):3800–3807. https://pubmed.ncbi.nlm.nih.gov/31074665/

Su J, Fu H, Xie B, Lu W, Li W, Wei Y, Zhang Q, Wei S, Chen Q, Lu Y, Jiang T (2019) Prenatal diagnosis of cri-du-chat syndrome by SNP array: report of twelve cases and review of the literature. Mol Cytogenet 12(1):1–6. https://pubmed.ncbi.nlm.nih.gov/31827621/

Takataya K, Yamazaki Y, Mizuno E (2016) Perceptions and feelings of fathers of children with down syndrome. Arch Psychiatr Nurs 30(5):544–551. https://pubmed.ncbi.nlm.nih.gov/27654235/

van Schendel RV, Page-Christiaens GCML, Beulen L, Bilardo CM, de Boer MA, Coumans ABC, Faas BHW, van Langen IM, Lichtenbelt KD, van Maarle MC, Macville MVE, Oepkes D, Pajkrt E, Henneman L (2017) Women's experience with non-invasive prenatal testing and emotional well-being and satisfaction after test-results. J Genet Counsel 26:1348–1356. https://doi.org/10.1007/s10897-017-0118-3

van Vliet D, van Wegberg AMJ, Ahring K, Bik-Multanowski M, Blau N, Bulut FD, Casas K, Didycz B, Djordjevic M, Federico A, Feillet F, Gizewska M, Gramer G, Hertecant JL, Hollak CEM, Jørgensen JV, Karall D, Landau Y, Leuzzi V, Mathisen P (2018) Can untreated PKU patients escape from intellectual disability? A systematic review. Orphanet J Rare Dis 13(1):149. https://doi.org/10.1186/s13023-018-0890-7

Vasudevan P, Suri M (2017) A clinical approach to developmental delay and intellectual disability. Clin Med 17(6):558–561. https://www.rcpjournals.org/content/clinmedicine/17/6/558

Vogel I, Tabor A, Ekelund C, Lou S, Hyett J, Petersen OB, Danish Fetal Medicine Study Group and Danish Cytogenetic Study Group (2019) Population-based screening for trisomies and atypical chromosomal abnormalities: improving efficacy using the combined first trimester screening algorithm as well as individual risk parameters. Fetal Diagn Ther 45(6):424–429. https://pubmed.ncbi.nlm.nih.gov/30199859/

Wolfe K, Stueber K, McQuillin A, Jichi F, Patch C, Flinter F, Strydom A, Bass N (2017) Genetic testing in intellectual disability psychiatry: opinions and practices of UK child and intellectual disability psychiatrists. J Appl Res Intellect Disabil 31(2):273–284. https://pubmed.ncbi.nlm.nih.gov/28833975/

World Health Organization (2020) Alcohol consumption and sustainable development: fact sheet on Sustainable Development Goals (SDGs): health targets (No. WHO/EURO: 2020-2370-42125-58041). World Health Organization. Regional Office for Europe. https://apps.who.int/iris/bitstream/handle/10665/340806/WHO-EURO-2020-2370-42125-58041-eng.pdf?sequence=1&isAllowed=y

Xiol C, Heredia M, Pascual-Alonso A, Oyarzabal A, Armstrong J (2021) Technological improvements in the genetic diagnosis of Rett syndrome spectrum disorders. Int J Mol Sci 22(19):10375. https://www.mdpi.com/1422-0067/22/19/10375

Zampini L, Dall'Ara F, Silibello G, Ajmone PF, Monti F, Rigamonti C, Lalatta F, Costantino MA, Vizziello PG (2021) "Your son has Klinefelter syndrome." How parents react to a prenatal diagnosis. Child Health Care 50(3):324–337. https://doi.org/10.1080/0273961 5.2021.1903325?scroll=top&needAccess=true

Zollino M, Zweier C, Van Balkom ID, Sweetser DA, Alaimo J, Bijlsma EK, Cody J, Elsea SH, Giurgea I, Macchiaiolo M, Smigiel R, Thibert RL, Benoist I, Clayton-Smith J, De Winter CF, Deckers S, Gandhi A, Huisman S, Kempink D, Kruisinga F, Lamacchia V, Marangi G, Menke L, Mulder P, Nordgren A, Renieri A, Routledge S, Saunders CJ, Stembalska A, Van Balkom H, Whalen S, Hennekam RC (2019) Diagnosis and management in Pitt-Hopkins syndrome: first international consensus statement. Clin Genet 95(4):462–478. https://doi.org/10.1111/cge.13506

Children and Adolescents with Intellectual Disability

Carmel Doyle and Neil Kenny

Chapter Topics

- This chapter examines the subject of the child and adolescent with intellectual disability.
- An explanation of what is meant by the child or adolescent with intellectual disability is offered.
- It also focuses on the prevalence and presentation of intellectual disability in this cohort.
- Furthermore, it recognises the importance of key supports including:
  - Healthcare
  - Early intervention and education inclusion
  - School-aged children and inclusion
  - Challenges to educational inclusion
- The chapter explores deeper thinking with reflective exercises throughout to support the reader.

Introduction

Intellectual disability is among the most common forms of disability in children (McConkey et al. 2019). Various conditions are evident where there are limitations in the functioning of the brain or

C. Doyle (✉)
Trinity College Dublin, Dublin, Ireland
e-mail: doylec5@tcd.ie

N. Kenny
Dublin City University, Dublin, Ireland
e-mail: neil.kenny@dcu.ie

neuromuscular system encompassing congenital or acquired conditions, with a variety of neurological, genetic or metabolic aetiologies that manifest as delayed development and functional limitations, sometimes limiting lifespan (Health Service Executive, and Faculty of Paediatrics, RCPI 2016). Many children with intellectual disabilities have no formal diagnosis, while some will have more commonly known conditions such as chromosomal abnormalities, severe cerebral palsy and epilepsy (see Chap. 5 for more detail on diagnosis).

Intellectual disability is the most common form of developmental disability in children (Eddy 2013) while the WHO Working Group on the Classification of Intellectual Disabilities for ICD-11 use the term, intellectual developmental disorders, recognising intellectual disabilities as both a health condition and disability (Foster et al. 2015). The ICD-11 defines intellectual developmental disorders as a group of developmental conditions characterised by significant impairment of cognitive functions, associated with limitations of learning, adaptive behaviour and skills (WHO 2022). It is also acknowledged that disability depends not only on a child's health condition or impairment but also crucially on the extent to which environmental factors support the child's full participation and inclusion in society (WHO 2022).

While classification of intellectual disability into mild, moderate, severe and profound

© The Author(s), under exclusive license to Springer Nature Switzerland AG 2023
F. Sheerin, C. Doyle (eds.), *Intellectual Disabilities: Health and Social Care Across the Lifespan*,
https://doi.org/10.1007/978-3-031-27496-1_6

categories can be a negative prospect for some, it allows for assessment of need and delineation of support requirements. Children with a mild intellectual disability tend to function well in everyday life and may require assistance and support to benefit optimally from school and to live independently. Children with moderate intellectual disability will have language and functional skills possibly needing additional supports in everyday life especially in the school environment, while children with a severe intellectual disability would usually have limited language skills and poor social skills and attend a special class or school while living with supports in the community. Children with a profound intellectual disability would typically display multiple disabilities and be heavily dependent for daily activities requiring high support in daily life. While a child's level of intellectual disability can be defined by their IQ, the types and amount of support the child needs are often more diagnostic than a number (Eddy 2013). There is general agreement that children with severe and profound intellectual disabilities require additional individualised supports, and the care requirement is commonly seen to extend over longer period of times, from infancy through to adulthood (Murphy et al. 2021).

Prevalence of Intellectual Disability in the Child Population

It is estimated that 15% of the total world population experience some form of disability with a prevalence rate suggested to be around 1% (Maulik et al. 2011). However, McKenzie et al. (2016) argue that it may be anything from 0.05 to 1.55%. Still, figures for those children experiencing disability worldwide are vague and can vary considerably. International population census data does not always include questions relating to disability, and therefore, datasets don't capture the prevalence rates of childhood disability (McConkey et al. 2019). Ireland examined census prevalence rates and established there was an increase of 8% in the child population with intellectual disability between 2011 and 2016. When compared with census data from Northern Ireland, who used a broader definition of disability, it appears

Northern Ireland has a higher prevalence, while Ireland has a higher prevalence than Scotland.

Numbers of children surviving with disabilities have risen due to increased knowledge and capability to treat premature infants and genetic disorders (Brenner et al. 2021) in addition to increased survival rates following serious illnesses (Alexander et al. 2022). The survival rate of preterm babies is rising with improved neonatal care, but aligned with this, the disability rate appears to be increasing suggesting these children have more long-term neurological deficits and intellectual disabilities. Additionally, developments in healthcare have increased the lifespan of children with genetic disorders. Furthermore, the number of individuals with profound intellectual disabilities is increasing as a result of advanced medical input and the availability of complex equipment and medication (Pinney 2017; Doyle 2020, 2021, 2022).

Presentation of Intellectual Disability in Children

The age at which intellectual disability presents is dependent upon the complexity of presentation and presence of specific disorders or syndromes coupled with parental observation and alertness (Foster et al. 2015). Presentation at birth tends to be obvious in the case of recognisable malformations or syndromes such as Down syndrome. Within the first year of life, delayed motor development and associated hypotonia are sometimes the most obvious features of intellectual disability (Sheridan et al. 2014). More notably, individuals with profound intellectual disabilities are usually unable to walk, feed independently or communicate verbally and require prescription medications and often high levels of assistance in daily living (Doyle 2020, 2021, 2022). Children with profound intellectual disabilities often have more than one disability and usually will have difficulty communicating (Mencap 2012). It is common for these individuals to have sensory or physical disabilities coupled with mental health problems and complex health needs (Mencap 2012, Royal College Nursing (RCN) 2013, National Institute for Health and Care Excellence

(NICE) 2022). Children with intellectual disability have an overall risk of developing medical complications associated with their physical disabilities, and almost all of these children require regularly administered medication (Doyle 2020, 2021, 2022). The combination of disabilities can also affect behaviour. With each individual condition, a specific symptom profile may exist with unique identifying symptom experiences (Malcolm et al. 2011). Children with profound intellectual disabilities may possess limited motor function and experience significantly more health problems than the general population (Davis et al. 2014). They also have an overall risk of developing medical complications and almost all require regularly administered medication to include anti-epileptic drugs (AEDs), sleep medication or anti-reflux medication among others (Doyle 2020, 2021, 2022).

Apart from cognitive and motor dysfunctions, the number and severity of associated characteristics augment the difficulties these children experience. Health problems can include respiratory, gastrointestinal conditions and epilepsy with an increasing number of children regarded as technology dependent due to their need for oxygen, suction equipment and feeding tubes (Dunworth-Fitzgerald and Sweeney 2013). Visual impairments are more common than hearing impairments mainly due to increased survival rates of premature babies who have a predisposition to retinopathy of prematurity (Leung et al. 2018). Usually, children with severe and profound intellectual disabilities will require extensive supports for daily living and care is particularly challenging (NICE 2022).

Reflective Exercise 1

While intellectual disability is the most common form of developmental disability in children, it can present in many different ways. Presentation at birth can be obvious or a delay in meeting milestones can be the first sign. Can you recall some of the children with intellectual disabilities that you have met?

- Did they have an early presentation with a definitive diagnosis?
- Was delayed development the first sign?
- Consider the impact of both an early and a later presentation.

Supporting the Child with Intellectual Disabilities and Their Family

The presentation of intellectual disabilities and its severity impacts on the interventions and supports required for the individual child or adolescent. The most useful approach for children with intellectual disabilities consists of multidisciplinary efforts aimed at many aspects of the child's life such as education, social and recreational activities, management of behavioural issues and associated impairments. Medication is not of any benefit in treating the core symptoms of intellectual disability as no drug has been found to improve intellectual function but is often required in treating comorbidities and directed at specific symptoms such as epilepsy, gastrointestinal issues or neuropathic pain. A range of services may be required to maintain or improve health and functioning of children with severe or profound intellectual disabilities. These services can include specialised medical and nursing services, therapeutic services, family support services, equipment and medical supplies and other related services such as early intervention, special education and transportation among others. Additionally, it is essential that children are supported to enjoy opportunities that other children experience such as play and leisure, social activities and accessible education (Hewitt-Taylor 2010). Interdisciplinary professionals across health, education or social care may need to establish processes to ensure care is coordinated in a consistent approach.

Health Supports

Health problems are well documented in children with intellectual disabilities with many of these children experiencing health disparities (Nicholson et al. 2022). Prevalence of medical conditions can be high and include, for example, gastrointestinal feeding issues, seizures, pulmonary problems, orthopaedic issues and general malaise. These medical conditions often determine children's attendance at school or engagement in specific activities on a daily basis with many children missing these activities (Zijlstra and Vlaskamp 2005). A wide range of health issues have been identified especially in children with severe and profound intellectual disabilities with some children experiencing an average of 12 health issues at any one time, many of which require medication interventions: highest prevalence rates were found for constipation, visual impairment, epilepsy, spasticity, deformations, incontinence and reflux (van Timmeren et al. 2016). Hospital admission of children with intellectual disabilities is characterised by a variety of conditions requiring treatment such as upper respiratory tract conditions (Fitzgerald et al. 2013), fluid and electrolyte disorders (Lindgren et al. 2021) and nervous system disorders, which include epilepsy, convulsions and seizures (Kessler et al. 2020). Common presenting issues to emergency departments for adolescents with intellectual disabilities have been identified as convulsions, epilepsy, psychological concerns with depression, emotional disturbance and psychological or physical distress (Hand et al. 2019a, b). More recently, Doody et al. (2021) identified that nearly three quarters of the intellectual disability population admitted to hospital were under the age of 18 with the top five intellectual disability conditions identified as Down syndrome, chromosomal conditions, microcephaly, DiGeorge syndrome and tuberous sclerosis. While the health needs of children with intellectual disabilities often overshadow other needs such as communication, play, socialising and learning, the management of health needs impacts on the ability of a child to engage in all of the other activities.

The role of nursing and allied health professionals is central to quality healthcare provision (Law et al. 2011). It is acknowledged that engagement of the child with intellectual disabilities in so far as is possible in planning and decision-making around their health is important and a core recommendation of the NICE guidance (2022). However, healthcare provision based on diagnosis is problematic as it may exclude children without definitive diagnoses or halt access at an earlier stage. A thorough assessment of need is essential noting that children with the same diagnosis may need very different supports emphasising the need for real person-centred supports (NICE 2022).

Reasonable adjustments such as allowing more time at appointments to communicate with the child and their family or longer consultation times are recommended (NICE 2022). Furthermore, ensuring the child and family are well informed makes for easier decision-making. The issue of repeated storytelling with continual explanations is well documented by families of children with intellectual disabilities (WHO 2017). A mechanism for ensuring consistent passage of information is the use of a hospital passport, a document that contains key information regarding a child's health, communication and support needs (Northway et al. 2017). This document then accompanies the child on all appointments or hospital admissions and provides valuable information while enhancing safety and also reducing the need for repeated storytelling. The UK Council for Disabled Children proposes the use of passports such as that developed by the University Hospital Bristol (2011), while the National Autistic Society has tailored one specifically for those individuals with autism (2017).

Although acknowledging the stress of raising a child with intellectual disabilities, parents also report many positive aspects that are often disregarded in the literature (Beighton and Wills 2017, 2019) with hope and a positive view of the future being important for parents (George-Levi and Laslo-Roth 2021). These positive aspects include an increased sense of personal strength and confidence, changed priorities, greater appreciation of life, pleasure in the child's accomplishments, increased faith/spirituality, more meaningful relationships and the positive effect that the child has on the wider community. These positives enable parents to adapt successfully to the stressful experiences of raising their child. However,

Table 6.1 Supporting the child with intellectual disability and their family (adapted from NICE (2022))

The child and family must be involved in planning and implementing their care

Use a person-centred approach to care.

Appropriate communication mechanisms should be in place for decision-making and up-to-date information provision.

Using a hospital/communication passport will assist in ensuring a consistent approach is adopted across disciplines without repeated storytelling.

Consultation times should be longer for appointments.

Assessment of need should be timely and well coordinated across disciplines.

Health professionals increase their awareness of colleagues roles and the various skill sets and expertise with the common goal of seamless coordination of care.

In addition to interdisciplinary working, interagency consultation and communication should be in place especially across health, education and social care service provision.

Supporting the child and family should encompass training in healthcare tasks relevant to the child's care.

Health professionals should receive training that will assist them in working with the child and family, in particular around specific health needs and communication.

Preparation for transition to adult services should be well planned in a timely manner.

If key professionals involved need to change, handover should be organised to allow for seamless transition.

Reflective Exercise 2

Scenario

Max is a 5-year-old boy who experienced anoxia at birth resulting in development of a profound intellectual disability with associated cerebral palsy, quadriplegia and epilepsy. He is oxygen dependent and contracts pneumonia regularly. He is also gastrostomy fed with no suck, swallow or gag reflex and requires suctioning frequently throughout the day. Max is incontinent and immobile requiring 24-h care for his daily activities of living. His mother cares for him on a continuous basis assisted by his father (who also works full-time) and he also has a younger brother. While Max attends a special school, he is often not well enough to attend due to his multiple medical and nursing needs. He receives respite care from a disability service provider for 3 nights every 7 weeks and also requires a nurse at nighttime. Max is prescribed 15 daily medications and additional others depending on his health status requiring multiple medication administrations. He attends the hospital outpatient department regularly and requires hospital admission at times when his condition is unstable.

A child and family person-centred approach to care is adopted, acknowledging that caring for Max requires full-time commitment from his family.

Take a moment to consider each of the following questions:

• Can you identify what supports Max and his family might find useful?
• Would a hospital passport be beneficial here? If so, what information would you seek to include?
• Have you been involved in an appointment with a child or family? Is there anything you could adapt to enhance the experience?
• How can healthcare professionals ensure emotional support is offered to the family?
• Reflecting on your own practice, consider what if anything you could change to enhance the child and family experience.

the emotional demands on parents caring for a child with intellectual disabilities are often neglected by healthcare professionals with many parents of children with disability displaying heightened depression scores and compromised mental health (Bemister et al. 2014). Therefore, it is imperative that direction to emotional and practical support services are offered to include social work and voluntary providers.

There are many ways of supporting the child with intellectual disabilities and their family through healthcare interactions (see Table 6.1), and this plays an important role in tandem with other supports such as early intervention and education.

Early Intervention

Early identification of children with intellectual disabilities, with an understanding that such early profiling will facilitate access to appropriate early childhood intervention (ECI), has been shown to have significant positive impacts on outcomes for the child and their family that span further into their developmental trajectory (Guralnick 2017). Appropriate access to services improves children's developmental potential, their ability to socially participate and their long-term quality of life (Scherzer et al. 2012; Collins et al. 2017). There is a close and symbiotic relationship between identification of intellectual disability or development difference and early intervention (EI), which are two distinct but complementary processes. EI for intellectual disabilities among vulnerable children must precede and facilitate access to EI services. Appropriate EI ameliorates differences in developmental functions, helping the acquisition of new skills that strengthen further learning. However, the benefits of appropriate EI also have wider impacts on the families and caregivers of children with intellectual disabilities, such as augmenting knowledge, confidence and the development of appropriate coping strategies, with positive impacts for their mental health (Guralnick 2017).

The risks to delayed development among this vulnerable cohort of children are compounded as children with intellectual disabilities have been shown to potentially receive less stimulation engagements within their home environment and fewer learning opportunities through education or health services (Canavera et al. 2018). Such cycles perpetuate ongoing exclusion and developmental differences between children with intellectual disabilities and their age-matched peer group and foreground the importance of supporting children with disabilities during their early years (Guralnick 2017). Appropriate EI supports during this early period of development are critical as development in language, cognition, motor and socio-emotional domains occurs rapidly in these first years. While these different domains of learning are often discussed as being separate, in reality they do not operate or develop in isolation. They depend on each other in supporting the child's learning, enabling each other and mutually interacting as the child operates on their environment and becomes more independent (Smythe et al. 2021). In addition, biological, psychosocial (Walker et al. 2011) and environmental factors have significant roles in brain development, in both brain structure

and function, and are also critically important. A failure to access appropriate supports during the critical early period of development can have lifelong impacts on quality of life and well-being for children and their families (Guralnick 2017; Smythe et al. 2021).

Under the United Nations Convention of Rights for a Child (UN 1989) and the United Nations Convention of the Rights of Persons with Disabilities (UNCRPD) (UN 2006), it is a requirement that governments provide EI and education services that are inclusive of and available to all children. However, while it is clear that EI for children with intellectual disability is of vital importance, the planning and delivery of inclusive services for all children can be more complex than initially suspected. The role of early identification and assessment is also hugely important as accurate assessment is often what guides access to services for children with intellectual disability and their families (Smythe et al. 2021). However, the process of accessing assessment and processes by which families can apply for an assessment differ greatly across jurisdictions and geographic areas (Dosreis et al. 2006). These divergences can have significant impacts on service provision and clinical practice. In Ireland, for example, services for children with disabilities developed historically in an ad hoc manner characterised by regional differences in service delivery and capacity, an approach that leads to diverse patterns of assessment and support. Furthermore, the assessed prevalence of autism in the Republic of Ireland is 1.5% (Boilson et al. 2016), while its prevalence in Northern Ireland is stated as being 4.5% (Rodgers and McCluney 2021), the differences reported being mostly likely explained by differences in clinical practice and service provision. Assessment and diagnosis are achieved through referral to professional psychiatric or psychological services, most typically in Ireland via the Health Service Executive (HSE) and Child and Adolescent Mental Health Services (CAMHS), although increasingly parents are seeking private assessment due to significant waiting lists attached to the Assessment of Need (AON) process (Government of Ireland 2005) via the HSE.

In the UK, there is a legal requirement for local authorities to identify children who are suspected as presenting with a disability as early as possible. The particular clinical commissioning group, NHS trust or NHS foundation then has a responsibility to engage with the parents of the child and inform the appropriate local authority, commencing arrangement of an appropriate assessment to take place. Transforming Care Partnerships are a mechanism to ensure that the identification of children with intellectual disability in accordance with the Healthy Child Pathway takes place at an early stage as possible.

It should be noted, however, that there is an international trend towards compartmentalising conditions such as intellectual disabilities, autism or mental health and separating service provision into 'specialist' discrete service teams for diagnosis and support (Gillberg 2010). This can lead to lengthy diagnosis journeys for some individuals who present with complex profiles or where there is a range of comorbid diagnosis with psychiatric conditions (Gillberg 2010; Green et al. 2018). For example, research has found that the rates of routine assessment screening for autistic children were significantly lower relative to other developmental disabilities due to a lack of expertise or experience among clinicians in the use of autism-specific screening tools (Dosreis et al. 2006). In addition, a range of other service factors were identified as functioning as barriers to early assessment access, such as staff turnover, management changes and limited capacity of services to recognise developmental disabilities through developmental surveillance (Dosreis et al. 2006).

In Ireland, there are significant delays in accessing AON, which are geographically dispersed across Community Health Organisation (CHO) areas (Government of Ireland 2018). Furthermore, 'even after the delay in assessing a child, there were often further waiting times of several years to access additional services … families are not given sufficient information on the intervention pathways needed' (GOI 2018, p. 30). The introduction of the Progressing Children's Disability Services (PCDS) by the HSE in recent years is an effort to standardise the systems of services for children with disabilities and standardise system of service delivery across Ireland (Inclusion Ireland 2022). The HSE reconfigured the last of the 91 Children's Disability teams in December 2021. However, a recent study found half of participating families of children with a disability in Ireland had not received any services at all under the PCDS system, with 83% of respondents reporting lack of services as one of their top 3 issues when surveyed (Inclusion Ireland 2022). Additionally, 95% of respondents reported that their child was waiting on a list to avail of for more than a year (Inclusion Ireland 2022). It is clear from this recent data that pathways to assessment, diagnosis, suitable education placements and appropriate interventions may be complex, interrupted or long in duration, particularly for children with complex presentations.

Furthermore, nursing supports for children with intellectual disability while in the special education setting should be considered. The school nurse has an important role to play centred on care delivery providing intimate care, administrating medications and undertaking complex medical interventions (NCSE 2018). The school nurse also crucially evaluates whether a child has health concerns that are impacting learning and how health barriers might be reduced (Yonkaitis and Shannon 2017). Notably, without school nursing supports, many children with complex and integrated health needs are not able to attend school and thus cannot meet their educational needs.

Early Intervention and Education Inclusion

Participation in high-quality early childhood education has been identified by the EU as being a priority educational objective across the member states (Drakopoulou 2020). Learners with disabilities have been consistently shown to be less likely to complete primary, secondary and post-secondary education relative to the completion rates among the general student population without disabilities (Grammenos 2020). Early childhood education is important as many children are only identified as having a learning difference or difficulty when they commence their educational journey; thus it supports earlier identification of disability or support needs (Drakopoulou 2020). Additionally, research has indicated that access to quality early childhood education provides long-lasting positive outcomes for pupils across their developmental trajectory, with the benefits being even more pronounced among vulnerable pupils or those from a disadvantaged background (Frawley 2014).

Some governments have introduced a range of policy initiatives to support the achievement of the strategic framework for European cooperation in education and training (Council of the European Union 2009) benchmark of reaching a minimum of 95% participation in early childhood education (ECE) among children between the age of 4 and 6 years (Council of European Union 2009). For example, the Irish Government introduced a new curriculum for ECE, *Aistear*, in 2009, which provides guidelines for education of all children from birth to 6, including those with additional needs (National Council for Curriculum and Assessment 2009). They invested further in 2018 by increasing the Early Childhood Care and Education Scheme (ECCE) to a second year of free preschool for all children and implementing the Access and Inclusion Model (AIM) to provide supports for preschool children with special education needs (SENs), including autistic children (Inter-Departmental Group 2015; Early Childhood Ireland 2017). Recent legislation, policies and government reports rubber stamp the Irish Government's commitment to inclusive education for all, including preschoolers with disabilities. However, it must be noted that there is currently no national policy on specialist EI provision in Ireland (Twomey and Shevlin 2017). Currently in Ireland inclusive educational provision for preschool-aged pupils includes a continuum of provision with access to inclusive educational practices through home tuition, AIM support within mainstream preschools and autism-specific EI special classes in special and mainstream schools (Banks et al. 2016; Twomey 2016; NCSE 2019).

Launched in 2016, AIM is a programme that supports children with disabilities to access the ECCE—a universal 2-year preschool programme. AIM offers progressive support to children ranging from universal to targeted. The programme offers a comprehensive approach to inclusion, targeted both at enabling culture changes and funding additional support structures. AIM includes training provisions on inclusion for leaders and staff, information dissemination and special needs support training. Supports range from leveraging expert advice to providing additional assistance in the preschool room. Through an application system, the programme pairs educational experts with parents and preschool providers to better enable the participation of all children in early childhood education. Additional supports are provided through capital grants for appliances and minor alterations, health service provision and additional instructional assistance (Pobal 2018). A survey evaluation of AIM was conducted in 2018 with practitioners and staff at early learning care settings as well as parents and caregivers. Overall, both target groups indicated a high level of satisfaction with the programme (Department of Children and Youth Affairs, (DCYA) 2019).

This is evident in the Irish Government's current approach of best supporting the needs of preschool-aged children through the continued inclusion of a continuum of educational provision (DES 2019). However, with the exception of specialist EI classes for preschool autistic children, the transition from preschool education to school-aged education provision in Ireland remains a challenge (Shevlin and Banks 2021). For comparison, children who receive an early assessment of need where a potential intellectual disability is suspected are provided with an education, health and care (EHC) assessment plan. These assessments aim to provide a rounded picture of a child's strengths and needs such that support needs or requirements can be planned for to support progress. The EHC is intended to underpin planning for long-term aspirations, plan for transitions to primary school and include information on each child's strengths and achievements. Such an early centralised approach supports universal expectations across service provision contexts.

Reflective Exercise 3

Recent decades have brought increasing emphasis within policy towards providing access to early intervention for children with disabilities within mainstream education settings.

- Do you feel this policy emphasis on including children with intellectual disabilities within mainstream early years classrooms is advisable and appropriate? Why?
- Identify the benefits, in your own view, of such provision within mainstream education settings. What are the potential positive lifespan impacts for children with intellectual disabilities and their families?
- Given the diversity of presentations among children with intellectual disability, can you identify any challenges this may present within mainstream early childhood educations settings?
- What additional supports from outside the education system may also need to be considered in supporting diverse cohorts of children with intellectual disability to access early childhood education settings appropriately?

School-Aged Children and Inclusion

The Europe-wide focus on early identification of disability in children and an emphasis on support for inclusive education is a priority for the EU through ET 2020, the strategic framework for European cooperation in education and training and the European Disability Strategy 2010–2020 (European Commission 2010). Notably, much of the reports and literature refer to children with disabilities and do not delineate further into intellectual disabilities. In particular, the need to integrate children with disabilities within mainstream education settings through the provision of individualised support is one of the eight priority areas within this European Disability Strategy. The NCSE (2019) undertook a study on inclusive educational provision in Ireland and eight European countries. The results established that all had a similar continuum model of inclusive educational provision to Ireland, with supports in mainstream schools, special schools and special classes.

The provision of education for children with intellectual disability has historically been addressed in a variety of ways across jurisdictions, with an international policy trend moving towards inclusive models of provision becoming more prevalent across the OECD in recent decades (Kenny et al. 2020). The UN Convention on the Rights of the Child (UN 1989) introduced a rights-based perspective regarding education policy and provision for young people with disabilities. This was further clarified by the Salamanca Statement (UNESCO 1994), signed by 300 participants representing 92 governments, which aimed to further the objective of promoting inclusive education for learners with disabilities and special needs. Additionally, the UNCRPD (2006) led to many countries no longer considering separate special education settings to be inclusive educational provision, from an educational policy perspective (NCSE 2019). However, while policy has increasingly moved towards an emphasis on inclusive provision within mainstream schools, the concept of inclusion itself remains contested. There is no internationally agreed definition of the concept of inclusive education (Dyssegaard and Larsen 2013). While inclusion was initially conceived of as relating only to disability, more contemporary understandings of the concept of inclusive education see it more broadly as a response to diverse and complex societal dynamics (Booth and Ainscow 2002; OECD 2004).

The EASIE (2018, p.12) cross-country report on inclusive education classified inclusive and mainstream education as follows:

Inclusive setting refers to education where the learner with special education needs (SEN) follows education in mainstream classes alongside their mainstream peers for the largest part (80% or more) of the school week.

Mainstream education implies placement in a mainstream class or placement in a separate special class within a mainstream school. Those learners who are not in mainstream settings are in fully separate special schools.

Clough and Nutbrown (2006) described inclusion as 'the drive towards maximal participation in and minimal exclusion from early year settings, from schools and from society' (p. 3).

Social models of disability would advocate for inclusion to be seen as emphasising the need for educational settings to change to successfully provide for the individual with disabilities rather than the individual pupil being forced to change to suit the school (Milton and Moon 2012; Banks and McCoy 2017; Goodall 2018). However, recent research suggests that, in the majority of EU countries, many students with disabilities still access education through placements in segregated settings (special classes or special schools) outside mainstream classes (Drakopoulou 2020). In contrast, some countries in the EU have made strides towards accessible and inclusive provision within mainstream education settings. For example, the rates of inclusion of students with disabilities within mainstream settings range from countries with high rates, such as Italy (99.12%), Malta (94.64%) and Iceland (91.81%), to countries with very low rates of access for these students, such as Sweden (11.21%) or Belgium (19.11%) (EASIE 2018). Indeed, even within the UK, there are wide divergences in participation for students with disabilities within mainstream settings, with Scotland reporting 94.65% of such learners are placed within mainstream settings, while England (53%) and Wales (46%) reported much lower rates of access (EASIE 2018). It is important to note that while there may be differences across countries in how inclusion is defined, there is clear evidence that their assessed form or degree of disability has an impact on their access to inclusive educational placements (Ferguson 2008). For example, research from the USA shows that while participation rates for pupils with intellectual disabilities in mainstream classrooms between 1989 and 2004 had grown from 31% to 52%, the participation rate for children with intellectual disabilities in mainstream classrooms only grew from 6.8% to 13% (Ferguson 2008).

There have been some efforts within the European Union to address the levels of diversity and difference in how prevalence rates are assessed across countries and how different jurisdictions support access to education for children with disabilities. The resulting approaches, within both policy and educational practice, are heavily influenced by the cultures, traditions and debates relating to education generally (and inclusive education specifically) within the specific countries. In the framework of ET 2020, the EU invited member states to develop more cooperation with learners with disabilities to promote inclusive education and personalised learning through support, as well as the early identification of additional learning needs (Council of the European Union 2009). This has led to the introduction of a range of national initiatives or policies to foster a greater focus on inclusive provision for children with disabilities within mainstream schools and greater engagement with them and their families.

As has been true in many OECD countries, Irish education policy has been seeking to shift provision for students with disabilities from segregated to mainstream provision in recent years; however this process has been hampered by the ad hoc manner in which the provision for pupils with disabilities developed over the decades (Shevlin and Banks 2021). Ireland's approach to the provision of education for pupils with disabilities is described as a 'multitrack' system that comprises a multiplicity of approaches and a variety of services between the mainstream and special systems (European Agency for Development in Special Needs Education 2003). While there remains a range of segregated specialist education settings, such as special schools, the majority of children with disabilities access education within mainstream schools (Kenny et al. 2020). Within these mainstream schools, pupils can be placed in either a special class designated for a particular disability (or range of disabilities) or they can access mainstream classes with their peer group pupils where they may also receive supplementary teaching (McCoy et al. 2014). In common with other countries, the number of children and young people identified with disabilities has increased dramatically over the past two decades making up over a quarter of the school population today (McCoy et al. 2020).

While Ireland's system of special education has undergone unprecedented change over the last three decades, it remains heavily influenced by a highly prescriptive national curriculum where standardised assessment of student performance on key stages is audited and used to profile schools (Department of Education and Skills 2017). This can lead to a range of barriers or challenges to inclusive education (Banks and McCoy 2017; Shevlin and Banks 2021). However, such challenge to inclusive access and provision also exists across many European countries and systems.

Challenges to Educational Inclusion

One of the major challenges facing inclusive education for children with disabilities across Europe relates to the reality that national frameworks are significantly heterogeneous and are heavily influenced by the differing cultural backgrounds or approaches to disability within each country (Genova 2015). Historic, political, social and cultural features diverge greatly across countries and significantly contribute educational policy development and enactment but also can underpin barriers to equitable access to education within countries (Bhaskar and Danermark 2006; Gabel and Miskovic 2014). This leads to wide divergence in approaches across differing countries, with differing levels of alignment with inclusive policy frameworks. Another key issue that can heavily impact access to inclusive educational placements for children with disabilities relates to the relatively recent enactment of legislative provision of access to free and compulsory education for children with disabilities in some countries. For example, such access has been enacted in Spain since 1980s, but only since 1998 in Lithuania and since 2008 in Greece.

These legal and policy developments have occurred simultaneously with a significant increase in the number of learners with disabilities being enrolled in mainstream school settings in recent decades (Shevlin and Banks 2021). In Europe, recent estimates place the number of children with disabilities or special needs at 15 million, with differences in levels of support to access educational inclusion being provided across differing countries (European Commission 2012). For example, in Ireland between 2011 and 2014, the number of students entitled to receive teaching

supports for 'low incidence' special needs in mainstream schools increased from 38,000 to 45,700. Indeed, the total expenditure on special education allocated by the Department of Education and Skills grew from €468 million to €1.5 billion between 2004 and 2016 (Department of Education and Skills 2016), with a rapid increase in the number of applications for additional supports outside of the General Allocation Model for education being a significant factor. For example, applications for additional resource-teaching hours for individual students increased to over 13,000 applications per year (Department of Education and Skills 2016). These changes continued across the decade, with, for example, the number of children with autism in receipt of special needs assistance (SNA) support in mainstream schools increasing by 83% in the 5-year period between 2011 and 2016 (Campbell et al. 2017).

Reflective Exercise 4
Figure 6.1 Below illustrates the continuum of support, the model for inclusion of children with disabilities in schools in Ireland
Given many children with intellectual disability will likely be accommodated within the highest level of support outlined in the continuum of support model, the school support-plus, there are likely to be implications for schools, teachers and school leaders. Consider some implications for inclusion of these children:

- Individualised and specialised assessment of areas of strength or priority areas for support will be a necessity for planning. Will such specialist skills or resource be available within school settings?
- Differentiation of teaching and learning approaches or curricular resources will be a valuable support to facilitate access for pupils with intellectual disability. Will schools have access to specialised and appropriate resources or funding to access such resources?
- Will teaching staff and special needs assistant staff have access to appropriate continuous professional development to develop skills and capacity within the school staff team? How can this be facilitated and resourced?
- How will school leaders be supported in planning the inclusion of pupils with complex individualised support needs and the management of additional support staff or specialised class settings/buildings?
- How can schools support the important role parents play in the process of supporting appropriate access to education for pupils with intellectual disability?

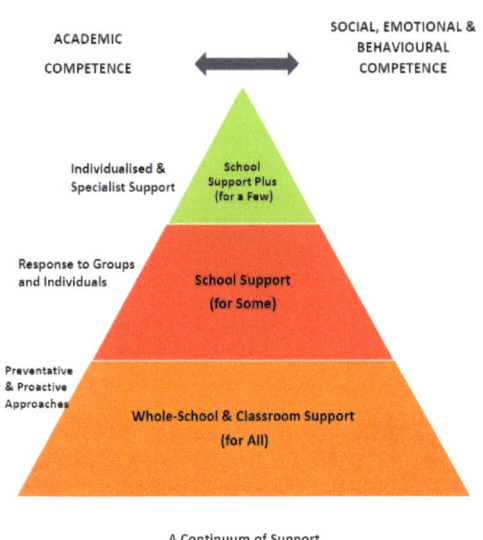

ACADEMIC COMPETENCE ⟷ SOCIAL, EMOTIONAL & BEHAVIOURAL COMPETENCE

Individualised & Specialist Support — School Support Plus (for a Few)

Response to Groups and Individuals — School Support (for Some)

Preventative & Proactive Approaches — Whole-School & Classroom Support (for All)

A Continuum of Support

Fig. 6.1 The Continuum of Support for children with special educational needs (DES 2019)

These changes have led to significant funding increases in order to resource the increased level of need within mainstream school settings. In 2017, Irish Government expenditure resourcing disability and special education support across several domains (education, health, social protection) accounted for 13.4% of total expenditure. Additionally, overall expenditure on this domain increased by 16.7% between 2011 and 2017 (Kenny et al. 2020). Special educational needs expenditure in 2017 reached €1683 million having increased by 38% from 2011 until that time (Campbell et al. 2017). These increases have funded, for example, an increase of increase 74% in SNAs in mainstream schools (from 8521 in 2014 to 14,877 in 2018). It should be recognised, however, that access to a placement within a mainstream education setting does not, of itself, facilitate high quality in education.

The school buildings, architecture features and levels of physical accessibility remain a significant issue for many children with disabilities within schools across the UK and Europe (Genova 2015). This is potentially another costly and challenging barrier that may prove slow to address. Despite the UNCRPD and the EU policy, transport systems and public school buildings still present physical access and sensory experience barriers to many children with disabilities or complex profiles. In addition, prejudice, ableism and negative stereotypes can still be strongly associated with provision of inclusive education for children with disability that can lead to policy and political barriers to the enactment of rights-based inclusive education frameworks that align with the UN CRPD and EU education policy (Portero 2012). In Ireland, for example, mirroring the overt barriers faced by government in the delivery of services to support children with disabilities and their families, there have been major delays in the enactment of these radical legislative and rights-based laws in Ireland. While the UNCRPD was 'adopted' in 2006, it was only signed into law in 2018 triggering the obligation to enact the radical structural changes it specifies in the education system (Kenny et al. 2020). Similarly, while the EPSEN act was signed into law in 2004, there remains an ongoing failure to also implement some aspects of the act, specifically regarding legal mandates to conduct assessments and provide services within a timely manner.

Forms of teaching being provided to children with disabilities within schools may also function as a barrier in many cases. Inappropriate or inflexible teaching or approaches have been shown to negatively impact pupil well-being and to impact levels of engagement among children (OECD 2016). For example, one study found that appropriate differentiation of instruction by teachers, individualising it to be appropriate to pupil profiles within a particular class, resulted in pupil anxiety decreasing by 5%. Pupil knowledge was also increased by 4% when teachers provided individual help to learners having difficulties in understanding a topic or task (OECD 2016).

A domain of particular focus is the appropriate and effective preparation of teachers to meet the needs of pupils with disabilities (and other diverse learners) within the school system. Some research pre-service teacher education may function as a further 'hidden' barrier to the enactment of inclusive practice within schools for learners with disabilities. According to the United Nations

Educational, Scientific and Cultural Organization (UNESCO) (1994) and Jenson (2018), children with disabilities have a right to an education suitable to their individual needs which should, where possible, be provided within their local mainstream schools alongside their peers. However, some researchers question this view that successful inclusion equals mainstream education unless appropriate pre-service and continuing professional development (CPD) education is available for teachers working with these children (Reed et al. 2012; Waddington and Reed 2017). Recent research suggests a lack of confidence among pre-service teachers in their knowledge and ability to implement inclusive practices in schools and a desire for more support in this area (NCSE 2017). Given inclusive education practice is among the core domains of teacher education in many countries, there is a concern that teachers leave teacher education under-prepared to support the education of children with disabilities (McCormack 2019). These issues matter as research illustrates there remains a close link between teacher education and access to CPD among teachers and their attitudes to the inclusion of children with disabilities within their class settings. For example, Kim et al. (2020) completed a mixed method study into early childhood teachers' experiences, attitudes and perceptions of inclusion. The study found that most teachers had positive attitudes towards inclusion but identified significant barriers to practices of inclusion within early years settings including lack of teacher and para-professional SEN inclusion training, resources and funding and support through expertise mentoring and collaborative approaches to support inclusion among staff. Further studies found that the nature and severity of the pupil's disability affected teachers' attitudes towards inclusion and inclusive practices, similar to Clough's (1999) description of 'hierarchies of tolerance' among teachers' perspectives of inclusion (Avramidis and Norwich 2002; Ryndak et al. 2000). These included a range of 'global teacher-related factors', such as teacher self-efficacy, training and SEN experience (Jenson 2018, p.5). Avramidis and Norwich (2002) discussed teacher-related factors as influential elements to teachers' confidence, experiences and attitudes to inclusive education policy and practice.

Conclusion

This chapter has explored the subject of the child and adolescent with intellectual disability, highlighting it as one of the most common forms of disability in children. Evidence shows prevalence has been increasing in recent decades, with increasing life expectancy among children and adolescents varying degrees of intellectual disabilities. Of concern, however, is that many children have no formal diagnosis. The age at which intellectual disability presents is dependent on a number of factors such as presence of specific conditions or observation of delayed developmental milestones. It is clear that a coordinated consistent person-centred approach is required of interdisciplinary professionals across health, education and social care. The necessary health supports are discussed, while the importance of EI is highlighted. EI is considered alongside inclusive education for school-aged children, areas which have both shown significant policy change in recent years. Many challenges exist in supporting inclusive education with differing cultures and approaches to disabilities in different countries worldwide. Understanding the various concepts around the child and adolescent with intellectual disability is important. With this in mind, the chapter explores deeper thinking with reflective exercises throughout to support the reader.

Key Concepts Discussed
- Prevalence of intellectual disability in the child population
- Presentation of intellectual disability in children
- Supporting the child with intellectual disabilities and their family
- Health supports
- Early intervention and education inclusion
- School-aged children and inclusion
- Challenges to educational inclusion

References

Alexander D, Quirke MB, Doyle C et al (2022) The meaning given to bioethics as a source of support by physicians who care for children who require long-term ventilation. Qual Health Res 32(6):916–928. https://doi.org/10.1177/10497323221083744

Avramidis E, Norwich B (2002) Teachers' attitudes towards integration/inclusion: A review of the literature. Eur J Spec Needs Educ 17:129–147. https://doi.org/10.1080/08856250210129056

Banks J, McCoy S, Frawley D, Kingston G, Shevlin M, Smyth F (2016) Special classes in Irish schools phase 2: a qualitative study. Economic and Social Research Institute (ESRI) Research Series. (Research Report No. 24; Economic and Social Research Institute (ERSI) Research Series). NCSE, Dublin

Banks J, McCoy S (2017) An Irish solution…? Questioning the expansion of special classes in an era of inclusive education. Econ Soc Rev 48:441–461

Beighton C, Wills J (2017) Are parents identifying positive aspects to parenting their child with an intellectual disability or are they just coping? A qualitative exploration. J Intellect Disabil 21(4):325–345

Beighton C, Wills J (2019) How parents describe the positive aspects of parenting their child who has intellectual disabilities: a systematic review and narrative synthesis. J Appl Res Intellect Disabil 32:1255–1279

Bemister TB, Brooks BL, Dyck RH et al (2014) Parent and family impact of raising a child with perinatal stroke. BMC Pediatr 14(182):11

Bhaskar R, Danermark R (2006) Metatheory, interdisciplinarity and disability research – a critical realist perspective. Scand J Disabil Res 8(4):287–297

Boilson AM, Staines A, Ramirez A et al (2016) Operationalisation of the European protocol for autism prevalence (EPAP) for autism spectrum disorder prevalence measurement in Ireland. J Autism Dev Disord 46(9):3054–3067

Booth T, Ainscow M (2002) Index for inclusion: developing learning and participation in schools. Centre for Studies on Inclusive Education (CSIE), Bristol

Brenner M, Greene J, Doyle C et al (2021) Increasing the focus on children's complex and integrated care needs: a position paper of the European academy of pediatrics. Front Pediatr 9:758415. https://doi.org/10.3389/fped.2021.758415

Campbell T, de Barra S, Duffy R et al (2017) Spending Review 2017. Disability and special education related expenditure. Department of Public Expenditure and Reform, Dublin

Canavera K, Johnson LM, Harman J (2018) Beyond parenting: the responsibility of multidisciplinary health care providers in early intervention policy guidance. Am J Bioeth 18(11):58–60. https://doi.org/10.1080/15265161.2018.1523499

Clough P (1999) Exclusive tendencies: concepts, consciousness and curriculum in the project of inclusion. Int J Incl Educ 3(1):63–73

Clough P, Nutbrown C (2006) Inclusion in the early years: critical analyses and enabling narrative. Sage Publications, UK

Collins PY, Pringle B, Alexander C et al (2017) Global services and support for children with developmental delays and disabilities: bridging research and policy gaps. PLoS Med 14(9):e1002393. https://doi.org/10.1371/journal.pmed.1002393

Council of the European Union (2009) 'Council conclusions of 12 May 2009 on a strategic framework for European cooperation in education and training ('ET 2020')', 2009/C 119/02, Official Journal of the European Union 2–10. https://eur-lex.europa.eu/legal-content/EN/ALL/?uri=celex%3A52009XG0528%2801%29

Davis R, Proulx R, van Schrojenstein Lantman-de Valk H (2014) Health issues for people with intellectual disabilities: the evidence base. In: Taggart L, Cousins W (eds) Health promotion for people with intellectual and developmental disabilities. Open University Press, Berkshire, pp 7–16

Department of Children and Youth Affairs (2019) Department of children, equality, disability, integration and youth annual reports. Stationary Office, Dublin. https://www.gov.ie/en/collection/24aea9-department-of-children-and-youth-affairs-annual-reports/

Department of Education and Skills (2016) Review of the pilot of a new model for allocating teaching resources to mainstream schools to support pupils with special educational needs. https://www.sess.ie/sites/default/files/inline-files/Review_Pilot_New_Model_SEN_18.01.17.pdf

Department of Education and Skills (2017) Guidelines for Primary Schools Supporting Pupils with Special Educational Needs in Mainstream Schools. Accessed at: https://www.education.ie/en/The-Education-System/Special-Education/Guidelines-for-Primary-Schools-Supporting-Pupils-with-Special-Educational-Needs-in-Mainstream-Schools.pdf

Department of Education and Skills (2019) Guidelines for primary schools supporting pupils with special educational needs in mainstream schools. https://www.gov.ie/en/collection/dca316-special-education-needs-a-continuum-of-support/

Doody O, McMahon J, Lyons R et al (2021) Presenting problem/conditions which result in people with an intellectual disability being admitted to acute hospitals in the Republic of Ireland: an analysis of NQAIS clinical data from 2016–2020. University of Limerick and Office of the Nursing and Midwifery Service Director, Health Service Executive, Ireland, Limerick

Dosreis S, Weiner CL, Johnson L (2006) Autism spectrum disorder screening and management practices among general pediatric providers. J Dev Behav Pediatr 27(2):88–94

Doyle C (2020) The importance of supportive relationships with general practitioners, hospitals and pharmacists for mothers who 'give medicines' to children with severe and profound intellectual disabilities. J Intellect Disabil 26(1):29–49

Doyle C (2021) 'Just knowing' and the challenges of giving medicines to children with severe and profound intellectual disabilities: a hermeneutic inquiry. Br J Learn Disabil 49(1):3–12

Doyle C (2022) Mothers' experiences of giving medicines to children with severe and profound intellectual disabilities – the impact on time. Child Care Health Dev 48(4):558–658

Drakopoulou E (2020) Inclusive Education and the Impact of COVID-19 on learners with disabilities. https://www.edf-feph.org/content/uploads/2021/06/Inclusive-Education-and-COVID-19_Eleni-Drakopoulou.docx

Dunworth-Fitzgerald M, Sweeney J (2013) Care of adults with profound intellectual and multiple disabilities. Learn Disabil Pract 16(8):32–37

Dyssegaard CB, Larsen MS (2013) Evidence on inclusion. Danish Clearinghouse for Educational Research, Copenhagen. https://edu.au.dk/fileadmin/edu/Udgivelser/Clearinghouse/Evidence_on_Inclusion.pdf

Early Childhood Ireland (2017) The ECCE Scheme. Early Childhood Ireland—Inspiring and Enabling Members to Provide Quality Experiences for Young Children and Their Families. The ECCE Scheme - Early Childhood Ireland

Eddy L (2013) Caring for children with special healthcare needs and their families. Wiley Blackwell, Chichester

European Agency for Special Needs and Inclusive Education - EASIE (2018) Dataset Cross-Country Report, focusing on the 2016/2017 school year. https://www.european-agency.org/data/cross-country-reports

European Agency for Development in Special Needs Education (2003) Thematic education. EADSNE, Brussels

European Commission (2010) Communication from the Commission to the European Parliament, the Council, the European Economic and Social Committee and the Committee of the Regions, European Disability Strategy 2010-2020: A Renewed Commitment to a Barrier-Free Europe. European Commission, Brussels

European Commission (2012) 'Special Needs Children and Disabled Adults Still Getting a Raw Deal from Education, says report. Commission Press Release (July). http://europa.eu/rapid/

Ferguson DL (2008) International trends in inclusive education: the continuing challenge to teach each one and everyone. Eur J Spec Needs Educ 23(2):109–120. https://doi.org/10.1080/08856250801946236

Fitzgerald P, Leonard H, Pikora TJ et al (2013) Hospital admissions in children with down syndrome: experience of a population-based cohort followed from birth. PLoS One 8(8):e70401

Foster A, Titheradge H, Morton J (2015) Genetics of learning disability. Paediatr Child Health 25(10):450–457

Frawley D (2014) Combating educational disadvantage through early years and primary school investment. Irish Educ Stud 33(2):155–171. https://doi.org/10.1080/03323315.2014.920608

Gabel SL, Miskovic M (2014) Discourse and the containment of disability in higher education: an institutional

analysis. Disabil Soc 29(7):1145–1158. https://doi.org/10.1080/09687599.2014.910109

Genova A (2015) Barriers to inclusive education in Greece, Spain and Lithuania: results from emancipatory disability research. Disabil Soc 30(7):1042–1054. https://doi.org/10.1080/09687599.2015.1075867

George-Levi S, Laslo-Roth R (2021) Entitlement, hope, and life satisfaction among mothers of children with developmental disabilities. J Autism Dev Disord 51(11):3818–3828

Gillberg C (2010) The ESSENCE in child psychiatry: early symptomatic syndromes eliciting neurodevelopmental clinical examinations. Res Dev Disabil 31(6):1543–1551. https://doi.org/10.1016/j.ridd.2010.06.002

Goodall C (2018) 'I felt closed in and like I couldn't breathe': a qualitative study exploring the mainstream educational experiences of autistic young people. Autism Dev Language Impairments 3. https://doi.org/10.1177/2396941518804407

Government of Ireland (2005) Disability act. Stationery Office, Dublin. https://www.irishstatutebook.ie/eli/2005/act/14/enacted/en/print.html

Government of Ireland (2018) Houses of the Oireachtas Joint Committee on Education and Skills Report on the provision of Autistic Spectrum Disorders and Special Classes in mainstream schools. https://data.oireachtas.ie/ie/oireachtas/committee/dail/32/joint_committee_on_education_and_skills/reports/2018/2018-10-25_report-on-the-provision-of-autistic-spectrum-disorders-asd-and-special-classes-in-mainstream-schools_en.pdf

Grammenos S (2020) European comparative data on Europe 2020 and persons with disabilities, labour market, education, poverty and health, analysis and trends. European Commission. https://op.europa.eu/en/publication-detail/-/publication/1f1a8b2c-e44d-11eb-895a-01aa75ed71a1/language-en

Green JM, Absoud V, Grahame O et al (2018) Pathological demand avoidance: symptoms but not a syndrome. Lancet 2(6):455–464. https://doi.org/10.1016/S2352-4642(18)30044-0

Guralnick MJ (2017) Early intervention for children with intellectual disabilities: an update. J Appl Res Intellect Disabil 30(2):211–229

Hand BN, Boan AD, Bradley CC et al (2019a) Emergency department utilization and monetary charges in adolescents with autism spectrum disorder, intellectual disability, and a population comparison group. Autism Res 12(7):1129–1138

Hand BN, Boan AD, Bradley CC et al (2019b) Ambulatory care sensitive admissions in individuals with autism spectrum disorder, intellectual disability, and population controls. Autism Res 12(2):295–302

Health Service Executive & Faculty of Paediatrics (2016) 'Neurodisability.' In A National Model of Care for Paediatric Healthcare Services in Ireland, Health Service Executive & Faculty of Paediatrics, Dublin. Chapter 33

Hewitt-Taylor J (2010) Supporting children with complex health needs. Nurs Stand 24(19):50–56

Inclusion Ireland (2022) Progressing disability services for children and young people parent experience survey report. https://inclusionireland.ie/wp-content/uploads/2022/03/Inclusion-Ireland-Progressing-Disability-Services-Report-March-2022.pdf

Inter-Departmental Group (2015) Inter- Departmental Group Report. https://aim.gov.ie/app/uploads/2021/05/Inter-Departmental-Group-Report-launched-Nov-2015.pdf

Jenson K (2018) A global perspective on teacher attitudes towards inclusion: literature review. ERIC https://eric.ed.gov/?id=ED585094

Kenny N, McCoy S, Mihut G (2020) Special education reforms in Ireland: changing systems, changing schools. Int J Incl Educ:1–20. https://doi.org/10.1080/13603116.2020.1821447

Kessler SK, Blank LJ, Glusman J et al (2020) Unplanned readmissions of children with epilepsy in the United States. Pediatr Neurol 108:93–98

Kim S, Cambray-Engstrom E, Wang J, Kang VY, Choi Y-J, Coba-Rodriguez S (2020) Teachers' experiences, attitudes, and perceptions towards early inclusion in urban settings. Inc 8(3):222–240

Law J, McCann D, O'May F (2011) Managing change in the care of children with complex needs: healthcare providers' perspectives. J Adv Nurs 67(12):2551–2560

Leung MP, Thompson B, Black J, Dai S, Alsweiler JM (2018) The effects of preterm birth on visual development. Clin Exp Optom 101:4–12. https://doi.org/10.1111/cxo.12578

Lindgren S, Lauer E, Momany E et al (2021) Disability, hospital care, and cost: utilization of emergency and in-patient care by a cohort of children with intellectual and developmental disabilities. J Pediatr 229:259–266

Malcolm C, Adams S, Anderson G et al (2011) The symptom profile and experience of children with rare life-limiting conditions: perspectives of their families and key health professionals. Cancer Care Research Centre, University of Stirling

Maulik PK, Macarenhas MN, Mathers CD et al (2011) Prevalence of intellectual disability: a meta-analysis of population-based studies. Res Dev Disabil 32(2):419–436

McConkey R, Craig S, Kelly C (2019) The prevalence of intellectual disability: a comparison of national census and register records. Res Dev Disabil 89:69–75. https://doi.org/10.1016/j.ridd.2019.03.009

McCormack P (2019) Educating students with autism spectrum disorder (ASD) through the ASD class model: a qualitative study exploring the experiences of ASD class teachers and principals in Irish primary schools. Dublin City University, Dublin

McCoy S, Banks J, Frawley D et al (2014) Understanding special class provision in Ireland. Phase 1: findings from a national survey of schools. NCSE, Dublin. http://ncse.ie/wp-content/uploads/2014/10/Report_16_special_classes_30_04_14.pdf

McCoy S, Shevlin M, Rose R (2020) Secondary school transition for students with special educational needs in Ireland. Eur J Spec Needs Educ 35(2):154–170. https://doi.org/10.1080/08856257.2019.1628338

McKenzie K, Milton M, Smith G et al (2016) Systematic review of the prevalence and incidence of intellectual disabilities: current trends and issues. Curr Dev Disord Rep 3:104–115

Mencap (2012) About profound and multiple learning disabilities. Mencap, Wales

Milton D, Moon L (2012) The normalisation agenda and the psycho-emotional disablement of autistic people. Autonomy 1(1):Article 1

Murphy M, Hill K, Begley T et al (2021) Respite care for children with complex care needs: a literature review. Compr Child Adolesc Nurs. https://doi.org/10.1080/24694193.2021.1885523

National Autistic Society (2017) My hospital passport for autistic people. The National Autistic Society, London

National Council for Curriculum and Assessment (NCCA) (2009) Aistear, the early childhood curriculum framework. National Council for Curriculum and Assessment, Dublin

National Council for Special Education (2017) NCSE Press Release 18th January 2017 NCSE Welcomes a Better and More Equitable Way of Allocating Teaching Resources for Special Needs. Trim: NCSE. NCSE--Press-Release-18th-January-2017final-for-web.pdf

National Council for Special Education (2018) Report of the cross sectoral team working group on nursing supports. NCSE, Ireland

National Council for Special Education (2019) Policy advice on special schools and classes: an inclusive education for an inclusive society? Trim, NCSE

NICE (2022) Disabled children and young people up to 25 with severe complex needs: integrated service delivery and organisation across health, social care and education (NG213). NICE, London

Nicholson E, Doherty E, Guerin S et al (2022) Healthcare utilisation and unmet health needs in children with intellectual disability: a propensity score matching approach using longitudinal cohort data. J Intellect Disabil Res Adv 66(5):442–453. https://doi.org/10.1111/jir.12927

Northway R, Rees S, Davies M et al (2017) Hospital passports, patient safety and person-centred care: a review of documents currently used for people with intellectual disabilities in the UK. J Clin Nurs 26(23–24):5160–5168

OECD (2004) Equity in education: students with disabilities, learning difficulties and disadvantages. OECD Publishing, Paris

OECD (2016) Netherlands 2016: foundations for the future. OECD Publishing, Paris

Pinney A (2017) Understanding the needs of disabled children with complex needs or life-limiting conditions. Council for Disabled Children and True Colours Trust, London

Pobal (2018) Access and Inclusion Model. Annual Report 2016–2017. Pobal, Dublin. https://www.pobal.ie/app/uploads/2018/12/AIM-Annual-Report-2016_2017.pdf

Portero BI (2012) Are there rights in a time of crisis? Disabil Soc 27(4):581–585. https://doi.org/10.1080/0968 7599.2012.659461

Reed P, Osborne LA, Waddington EM (2012) A comparative study of the impact of mainstream and special school placement on the behaviour of children with autism spectrum disorders. Br Educ Res J 38(0):749–763. https://doi.org/10.1080/01411926.2011.580048

Rodgers HR, McCluney J (2021) Prevalence of autism (including asperger syndrome) in school age children in Northern Ireland: annual report 2021. https://dera.ioe.ac.uk//36713/1/asd-children-ni-2020.pdf

Royal College of Nursing (2013) Meeting the health needs of people with learning disabilities, RCN guidance for nursing staff. Royal College of Nursing, London

Ryndak D, Jackson L, Billingsley F (2000) Defining school inclusion for students with moderate to severe disabilities: what do experts say? Exceptionality 8:101–116. https://doi.org/10.1207/S15327035EX0802_2

Scherzer AL, Chhagan M, Kauchali S et al (2012) Global perspective on early diagnosis and intervention for children with developmental delays and disabilities: review. Dev Med Child Neurol 54(12): 1079–1084

Sheridan M, Sharma A, Cockerill H (2014) From birth to five years, children's developmental Progress, 4th edn. Taylor & Francis, UK

Shevlin M, Banks J (2021) Inclusion at a crossroads: dismantling Ireland's system of special education. Educ Sci 11(4):161. https://doi.org/10.3390/educsci11040161

Smythe T, Zuurmond M, Tann CJ et al (2021) Early intervention for children with developmental disabilities in low and middle-income countries – the case for action. Int Health 13(3):222–231. https://doi.org/10.1093/inthealth/ihaa044

Twomey M (2016) Transitions: space and place. Children's Res Dig 3(2)

Twomey M, Shevlin M (2017) Parenting, autism spectrum disorders and inner journeys. J Res Spec Educ Needs 17(3):157–167

UNESCO (1994) The Salamanca statement and framework for action on special needs education: adopted by the world conference on special needs education; access and quality. Salamanca, Spain, 7–10 June

University Hospital Bristol (2011) My hospital passport. University Hospital Bristol, Bristol

United Nations (1989) Convention on the rights of the child. United Nations Treaty Ser 1577(3):1–23

United Nations (2006) Convention on the rights of persons with disabilities. Treaty Ser 2515:3. https://www.un.org/development/desa/disabilities/convention-on-the-rights-of-persons-with-disabilities/convention-on-the-rights-of-persons-with-disabilities-2.html

van Timmeren EA, van der Putten AAJ, van Schrojenstein Lantma-de Valk HMJ et al (2016) Prevalence of reported physical health problems in people with severe or profound intellectual and motor disabilities: a cross-sectional study of medical records and care plans. J Intellect Disabil Res 67: 28–33

Waddington EM, Reed P (2017) Comparison of the effects of mainstream and special school on National Curriculum outcomes in children with autism spectrum disorder: an archive-based analysis. J Res Spec Educ Needs 17(2):132–142. https://doi.org/10.1111/1471-3802.12368

World Health Organization (2017) Medication without harm: WHO global patient safety challenge. WHO, Geneva

World Health Organisation (WHO) (2022) Definition: intellectual disability. WHO, Denmark. http://www.euro.who.int/en/health-topics/noncommunicable-diseases/mental-health/news/news/2010/15/childrens-right-to-family-life/definition-intellectual-disability

Walker SP, Wachs TD, Grantham-McGregor S et al (2011) Inequality in early childhood: risk and protective factors for early child development. Lancet 378(9799):1325–1338. https://doi.org/10.1016/S0140-6736(11)60555-2

Yonkaitis CF, Shannon RA (2017) The role of the school nurse in the special education process: part I: student identification and evaluation. NASN Sch Nurse 32(3):178–184. https://doi.org/10.1177/19426 02X17700677

Zijlstra HP, Vlaskamp C (2005) The impact of medical health conditions of children with profound intellectual and multiple disabilities. J Appl Res Intellect Disabil 18:151–161

Intellectual and Developmental Disabilities and Rare Diseases

Suja Somanadhan, Norah L. Johnson, Bernadette Sheehan Gilroy, Anne Lawlor, and Jerry Vockley

Chapter Topics

- This chapter provides an overview of rare diseases/disorders.
- The aetiological classifications of rare diseases are identified.
- A discussion on rare diseases in the context of preventable intellectual and developmental disabilities is presented.
- Impact of rare metabolic diseases across the lifespan.
- The implications for an informal carer and the professional focus required are highlighted.
- A vignette addressing key issues discussed in the chapter is presented.

S. Somanadhan (✉)
UCD School of Nursing Midwifery and Health Systems, UCD Centre for Interdisciplinary Research, Education and Innovation in Health Systems (UCD IRIS), University College Dublin, Belfield, Dublin, Ireland
e-mail: suja.somanadhan@ucd.ie

N. L. Johnson
Marquette University College of Nursing, Milwaukee, WI, USA
e-mail: norah.johnson@marquette.edu

B. S. Gilroy
PKU Association of Ireland, Dublin, Ireland

A. Lawlor
22Q11 Ireland, Dublin, Ireland

J. Vockley
Department of Pediatrics, University of Pittsburgh School of Medicine, Center for Rare Disease Therapy, UPMC Children's Hospital of Pittsburgh, Pittsburgh, PA, USA

Introduction

Rare disease is a collective term for a group of predominantly genetic disorders (approximately 80% genetic in origin) with a broad diversity of signs and symptoms. Each disorder is usually defined by the respective rarity of the incidence in the population. In the USA, it is called a rare disease, and the incidence affects less than 200,000 people, and in Europe, no more than 1 person in 2000 is called a rare disease. The term 'ultra-rare' is used to describe genetic disorders with the lowest incidences (typically <1000–5000). Most rare diseases are present at birth and can affect the trajectory of the individual's physical, intellectual, and/or emotional development. Early detection, diagnosis, and intervention can prevent early death or disability and enable children to reach their full potential. Rare diseases pose medical, financial, and psychological challenges for those who live with associated health challenges, with or without intellectual and developmental disabilities. While each rare disease affects a limited number of individuals, rare conditions have a total prevalence of approximately 6–8% combined in the global population. Around 450 million people worldwide are affected by 1 out of 5000–8000 rare diseases, half of whom are children.

© The Author(s), under exclusive license to Springer Nature Switzerland AG 2023
F. Sheerin, C. Doyle (eds.), *Intellectual Disabilities: Health and Social Care Across the Lifespan*,
https://doi.org/10.1007/978-3-031-27496-1_7

General Aspects of Intellectual Disability and Rare Disorders

This section focuses on those with a rare condition associated with complex needs, intellectual and developmental disabilities, and/or physical disability.

Defining Intellectual and Developmental Disabilities

Intellectual disabilities are characterised by significant limitations in intellectual functioning and adaptive behaviour as expressed in conceptual, social, and practical adaptive skills (American Association on Intellectual and Developmental Disabilities (AAIDD) 2022). This disability originates before the age of 18 years. Functional limitations are broad, including language development, social interaction, motor skills, and self-care. Depending on the level of impairment, children will have varying support needs, ranging from modified academic instruction and functional assistance to full-time care for activities of daily living (Zablotsky et al. 2019). Developmental disabilities refer to those children with intellectual disabilities but also other disabilities that may be physical, learning, language, or behavior in nature (AAIDD 2022).

Defining Rare Diseases/Disorders

Rare disease constitutes a large and heterogeneous group of diagnoses, which may cause intellectual and developmental disabilities with a significant impact on the lives of affected individuals, their families, and the healthcare system (Boyle et al. 2011; Castro et al. 2017; Kvarnung and Nordgren 2017). These complex conditions tend to be chronic, debilitating, and multisystemic, often associated with physical, sensory, and intellectual disability (Ward et al. 2022). Rare diseases are significantly associated with mortality, morbidity, and disability, affecting population health outcomes. Many people worldwide are struggling in search of a diagnosis for a

rare disease (Isono et al. 2022). There are different groups of undiagnosed patients, such as 'not yet diagnosed' or undiagnosed. In recent years, rare diseases have become a global public health and national policy priority (Non-Governmental Organisation (NGO) 2019).

There is a disparity in the international definition of rare diseases, with some definitions depending solely on the number of people living with certain diseases. Rare diseases (RD) are diseases or conditions affecting fewer than 200,000 individuals or approximately 1/15000 in the USA, according to the US Orphan Drug Act (2013). In contrast, an RD is a condition with less than 5 affected persons per 10,000 in Europe (European Commission (EC) 1999). They are often life-threatening or chronically debilitating diseases and are mostly inherited. A rare disease may affect only a handful of individuals, often known as 'ultra-rare', with a prevalence <1 per 50,000 persons (NICE 2004), for example, lysosomal storage diseases (LSD). Some diseases are 'rare' in some demographics or regions but not others, e.g. sickle cell diseases. Another example is tuberculosis (TB), which is rare in Europe or the USA but is one of the top 10 causes of death worldwide (WHO 2021). There are estimated to be between 6000 and 8000 rare diseases, making their cumulative prevalence common (Dawkins et al. 2018), and new conditions are regularly described in the medical literature.

Prevalence of Rare Diseases

Globally, it is estimated that over 450 million people (6%–8%) of the world population have a rare disease (Repetto and Rebolledo-Jaramillo 2020). Rare diseases affect around three million people in the UK (The UK Rare Diseases Framework (2021), approximately 300,000 people in Ireland (HSE 2022a, b), and about 30 million people in the USA (U.S. GAO 2021). Thus, while rare diseases are individually rare, collectively they are common in society and as such deserve public health attention needed for optimal health outcomes for those affected. The large cumulative incidence across rare diseases and the extensive variety of disorders create a significant public health crisis worldwide (McMullan et al. 2021).

The most debilitating part of rare diseases is the intellectual and developmental disabilities that are estimated to affect 1–3% of the population (Maenner et al. 2016; Purugganan 2018). The prevalence of developmental disability amongst children from the USA aged 3–17 years increased between 2009 and 2017 (Zablotsky et al. 2019). Measuring the prevalence of developmental disabilities in the population helps gauge the adequacy of available services and interventions. The percentage of children diagnosed with both an intellectual disability and a developmental disability also increased significantly between 2009 and 2017, resulting in a growing population of children (one out of every six) with one or more displaying developmental disabilities (Zablotsky et al. 2019).

Aetiological Classifications

Classification of Rare Diseases

There are a variety of sources that classify rare diseases. Orphanet (www.orpha.net) is a European portal for rare disease information co-funded by the European Commission. Orphanet aims to increase knowledge of rare diseases in order to improve the diagnosis, care, and treatment of people with rare diseases (Orphanet 2018). The Genetic and Rare Diseases Information Center (GARD) information specialists also assign rare disease categories. This programme is funded by two institutes of the National Institutes of Health (NIH): National Center for Advancing Translational Sciences (NCATS) and the National Human Genome Research Institute (NHGRI). Rare diseases are often included in more than one category if they affect multiple body parts. Searching for disease allows a view of the position of a given condition in a classification. Selecting the disease of interest in the search results displays a list of all classifications containing the chosen disorder. Rare diseases are often included in more than one category if they affect multiple body parts, though practices

vary from country to country in implementing policy and practice. For example, in Ireland, the HSE (HSE 2019) proposed transition services for (1) those with a chronic but relatively stable condition for which normal or near-normal life expectancy is anticipated, (2) those with a rare life-limiting condition, and (3) those with a rare condition associated with complex needs (intellectual and/or physical disability). A nosology of inborn errors of metabolism has recently been published that provides a framework for characterising these disorders (Ferreira et al. 2019).

Classification of Intellectual and Developmental Disabilities

The diagnosis of a rare disease and the management of children with rare diseases are complex. Thorough clinical evaluation and investigation of both nongenetic and genetic aetiologies can yield definitive diagnoses for many individuals with intellectual and developmental disabilities. Males are affected by X-linked recessive disorders much more frequently than females, and approximately 40% of boys with genetic disorders have been reported to have intellectual disability, primarily attributable to X-linked genetic disorders (Yeargin-Allxopp et al. 1997; Leonard and Wen 2002). X-linked syndromes include Lowe syndrome, Hunter syndrome, Menkes syndrome, Duchenne muscular dystrophy, and Rett syndrome. However, not everyone with an intellectual and developmental disability have received such an assessment, identifying an opportunity for healthcare providers to advocate for genetic consultation for undiagnosed individuals with co-occurring intellectual and developmental disabilities.

Obtaining a genetic diagnosis can help an individual and their family explain a lifelong disabling cognitive disorder, guide prognosis, and highlight medical comorbidities. Multiple factors are involved in intellectual disability, including genetic inheritance and environmental conditions (Ilyas et al. 2020). Studies suggest that up to 40% of intellectual and developmental disabilities have a genetic basis (Kaufman et al. 2010;

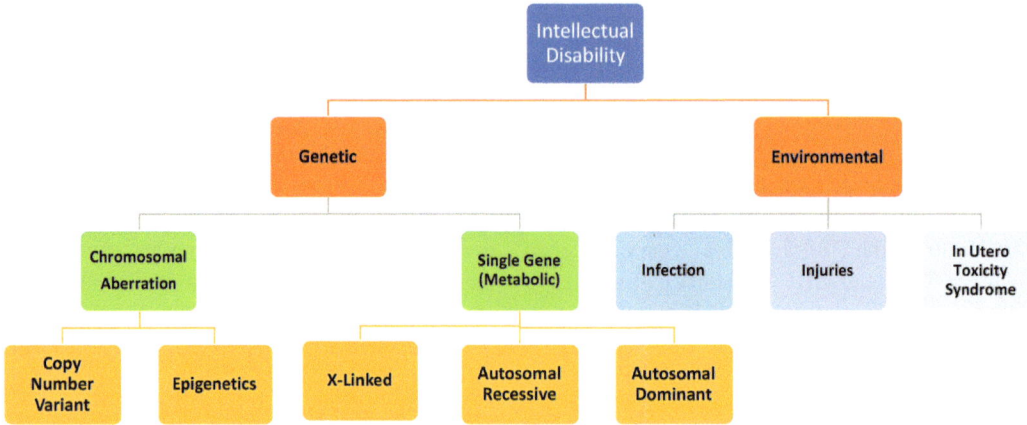

Fig. 7.1 Aetiological classification of intellectual disability

Langenfeld et al. 2021). The aetiological classification of intellectual disability is broad and is one of several conditions collectively known as developmental disability (AAIDD 2022). It has been divided into genetic causes and environmental exposure (Ilyas et al. 2020; Lee et al. 2022). The aetiological classification of intellectual disability that falls within the category of rare diseases is outlined in Fig. 7.1.

Inborn Error of Metabolism (IEM)

Inborn errors of metabolism (IEMs) describe those diseases caused by a block in a metabolic pathway due to the deficient activity of a specific enzyme (Gilbert-Barness and Farrell 2016; Guerrero et al. 2018). In IEMs, symptoms are caused by the accumulation of toxic by-products because of the block or the lack of a critical metabolite past it, often leading to intellectual and developmental disabilities and additional behavioural problems. IEMs typically occur as single-gene disorders. While IEMs can be inherited in an autosomal-dominant, autosomal recessive or X-linked fashion, autosomal recessive IEMs are most common. Phenylketonuria (PKU) is an example of an inherited autosomal recessive disorder of phenylalanine metabolism, in which especially high phenylalanine concentrations can cause brain dysfunction if untreated. This brain dysfunction results in severe intellectual

disability, epilepsy, and behavioural problems (Lee et al. 2022). Metabolic and molecular genetic testing is necessary to assess all individuals with intellectual and developmental disabilities.

Diagnosis of Rare Disorders

Diagnosis and management of children with rare disorders are complex due to the heterogeneity of the diseases that cause intellectual and developmental disabilities. However, making a diagnosis is critical due to the impact on the lives of affected individuals, their families, and the healthcare system (Kvarnung and Nordgren 2017). The presence of an aetiological diagnosis is key for both paediatric primary care providers and families. Moeschler and Shevell (2014) provided a comprehensive list of the purposes of the medical genetics evaluation of children with intellectual and developmental disabilities.

Evidence suggests that the percentage of individuals with identifiable metabolic disorders as a cause of intellectual disability ranges from 1% to 5% (Van Karnebeek et al. 2005; Lion-Francois et al. 2006; Engbers et al. 2009). The chromosomal abnormalities may be observed in about 25–30% of people with intellectual and developmental disabilities though they are rare in metabolic disorders (Moeschler and Shevell 2014). Of 81 treatable genetic metabolic diseases

Table 7.1 Metabolic screening tests

Specimen	Test
Blood	Amino acids
	Homocysteine
	Acylcarnitine profile
	Glycosylation
Urine	Organic acids
	GAA/creatine metabolites
	Purines and pyrimidines
	Mucopolysaccharide screen
	Oligosaccharide screen

presenting with intellectual disability, 50 (62%) were identified by routinely available metabolic screening tests (Table 7.1) and 55 (69%) of the treatable IEMs had a non-neurologic feature as a prominent part of the phenotype (van Karnebeek and Stockler 2012). The non-neurologic features affect anatomic/organ systems, bones and joints, dermatology, endocrinology, eye, facial dysmorphism, growth and stature, heart, gastrointestinal, haematology, immunology, kidney, liver, and odour. Thus, non-neurologic features noted here should be concerning phenotypic findings deserving of aetiological investigation for a possible genetic aetiology.

As many metabolic disorders are treatable conditions, early recognition and intervention are critical, especially for disorders that cause early intellectual and developmental disabilities (van Karnebeek and Stockler 2012; Liao et al. 2019; Almannai et al. 2021). Accessing digital information tools for clinicians such as http://www.treatable-id.org helps to improve early recognition and intervention for such conditions (Hoytema van Konijnenburg et al. 2021). This tool adopts a diagnostic algorithm with strategies to facilitate a practical guide for biochemical and genetic/genomic diagnosis. The IEMs are grouped according to diagnosis via 'metabolic screening tests' (first tier) versus IEMs diagnosed via a 'single test per single disease' (second tier) approach. First, their screening tests were defined as tests in blood and urine that are readily available in biochemical laboratories in most developed countries. A considerable proportion of preventable intellectual disabilities (62%) can be reliably detected through a panel of metabolic screening tests on blood and urine.

Metabolic tests in the second tier group evaluate preventable intellectual disabilities for which biochemical markers are difficult to interpret, and/or conventional diagnostic approach requires an invasive procedure or poorly accessible test (i.e. only performed in a few centres worldwide). Genetic testing (targeted molecular analysis as well as exome sequencing) can be performed in parallel. They are translated into a stepwise algorithm and are available via http://www.treatable-id.org, freely downloadable for all interested individuals.

Liao et al. (2019) conducted a retrospective study of the aetiological characteristics of 1051 children with intellectual and developmental disabilities in central China. They investigated the role of genetic analysis to explore the aetiology where the cause of the disease was uncertain. Children had mild (367, 34.9%), moderate (301, 28.6%), severe (310, 29.5%), and profoundly severe (73, 6.9%) intellectual and developmental disabilities. In this study, inherited metabolic disease accounted for 0.8% (8/1051) of aetiology, close to the figure of 0.2% to 8.4% reported previously by van Karnebeek and Stockler (2012).

Despite multiple recommendations and guidelines from the USA and Europe, the diagnostic practices for investigating people with unexplained intellectual and developmental disabilities vary from country to country. For example, O'Byrne et al. (2016) provided an overview of a protocol for first-line assessment and investigations for unexplained developmental delay/learning disability. Miclea et al. (2015) argued for the necessity of implementing a standard practice due to (1) the high prevalence of developmental disabilities (3% of the population), (2) the high genetic contribution to this type of pathology, and (3) insufficient referral for genetic consultation. Identifying the intellectual and developmental delay is an important preliminary step in strategising investigations (Moeschler and Shevell 2014). These disorders should be investigated in children younger than 2–3 years old and preferably as part of the newborn screening programme (NBS) to receive a timely diagnosis and appropriate treatment to avoid developing intellectual and developmental disabilities.

Early detection, diagnosis, and intervention can prevent death or disability and enable children to reach their full potential (CDC 2012). NBS form part of a public health screening of infants shortly after birth. The goal of NBS is the pre-symptomatic detection of infants with congenital conditions and metabolic disorders, aimed at the earliest possible recognition and management of affected newborns to prevent the morbidity, mortality, and disabilities associated with an inherited metabolic disease (Kelly et al. 2016), so that treatment may be commenced as early as possible to prevent, or ameliorate, the long-term consequences of the condition. NBS primarily aims to identify treatable rare genetic disorders with risks of developmental delay, severe disability, or premature death (McCandless and Wright 2020).

The testing involved in NBS is primarily performed by measuring metabolites, enzyme activity, or other biochemicals in samples of blood collected on filter paper obtained from a heel prick (HSE 2022a, b). For example, in the USA, about four million babies born annually are tested for at least 29 treatable genetic, metabolic, endocrine, and infectious diseases within the first week of life (CDC 2012; NIH 2022). In Ireland, a newborn screening programme currently tests nine inherited conditions: phenylketonuria (PKU), homocystinuria, maple syrup urine disease (MSUD), classical galactosaemia, congenital hypothyroidism, cystic fibrosis, medium-chain acyl-CoA dehydrogenase deficiency (MCADD), glutaric aciduria type 1 (GA1), and adenosine deaminase deficiency severe combined immunodeficiency (ADA-SCID) (HSE 2022a, b). NBS results should be followed up with definitive diagnostic testing.

The methods for establishing an aetiological diagnosis in individuals with rare disorders have improved dramatically, as a precise molecular diagnosis is essential for efficient management and treatment (Boycott et al. 2017). See Table 7.2 for examples of diagnostic testing.

Table 7.2 Diagnostic testing

Cytogenetics

Cytogenetic testing is used when a chromosome abnormality is suspected. It involves the analysis of cells in a sample of blood, tissue, amniotic fluid, bone marrow, or cerebrovascular fluid to identify any changes in an individual's chromosomes. It can be performed prenatally after biochemical screening or ultrasound with abnormal findings. It is also used for parents with multiple miscarriages or significant results in their pedigree analysis. Postnatally, cytogenetic testing plays a role in distinguishing people with mosaicism, intellectual disability, autism, or developmental delays (Boycott et al. 2017). Older technology relied on karyotypic analysis of stimulated lymphocytes from peripheral blood or chorionic villus sampling. More recently, molecular testing relies on single-nucleotide polymorphism (SNP) microarrays that allow the detection of smaller copy number variants.

Next-generation sequencing (NGS) panels

NGS is a relatively new technique for genetic testing. NGS has the advantage compared to traditional Sanger DNA sequencing of higher throughput, lower cost, and the ability to sequence multiple genes at one time, allowing the identification of causal mutations, including de novo, novel, and familial mutations, associated with syndromes. The broad application of NGS panels has led to the recognition of a broader phenotypic spectrum of many disorders, providing vastly improved diagnosis for variant presentations (Dunn et al. 2018).

Whole exome sequencing (WES)

Whole exome sequencing refers to the sequencing of all protein-coding regions (exons) of the genome using NGS techniques. It is a more cost- and time-effective diagnostic tool than traditional stepwise evaluation when a clinical diagnosis is not apparent (Dunn et al. 2018; Manickam et al. 2021).

Whole genome sequencing (WGS)

Whole genome sequencing provides greater genome coverage, including non-coding regions, and can be completed more rapidly compared to whole exome sequencing and gene panels. However, current analytical techniques still emphasise exons and intron/exon boundaries, minimising the increase in diagnostic yield. Incorporation into newborn screening has been proposed (Dunn et al. 2018; Woerner et al. 2021).

Clinical Presentations

The low prevalence and considerable heterogeneity of rare diseases make it challenging to focus specifically on individual rare conditions. Rare diseases with a genetic inheritance can cause intellectual and developmental disabilities with a

Table 7.3 Neurological features and other red flags suggestive of IEM

- Family history of IEM or unexplained infant death
- Consanguinity
- Failure to thrive
- Head circumference > 2 SD above or 2 SD below mean
- Recurrent episodes of vomiting, ataxia, seizures, lethargy, and coma
- History of being severely symptomatic and needing longer to recover from inter-current (viral) illness
- Unusual dietary preferences
- Regression in developmental milestones
- Developmental delay or intellectual disability
- Severe hypotonia, dystonia, seizures, and abnormal hypertonia (spasticity)
- Neuroimaging abnormalities

significant impact on the lives of affected individuals and their families and the healthcare system (Kvarnung and Nordgren 2017). The clinical presentation of rare disorders includes broad, diverse signs and symptoms involving multiple systems, the nervous system, intellectual disability, neuropsychiatric disorders, epilepsy, and motor dysfunction (Kvarnung and Nordgren 2017). For many rare diseases, signs may be observed at birth or in childhood (Table 7.3).

Rare diseases pose challenges for affected individuals and their families regarding the diagnostic process and getting the correct diagnosis, treatment, and optimal care. Clinicians who care for affected individuals with rare diseases face numerous challenges, such as gaining knowledge and experience in caring for such individuals and the availability of local experts and expert clinical guidelines. Even in rare disorders where the fundamental biochemical defect is known, such as PKU and other enzyme defects, the exact basis for brain dysfunction is uncertain. The outcome for treated PKU, MSUD, galactosemia, homocystinuria, and lysosomal storage disorders is not yet optimal. Some rare metabolic diseases cause intellectual disabilities that may worsen throughout a person's life. Treatment often requires the lifelong maintenance of a medical diet that avoids substances that cannot be appropriately metabolised.

At an EU level, there are 24 European Reference Networks (ERNs) focusing on rare disorders enabling virtual interaction of healthcare providers across Europe. They aim to facilitate discussion on complex or rare disease knowledge, treatment, and resources (European Commission (2022). Conversely, in the USA, the National Organization for Rare Disorders (NORD) Rare Disease Centers of Excellence (CoE) Program brings together 31 clinical expert centres in a nationwide network across the USA. They bring cutting-edge facilities to provide specialised care and disease management standards for people living with a rare disease and their families (NORD 2022).

Therapies for Inborn Error of Metabolism (IEM)

Treatable IEMs present with a wide variety of symptoms, including intellectual and developmental disabilities as a significant feature (van Karnebeek and Stockler 2012; Liao et al. 2019). For many IEMs, treatment is mainly supportive and based on clinical symptoms. However, focused treatment exists for some disorders based on manipulation of substrate or products, replacement of missing enzymes, and activation of alternative metabolic pathways (Ginocchio and Brunetti-Pierri 2016). Based on these mechanisms, IEMs have traditionally been treated and managed by restricting upstream nutrients to avoid intoxication, supplementing downstream nutrients to avoid secondary deficiency, stimulating alternative routes for precursor metabolite disposal, or replacing the defective enzyme with intravenous protein infusions (Ginocchio and Brunetti-Pierri 2016). Some chemicals can act as chaperonins that enhance the stability of mutant proteins. Gene replacement or substitution therapy is rapidly becoming a possibility for some disorders, while mRNA therapy can provide an alternative source of enzyme in some conditions.

Figure 7.2 provides an overview of the therapies associated with inherited metabolic disorders.

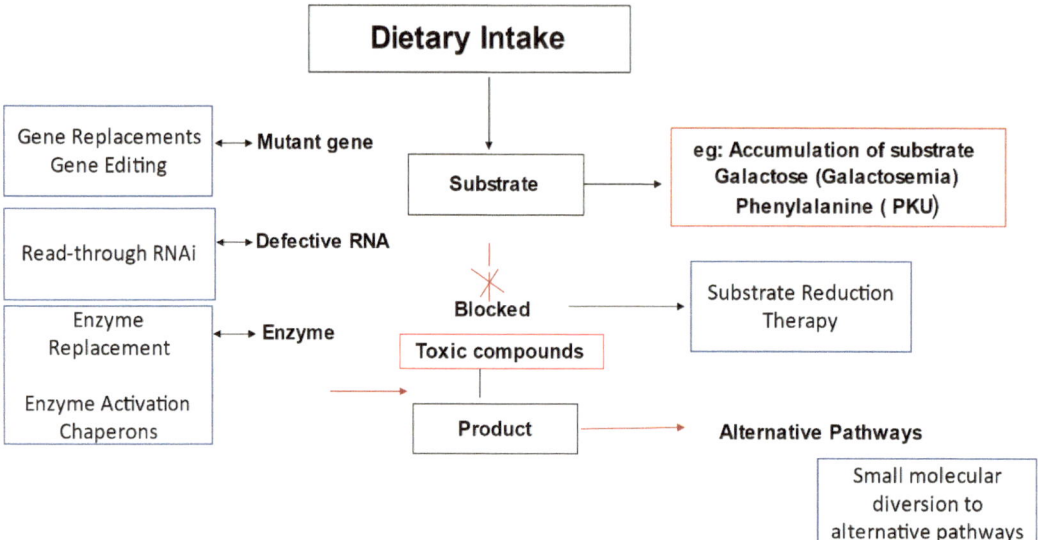

Fig. 7.2 Therapies for inherited metabolic disorders

Impact of Rare Metabolic Diseases Across the Lifespan

Advances in screening, diagnosis, treatment, and management of IEMs have led to improved health outcomes and increased life expectancy, with most individuals now surviving into adulthood (Stepien et al. 2021; Gold et al. 2022). The individual living with rare metabolic diseases may show signs and symptoms across their lifespan. Most paediatric rare diseases involve complex medical issues, requiring lifelong, highly specialised and coordinated care (Gunne et al. 2020). However, there are challenges to all dimensions of the individual and family's life. As they grow up, the care of individuals with IEM should be transferred from paediatric to adult healthcare settings. Stepien et al. (2021) conducted a European-wide survey to identify unmet needs regarding the transition process in rare metabolic diseases. Most centres ($n = 67\%$) have no designated transition or care coordinator. in 77% of centres, paediatricians share a medical summary, transition letter, and emergency plan with the adult team and the individual and percentage of individuals remain under paediatric care throughout their life. The main challenges identified by healthcare professionals (HCPs) in

managing transition are lack of time and shortage of adult metabolic physician positions. Gold et al. (2022) carried out current care practices for adults with IEMs in the USA. Ninety-one providers from 73 institutions completed the survey. Most adults with IEM disorders receive lifelong care from a single metabolic clinician, predominantly in paediatric clinic settings. Adults receive comprehensive ambulatory metabolic care, but fewer trainees participate compared with paediatric visits. Most acute IEM management occurs in paediatric hospitals. The transition from children's services to adult rare disease services was seen as a significant barrier to achieving good care outcomes.

Due to the complexity and heterogenicity of rare metabolic diseases and related intellectual and developmental disabilities, there are challenges to all dimensions of the individual and family's life. Evidence indicates that rare diseases can significantly reduce the quality of life for individuals and their families. The impact can be diverse and include loss of physical function, cognitive and communication impairments, emotional problems, and social isolation (Somanadhan and Larkin 2016; Slade et al. 2018; Somanadhan et al. 2021). As specialist expertise is scarce, the individual and their families may find it challenging to gain access to services to address day-to-day caring needs, including transition, self-management, and integrated care (care closer to home). People living with a rare disease also face discrimination at work, school, and leisure. Very little is known about the experience of living with a rare disease with a focus on equality, diversity, and inclusion (EDI) as a method to promote transition, self-management, and independent living, especially amongst the paediatric population (von der Lippe et al. 2017). It is essential that the specific ways in which individual and family-focused experiences living with a rare disease and its impact on their life across the lifespan be explored and targeted, ensuring that people living with a rare disease have access to social, educational, and leisure inclusion on equal footing with other citizens (EURORDIS 2019). Rare diseases pose challenges not only to affected individuals (Stoller 2018) but also to those who care for them and broadly for the health and social systems of each nation (Hedley et al. 2021). This complex nature of rare diseases disrupts family roles, relationships, functional status, quality of life, day-to-day family management, and mental health and well-being. An individual and family-centred approach is vital to plan, deliver, and evaluate healthcare grounded in mutually beneficial partnerships amongst healthcare providers, individuals, and families (IPFCC 2022).

The Implications for an Informal Carer and the Professional Focus

Rare metabolic disorders are often multi-systemic disorders. This means this condition affects multiple organs in the body. Individuals may show signs and symptoms across their lifespan that reflect the underlying metabolic disorder. Preventing intellectual and developmental disability is the ultimate goal for some disorders but is often not possible, even with early diagnosis.

Nurses and midwives are trusted and in close contact with parents after birth and throughout the child's early years. NBS for rare diseases is crucial because it helps families anticipate symptoms and identify treatments that improve a child's chance at the best outcomes and quality of life. Thus, it is important to include the awareness of the opportunities for and goals of NBS in nursing education and to always check the screening results for individuals. It is also important for nurses to understand that only some rare disorders are identified by NBS. Thus, recognising children's developmental or other unexplained clinical concerns is an important first step to identifying and treating a rare disease. This can be accomplished using such tools as developmental screening instruments (such as the Denver Developmental Scale) and obtaining family histories, integrating genetics and genomics into nursing care (Johnson et al. 2013). Maintaining open communication with families can allow a nurse to be a critical touch point for families worried about their child and lead to consideration and diagnosis of a rare disease. Early detection and prompt management of metabolic crises are crucial to achieving favourable outcomes for which treatable options are available (Smith 2008).

Most children and young people living with rare metabolic diseases can have their own regimens. As an informal carer or nurse, it's important to have open communication and always ask the individual if they can answer your question or ask their parents or healthcare professionals. Genetic and genomic education and awareness can help the understanding of diagnoses and why the disease occurred, potential risks of developing the other illness, and medical interventions and treatment options to reduce disease development or progression (Ginsburg et al. 2019). Integrating a standardised and high-quality family history assessment increases the likelihood of detecting carriers for rare genetic diseases. Evidence suggests that nurses lack sufficient knowledge to incorporate genomic applications in clinical settings (Bashore et al. 2018). Therefore, providing clinically relevant education and training in genetics and genomics is paramount for nursing education to develop appropriate skills and knowledge that will enable them to provide optimal care to individuals and their families (Tonkin et al. 2011).

To promote early intervention, nurses will benefit from genetics and genomics knowledge related to rare genetic diseases' early identi-fication, diagnosis, and implications for the individuals and families (Johnson et al. 2013). Families with a child with a rare metabolic disorder will require nursing support to advo-cate for optimal health outcomes. Nurses play a key role in the daily illness management in the hospital setting, which includes assessment, medication management, coordination of mul-tidisciplinary management, parent education, and support. Since rare metabolic diseases are multi-systemic diseases, the day-to-manage-ment and treatment require input from health-care disciplines such as dietetics, psychology, social workers, play specialists, medicine, and nursing. Dieticians educate individuals, par-ents, carers, and other healthcare profession-als on dietary management of these disorders. Psychologists play a key role during diagnosis in meeting with families and are then available for help when needed afterwards. Examples of support they can offer include developmental assessments where there are concerns regard-ing the development, advice and support on managing aspects of a child's behaviour that are causing concern from time to time, and psy-chological assessments when there is a concern about a child's progress in school (NCIMD 2022). Medical social workers focus on the social and emotional impact of illness on the lives of individuals and their families, while the physiotherapist will assess the child's physical development (NCIMD 2022).

Caring for a family member with rare dis-eases has a broad impact across all dimensions of the family's life (Malcolm et al. 2011; Grant et al. 2013; Somanadhan and Larkin 2016). The families must adapt to and support their child's intellectual and/or developmental needs, which can increase with age. Studies have consistently shown that having a rare disorder gives rise to difficulties in family dynamics, including strain on marital relationships, feelings of isolation, and additional financial pressures, as well as having a negative impact on healthy siblings (Malcolm et al. 2011; Grant et al. 2013; Somanadhan and Larkin 2016). Families report that transitions of being a parent with a rare disease and illness

trajectory create many challenges for their day-to-day life and traditional roles, leading to stig-matisation and isolation in society (Somanadhan et al. 2021).

Good communication skills with parents of young children allow a nurse to foster better care for individuals with rare diseases and parents' satisfaction. By maintaining compassion and curiosity along with an open mind, nurses can accomplish a short assessment of individual and family needs and address diagnostic and thera-peutic needs (Shajani and Snell 2019). Conversa-tions with parents when children have symptoms of rare diseases and an uncertain diagnosis are high-anxiety situations (Johnson et al. 2020). Individuals may have had multiple evaluations with no certainty and faced difficulty obtaining services, resulting in a loss of faith in care provid-ers. A nurse in this setting can be the difference between persistence on the part of the family in their diagnostic odyssey and an individual's loss to follow-up.

Vignette One

The following vignette exemplifies man-aging uncertainty associated with fami-lies' experience of living with a child with a rare metabolic condition called phenylketonuria (PKU).

We received our child's diagnosis of PKU via telephone when our daughter was 10 days old, and we were instructed to make our way to the expert metabolic cen-tre to confirm the diagnosis. We remained there for 1 week. During this time, we met with the specialist metabolic team who educated us on the condition, the blood spot technique, and how to get reimbursed for medical formula she would require. It was a very traumatic time. We were griev-ing for the child we never actually had… that child without PKU. With very little prior knowledge of the condition, we felt helpless, dependent, and very lost. It was emphasised how lucky we were to receive a diagnosis; however our family like many others could have greatly benefited from psychological support, a peer family support programme, appropriate on-site breastfeeding facilities, and parental sleeping accommodation. PKU dietary management was described to us as a lifestyle adjustment.

The initial years can be a very anxious time for families. Protein gives that feeling of fullness. Our child was never satisfied with synthetic protein formula and breast milk alone and woke regularly for feeds. If phenylalanine (PHE) levels were elevated due to cessation of a growth spurt, teething, or a childhood vaccination, our child tended to sleep for longer. Babies and toddlers sometimes refuse their synthetic protein formula due to teething or illness and lack of adherence to dietary management is very stressful for parents/carers. We were encouraged to progress from a bottle to a sippy cup when age-appropriate so our daughter could taste the unpalatable formula on their full palate. This transition is one of the most challenging for children and their families. To reduce the stress on the child and on us parents, we punctured small holes in the teat of her bottle, which kept everyone happy! We eventually progressed to a beaker and used a straw to reduce the risk of dental erosion due to the composition of the formula.

Those with greater protein tolerance post fortnightly or monthly blood spot cards. Results are received 3–5 days later via text message, and this determines dietary management for the following week. If the reading is out of range, we telephone the metabolic dietitians and await further instruction via telephone. Those attending adult services however wait up to 12 days to receive their blood PHE via telephone.

There needs to be an acknowledgement that PKU is a lifelong condition. Our community would greatly benefit from a handheld PHE monitoring device for a faster PHE result and to reduce stress and anxiety for families and caregivers.

The lack of awareness of PKU and dietary requirements of low-protein dietary management amongst the peripheral hospitals, pharmacies, and the food industry are particularly difficult for families. Some restaurants refuse to reheat a home-cooked meal or cook medical pasta at the same time as other meals, and most restaurants do not provide detailed menu ingredients. Many social occasions involve food and those living with PKU can be excluded. Adults often speak about feelings of guilt and shame as a result of breaking dietary management or buried frustrations watching others around them enjoy their food. Likewise, families too sometimes feel guilty enjoying their food experiences in front of their loved ones. When it comes to treatment, there needs to be more choice. Not all treatments suit all people living with the same condition.

Reflective Exercise
- Reflecting on this scenario, can you identify the key parental concerns on receiving the news their daughter had a diagnosis of PKU? Have you experienced these concerns in your area of practice?
- Can you identify supporting measures that should be put in place for this or other families when they receive the diagnosis of PKU?
- Can you discuss how nurses and other healthcare professionals can raise awareness of rare diseases?

Vignette Two

The following vignette exemplifies a rare disease journey of a family of an adult living with a 22q deletion syndrome.

In 1989 when my daughter was 6, she had a clinical psychology assessment, resulting in a diagnosis of 'mild mental retardation – cause unknown'. This was conducted on the advice of her first teacher, and this diagnosis resulted in a refusal by the school to take her back, and so began her journey into special needs education. My daughter had several disparate minor physical symptoms, present since birth, necessitating regular GP and hospital visits, both an inpatient and outpatient. The vague terms 'failure-to-thrive' and 'global development delay' were also terms I heard during her early years. There was an adoption of the 'wait-and-see' attitude when these delays were mentioned. Thankfully, processes have changed somewhat over time, and a better more streamlined service is now available for all children with the suspected diagnosis.

In 1998 my daughter was 15 and attending a special needs school full-time. At this time, the school medical doctor contacted me to ask if I would be interested in a new genetic test that 'might explain all her difficulties'. This fluorescent in situ hybridization (FISH) test revealed a micro-deletion on the 'q' arm of her 22nd chromosome and explained all of her difficulties; it was like putting the pieces of a jigsaw together and things began to make sense.

However, as her mother and a layperson with no medical, clinical, or genetic background, this rare disease diagnosis also confused me. There is nothing 'rare' about her symptoms and 'mild' is a misnomer to me as a parent. When taken together and over time, her minor disparate symptoms result in significant disability, which is not mild when you live with it. My daughter is now in her 30s and I can reveal that my

lived experience has taught me a lot and she has been my teacher. This is a lifespan condition needing a lifespan approach to care.

My other teaching has come from being involved in a parent support group and linking in with a global 22q network of families, clinicians, and researchers. I am also involved in a more collective 'rare' space. I have learnt that 22qDS is just one of a sizeable group of individually rare yet collectively common rare diseases; it is just one of many. In the case of chromosomal conditions, there are also many overlapping symptoms, e.g. feeding and gastrointestinal issues, speech and language difficulties, global developmental delay, hypotonia, ear-nose-throat, and respiratory and chest infections. In school, the symptoms extend to learning and behavioural differences like dyscalculia, dyspraxia, sensory processing disorder, anxiety, and autism spectrum disorders. It is important to note that as parents and families, we don't live with any one symptom; we live with a person who experiences several of these symptoms simultaneously.

Almost 200 anomalies are associated with 22q, and no two people with the condition will experience it the same way. Symptoms can vary from mild to severe, and this significant clinical variation continues to make 22qDS diagnostically challenging. In the absence of newborn screening for 22qDS, many families face a 'diagnostic odyssey' (this also pertains to other chromosomal conditions and to rare diseases in general).

Nurses, midwives, and other health and social care professionals are well placed to help in this instance. It is important to highlight the need for awareness of rare diseases amongst these professionals to help end or shorten the diagnostic odyssey. Adequate education of genetic/genomics information can help focus on what are relatively common symptoms and red flags for a rare disease. This could enable access to any available treatments helping to minimise any adverse impact on developmental, intellectual, and cognitive abilities. Most importantly, they could help support families on what can be a very isolating and confusing journey as they try to access medical, social care, and educational support for their children with complex care needs.

Reflective Exercises
- Reflecting on the information within this chapter, how might diagnosis differ today from what has been identified in this scenario?
- Discuss the nurse's or other health professional role from diagnosis to support. Can you identify key areas they can assist the individual and parent with? Think of your own role, how could you assist?
- Many children with rare conditions grow up and not out of their conditions. Can you identify key caring needs of these families that might change over time?

Conclusion

This chapter provides a basis for understanding the term rare disease/disorder and, in doing so, provides an overview of the prevalence of such conditions and the resultant intellectual and/or developmental disability. While multiple causes are existent, the detail here summarised the main causes and summarises the aetiological classification of such conditions. The impact of rare diseases/disorders is considered with implications for the child and family and carers pondered. The two vignettes presented provide some thoughtful insights for consideration and reflective questions are offered for the reader to think about also.

Key Concepts Discussed
- Overview and prevalence of rare diseases/disorders
- Aetiological classifications of rare diseases
- Rare diseases in the context of preventable intellectual and developmental disabilities
- Impact of rare metabolic diseases across the lifespan
- The implications for an informal carer and the professional focus
- A vignette addressing the diagnosis of a child with PKU and the impact of the same
- A vignette addressing the diagnosis of a child with a rare disease and the impact of the same

References

Almannai M, Al Mahmood RA, Mekki M, El-Hattab AW (2021) Metabolic seizures. Front Neurol 12. https://doi.org/10.3389/fneur.2021.640371

American Association on Intellectual and Developmental Disabilities (AAIDD) (2022) Defining Criteria for Intellectual Disability. https://www.aaidd.org/intellectual-disability/definition. Accessed 20 Apr 2022

Bashore LM, Daniels G, Borchers L, Howington LL, Cheek DJ (2018) Facilitating faculty competency to integrate genomics into nursing curriculum within a private US University. Nursing 8:9–14. https://doi.org/10.2147/nrr.s165852

Boycott KM, Rath A, Chong JX, Hartley T, Alkuraya FS, Baynam G, Brookes AJ, Brudno M, Carracedo A, den Dunnen JT, Dyke S, Estivill X, Goldblatt J, Gonthier C, Groft SC, Gut I, Hamosh A, Hieter P, Höhn S, Hurles ME, Lochmüller H (2017) International cooperation to enable the diagnosis of all rare genetic diseases. Am J Hum Genet 100(5):695–705. https://doi.org/10.1016/j.ajhg.2017.04.003

Boyle CA, Boulet S, Schieve LA, Cohen RA, Blumberg SJ, Yeargin-Allsopp M, Visser S, Kogan MD (2011) Trends in the prevalence of developmental disabilities in US children, 1997–2008. Pediatrics 127(6):1034–1042. https://doi.org/10.1542/peds.2010-2989

Castro R, Senecat J, de Chalendar M, Vajda I, Dan D, Boncz B, EURORDIS Social Policy Advisory Group (2017) Bridging the gap between health and social care for rare diseases: key issues and innovative solutions. Adv Exp Med Biol 605–627. https://doi.org/10.1007/978-3-319-67144-4_32

Centers for Disease Control and Prevention (CDC) (2012) CDC grand rounds: newborn screening and improved outcomes. MMWR Morb Mortal Wkly Rep 61(21):390–393

Dawkins H, Draghia-Akli R, Lasko P, Lau L, Jonker AH, Cutillo CM, Rath A, Boycott KM, Baynam G, Lochmüller H, Kaufmann P, Le Cam Y, Hivert V, Austin CP, International Rare Diseases Research Consortium (IRDiRC) (2018) Progress in rare diseases research 2010-2016: an IRDIRC perspective. Clin Transl Sci 11(1):11–20. https://doi.org/10.1111/cts.12501

Dunn P, Albury CL, Maksemous N, Benton MC, Sutherland HG, Smith RA, Haupt LM, Griffiths LR (2018) Next generation sequencing methods for diagnosis of epilepsy syndromes. Front Genet 9:20. https://doi.org/10.3389/fgene.2018.00020

Engbers HM, Berger R, Ven Hasselt P, De Koning T, Monique GMDSVDV, Kroes H, Visser G (2009) Metabolic evaluation in neurodevelopmental disabilities reply. Ann Neurol 65(4):484–484. https://doi.org/10.1002/ana.21701

European Commission (2022) Public health. European Reference Networks. https://health.ec.europa.eu/european-reference-networks/overview_en. Accessed 30 Oct 2022

European Council Regulation (EC) (1999) No 141/2000 on orphan medicinal products http://data.europa.eu/eli/reg/2000/141/oj. Accessed 30 Oct 2021

EURORDIS (2019) Position paper: achieving holistic person-centred care to leave no one behind. eurordis.org. https://www.eurordis.org/publications/position-paper-achieving-holistic-person-centred-care-to-leave-no-one-behind/. Accessed Jan 2021

Ferreira CR, van Karnebeek C, Vockley J, Blau N (2019) A proposed nosology of inborn errors of metabolism. Genet Med 21(1):102–106. https://doi.org/10.1038/s41436-018-0022-8

Gilbert-Barness E, Farrell PM (2016) Approach to diagnosis of metabolic diseases. Transl Sci Rare Dis 1(1):3–22. https://doi.org/10.3233/trd-160001

Ginocchio VM, Brunetti-Pierri N (2016) Progress toward improved therapies for inborn errors of metabolism. Hum Mol Genet 25(R1):R27–R35. https://doi.org/10.1093/hmg/ddv418

Ginsburg GS, Wu RR, Orlando LA (2019) Family health history: underused for actionable risk assessment. Lancet 394(10198):596–603. https://doi.org/10.1016/s0140-6736(19)31275-9

Gold JI, Gold NB, Strong A, Tully E, Xiao R, Schwartz LA, Ficicioglu C (2022) The current state of adult metabolic medicine in the United States: results of a nationwide survey. Genet Med 24(8):1722–1731. https://doi.org/10.1016/j.gim.2022.04.018

Grant S, Cross E, Wraith JE, Jones S, Mahon L, Lomax M, Bigger B, Hare D (2013) Parental social support, coping strategies, resilience factors, stress, anxiety and depression levels in parents of children with mps III (Sanfilippo syndrome) or children with intellectual disabilities (ID). J Inherit Metab Dis 36(2):281–291. https://doi.org/10.1007/s10545-012-9558-y

Guerrero RB, Salazar D, Tanpaiboon P (2018) Laboratory diagnostic approaches in metabolic disorders. Ann Transl Med 6(24):470–470. https://doi.org/10.21037/atm.2018.11.05

Gunne E, McGarvey C, Hamilton K, Tracey E, Lambert DM, Lynch SA (2020) A retrospective review of the contribution of rare diseases to paediatric mortality in Ireland. Orphanet J Rare Dis 15:1. https://doi.org/10.1186/s13023-020-01574-7

Health Service Executive (HSE) (2019) Model of Care for Rare Diseases, National Rare Diseases Office. https://www.hse.ie/eng/services/list/5/rarediseases/. Accessed 30 Mar 2021

Health Service Executive (HSE) (2022a) A practical guide to newborn bloodspot screening in Ireland, 9th edn. National Newborn Bloodspot Screening Laboratory, Children's Health Ireland, Dublin

Health Service Executive (HSE) (2022b) National Rare Diseases Office. https://www.hse.ie/eng/services/list/5/rarediseases/. Accessed 30 Mar 2021

Hedley V, Bottarelli V, Weinman A, Taruscio D (2021) Shaping national plans and strategies for rare diseases in Europe: past, present, and future. J Community Genet 12(2):207–216. https://doi.org/10.1007/s12687-021-00525-4

Hoytema van Konijnenburg EMM, Wortmann SB, Koelewijn M, Tseng LA, Houben R, Stockler-Ipsiroglu S, Ferreira CR, van Karnebeek CDM (2021) Treatable inherited metabolic disorders causing intellectual disability: 2021 review and digital app. Orphanet J Rare Dis 16(1):170. https://doi.org/10.1186/s13023-021-01727-2

Ilyas M, Mir A, Efthymiou S, Houlden H (2020) The genetics of intellectual disability: advancing technology and gene editing. F1000Research 9:22. https://doi.org/10.12688/f1000research.16315.1

Isono M, Kokado M, Kato K (2022) Why does it take so long for rare disease patients to get an accurate diagnosis? A qualitative investigation of patient experiences of hereditary angioedema. PLoS One 17:3. https://doi.org/10.1371/journal.pone.0265847

Johnson NL, Giarelli E, Lewis C, Rice CE (2013) Genomics and autism spectrum disorder. J Nurs Scholarsh 45(1):69–78. https://doi.org/10.1111/j.1547-5069.2012.01483.x

Johnson N, Sangasy P, Robinson K (2020) 'No one could calm him down': mothers' experience of autism diagnosis and obtainment of resources in an urban public school district. Fam Syst Health 38(3):255–264. https://doi.org/10.1037/fsh0000527

Kaufman L, Ayub M, Vincent JB (2010) The genetic basis of non-syndromic intellectual disability: a review. J Neurodev Disord 2(4):182–209. https://doi.org/10.1007/s11689-010-9055-2

Kelly N, Makarem DC, Wasserstein MP (2016) Screening of newborns for disorders with high benefit-risk ratios should be mandatory. J Law Med Ethics 44(2):231–240. https://doi.org/10.1177/1073110516654133

Kvarnung M, Nordgren A (2017) Intellectual disability & rare disorders: A diagnostic challenge. Adv Exp Med Biol 1031:39–54. https://doi.org/10.1007/978-3-319-67144-4_3

Langenfeld A, Schema L, Eckerle JK (2021) Genetic developmental disability diagnosed in adulthood:

a case report. J Med Case Rep 15(1):28. https://doi. org/10.1186/s13256-020-02590-8

Lee K, Cascella M, Marwaha R (2022) Intellectual disability. NIH National Library of Medicine. StatPearls Publishing, Treasure Island, FL. https://www.ncbi. nlm.nih.gov/books/NBK547654/. Accessed 10 May 2021

Leonard H, Wen X (2002) The epidemiology of mental retardation: challenges and opportunities in the new millennium. Ment Retard Dev Disabil Res Rev 8(3):117–134. https://doi.org/10.1002/mrdd.10031

Liao, L.H., Chen, C., Peng, J., Wu, L.W., He, F., Yang, L.F., Zhang, C.L/, Wang, G.L., Peng, P., Ma, Y.P., Miao, P. and Yin, F. (2019) Diagnosis of intellectual disability/global developmental delay via genetic analysis in a central region of China. Chin Med J, 132(13), 1533–1540. doi: https://doi.org/10.1097/ cm9.0000000000000295

Lion-Francois L, Cheillan D, Pitelet G, Acquaviva-Bourdain C, Bussy G, Cotton F, Guibaud L, Gérard D, Rivier C, Vianey-Saban C, Jakobs C, Salomons GS, des Portes, V. (2006) High frequency of creatine deficiency syndromes in patients with unexplained mental retardation. Neurology 67(9):1713–1714. https://doi. org/10.1212/01.wnl.0000239153.39710.81

Maenner MJ, Yeargin-Allsopp M, Naarden Braun KV, Christensen DL, Schieve LA (2016) Development of a machine learning algorithm for the surveillance of autism spectrum disorder. PLoS One 11(12). https:// doi.org/10.1371/journal.pone.0168224

Malcolm C, Forbat L, Anderson G, Gibson F, Hain R (2011) Challenging symptom profiles of life-limiting conditions in children: a survey of care professionals and families. Palliat Med 25(4):357–364. https://doi. org/10.1177/0269216310391346

Manickam K, McClain MR, Demmer LA, Biswas S, Kearney HM, Malinowski J, Massingham LJ, Miller D, Yu TW, Hisama FM, ACMG Board of Directors (2021) Exome and genome sequencing for pediatric patients with congenital anomalies or intellectual disability: an evidence-based clinical guideline of the American College of Medical Genetics and Genomics (ACMG). Genet Med 23(11):2029–2037. https://doi. org/10.1038/s41436-021-01242-6

McCandless SE, Wright EJ (2020) Mandatory newborn screening in the United States: history, current status, and existential challenges. Birth Defects Res 112(4):350–366. https://doi.org/10.1002/bdr2.1653

McMullan J, Crowe AL, Downes K, McAneney H, McKnight AJ (2021) Carer reported experiences: supporting someone with a rare disease. Health Soc Care Community 30(3):1097–1108. https://doi. org/10.1111/hsc.13336

Miclea D, Peca L, Cuzmici Z, Pop IV (2015) Genetic testing in patients with global developmental delay/ intellectual disabilities. A Review. Med Pharm Rep 88(3):288–292. https://doi.org/10.15386/cjmed-461

Moeschler JB, Shevell M, Committee on Genetics (2014) Comprehensive evaluation of the child with intellectual disability or global developmental delays.

Pediatrics 134(3):e903–e918. https://doi.org/10.1542/ peds.2014-1839

National Centre for Inherited Metabolic Disorders (NCIMD) (2022) National Centre for inherited metabolic disorders. Children's Health Ireland, Dublin

National Institute for Health and Clinical Excellence NICE (2004) Citizens council report ultra orphan drugs. Citizens Council Reports No 4. PMID: 28230958

National Institute of Health (NIH) (2022) How many newborns are screened in the United States? https:// www.nichd.nih.gov/health/topics/newborn/condition-info/infants-screened. Accessed 10 May 2022

Non-Governmental Organisation (NGO) Committee for Rare Diseases (2019) Non-Governmental Organisation (NGO) Committee for Rare Diseases. https:// www.ngocommitteeerarediseases.org/. Accessed 22 May 2022

Nord Rare Disease Centers of excellence (2022) NORD (National Organization for Rare Disorders). https:// rarediseases.org/centersofexcellence/. Accessed 12 Apr 2022

O'Byrne JJ, Lynch SA, Treacy EP, King MD, Betts DR, Mayne PD, Sharif F (2016) Unexplained developmental delay/learning disability: guidelines for best practice protocol for first-line assessment and genetic/ metabolic/radiological investigations. Ir J Med Sci 185:241–248

Orpha.net (2018) Activity report. https://www.orpha.net/ orphacom/cahiers/docs/GB/ActivityReport2017.pdf. Accessed 13 May 2022

Purugganan O (2018) Intellectual disabilities. Pediatr Rev 39(6):299–309. https://doi.org/10.1542/pir.2016-0116

Repetto GM, Rebolledo-Jaramillo B (2020) Chapter 3— Rare diseases: genomics and public health. In: Patrinos GP (ed) Applied genomics and public health. Academic Press, London, pp 37–51

Shajani Z, Snell D (2019) Wright & Leahey's nurses and families: a guide to family assessment and intervention, 7th edn. F.A. Davis Company, Philadelphia, PA

Slade A, Isa F, Kyte D, Pankhurst T, Kerecuk L, Ferguson J, Lipkin G, Calvert M (2018) Patient reported outcome measures in rare diseases: a narrative review. Orphanet J Rare Dis 13(1):61. https://doi.org/10.1186/ s13023-018-0810-x

Smith M (2008) Care of the infant with inherent metabolic disease. Paediatr Care 20(4):38–45. https://doi. org/10.7748/paed2008.05.20.4.38.c8254

Somanadhan S, Larkin PJ (2016) Parents' experiences of living with, and caring for children, adolescents and young adults with mucopolysaccharidosis (MPS). Orphanet J Rare Dis 11(1):138. https://doi. org/10.1186/s13023-016-0521-0

Somanadhan S, Brinkley A, Larkin PJ (2021) Living through liminality? Situating the transitional experience of parents of children with mucopolysaccharidoses. Scand J Caring Sci 36(3):614–624. https://doi. org/10.1111/scs.13026

Stepien KM, Kieć-Wilk B, Lampe C, Tangeraas T, Cefalo G, Belmatoug N, Francisco R, del Toro M, Wagner L, Lauridsen AG, Sestini S, Weinhold N, Hahn A,

Montanari C, Rovelli V, Bellettato CM, Paneghetti L, van Lingen C, Scarpa M (2021) Challenges in transition from childhood to adulthood care in rare metabolic diseases: results from the first multi-center european survey. Front Med 8:652358. https://doi.org/10.3389/fmed.2021.652358

Stoller JK (2018) The challenge of rare diseases. Chest 153(6):1309–1314. https://doi.org/10.1016/j.chest.2017.12.018

The Institute for Patient- and Family-Centered Care (IPFCC) (2022) About Us. https://www.ipfcc.org/about/index.html. Accessed 15 May 2022

The UK Rare Diseases Framework (2021) The UK rare diseases framework. Department of Health and Social Care. https://assets.publishing.service.gov.uk/government/uploads/system/uploads/attachment_data/file/950651/the-UK-rare-diseases-framework.pdf. Accessed 5 May 2022

Tonkin E, Calzone K, Jenkins J, Dale L, Prows C (2011) Genomic education resources for nursing faculty. J Nurs Scholarsh 43(4):330–340. https://doi.org/10.1111/j.1547-5069.2011.01415.x

US Government Accountability Office (US. GAO) (2021) Rare diseases: although limited, available evidence suggests medical and other costs can be substantial, rare diseases: although limited, available evidence suggests medical and other costs can be substantial | U.S. GAO. https://www.gao.gov/products/gao-22-104235. Accessed 12 May 2022

US Orphan Drug Act (2013) 78 FR 35117—Orphan Drug Regulations. https://www.govinfo.gov/app/details/FR-2013-06-12/2013-13930. Accessed 12 July 2022

van Karnebeek CDM, Stockler S (2012) Treatable inborn errors of metabolism causing intellectual disability: a systematic literature review. Mol Genet Metab 105(3):368–381. https://doi.org/10.1016/j.ymgme.2011.11.191

van Karnebeek CD, Scheper FY, Abeling NG, Alders M, Barth PG, Hoovers JM, Koevoets C, Wanders RJ, Hennekam RC (2005) Etiology of mental retardation in children referred to a tertiary care center: a prospective study. Am J Ment Retard 110(4):253–267. https://doi.org/10.1352/0895-8017(2005)110[253:EOMRIC]2.0.CO;2. PMID: 15941363

von der Lippe C, Diesen PS, Feragen KB (2017) Living with a rare disorder: a systematic review of the qualitative literature. Mol Genet Genomic Med 5(6):758–773. https://doi.org/10.1002/mgg3.315

Ward AJ, Murphy D, Marron R, McGrath V, Bolz-Johnson M, Cullen W, Daly A, Hardiman O, Lawlor A, Lynch SA, MacLachlan M, McBrien J, Ni Bhriain S, O'Byrne JJ, O'Connell SM, Turner J, Treacy EP (2022) Designing rare disease care pathways in the Republic of Ireland: a co-operative model. Orphanet J Rare Dis 17(1):162. https://doi.org/10.1186/s13023-022-02309-6

Woerner AC, Gallagher RC, Vockley J, Adhikari AN (2021) The use of whole genome and exome sequencing for newborn screening: challenges and opportunities for population health. Front Pediatr 9:663752. https://doi.org/10.3389/fped.2021.663752

World Health Organization (WHO) (2021) Tuberculosis. https://www.who.int/news-room/fact-sheets/detail/tuberculosis. Accessed 16 Aug 2022

Yeargin-Allxopp M, Murphy CC, Cordero JF, Decouflé P, Hollowell JG (1997) Reported biomedical causes and associated medical conditions for mental retardation among 10-year-old children, metropolitan Atlanta, 1985 to 1987. Dev Med Child Neurol 39(3):142–149. https://doi.org/10.1111/j.1469-8749.1997.tb07401.x

Zablotsky B, Black LI, Maenner MJ, Schieve LA, Danielson ML, Bitsko RH, Blumberg SJ, Kogan MD, Boyle CA (2019) Prevalence and trends of developmental disabilities among children in the United States: 2009–2017. Pediatrics 144(4):e20190811. https://doi.org/10.1542/peds.2019-0811

Other Related Neurodevelopmental Conditions

8

Caroline Dalton O'Connor
and Helena Isabel da Silva Reis

Chapter Topics

- Three distinctive conditions are explored: Down syndrome, Cerebral palsy and Autism Spectrum Disorder.
- The support needs of people with Down syndrome will be explored.
- An outline of the support needs of people with cerebral palsy will be presented.
- The support needs of people with autism and intellectual disability will also be identified.

Introduction

People with intellectual disabilities experience diverse neurodevelopmental conditions, which impact from a biopsychosocial perspective and impact their quality of life. This chapter will examine in detail three distinctive conditions, Down syndrome, cerebral palsy and autism spectrum disorder. This chapter will also focus on enhancing the readers knowledge of the aforementioned conditions and identifying the specific support needs of people with Down syndrome, cerebral palsy and autism, from a person-centred, right-based perspective.

C. D. O'Connor (✉)
University College Cork, Cork, Ireland
e-mail: c.doconnor@ucc.ie

H. I. da Silva Reis
Politechnico de Leira, Leiria, Portugal
e-mail: helena.s.reis@ipleiria.pt

Exploring Down Syndrome

Down syndrome is the most common chromosomal disorder associated with intellectual disability, occurring in all populations, irrespective of race, nationality or socioeconomic status. Down syndrome was originally described in 1886, by Dr. John Langdon Down, who observed similar features in some of his patients. Further exploration in 1959, by Dr. Jerome Lejeune, identified that the syndrome was caused by a third copy of chromosome 21.

Cause of Down Syndrome

Down syndrome is also referred to as Trisomy 21. Typically, a baby is born with 46 chromosomes; babies with Down syndrome have 47. There are three main forms of Down syndrome (see Table 8.1).

Table 8.1 Forms of Down syndrome

Form of Down syndrome	Prevalence	Description
Trisomy 21	95%	Three chromosomes 21 in every cell
Translocation	3–5%	Extra part of chromosome 21 attaches to another chromosome in every cell
Mosaicism	1–2%	An extra copy of chromosome 21 is present in some but not all cells

© The Author(s), under exclusive license to Springer Nature Switzerland AG 2023
F. Sheerin, C. Doyle (eds.), *Intellectual Disabilities: Health and Social Care Across the Lifespan*,
https://doi.org/10.1007/978-3-031-27496-1_8

Table 8.2 Maternal age and Down syndrome

Maternal age	Associated level of risk
20 years of age	1 in 1500 chance
30 years of age	1 in 800 chance
35 years of age	1 in 270 chance
40 years of age	1 in 100 chances
45 years of age	1 in 50 or greater chance

The presence of an extra chromosome 21 mainly results from nondisjunction, which occurs during meiosis. Nondisjunction occurs when paired chromosomes fail to separate during cell division. Two copies of the same chromosome then go to one daughter and cell and none to the other. Advanced maternal age is associated with an increased risk of issues arising during meiosis and has been identified as a risk factor for Down syndrome (see Table 8.2).

HSE (2020)

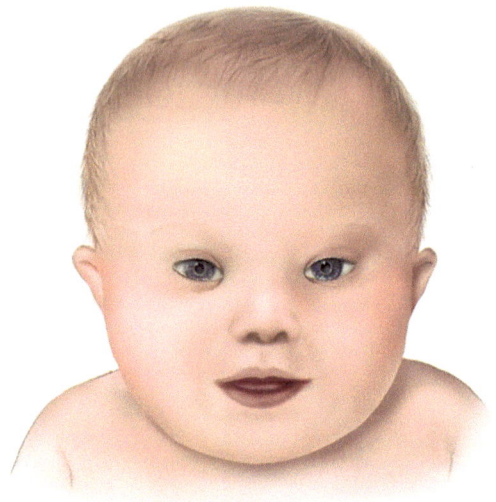

Fig. 8.1 Features of a baby with Down syndrome (source Wikimedia Commons)

Prevalence Rates

While the global prevalence rate for Down syndrome is difficult to identify (Antonarakis et al. 2020), it is estimated to occur in approximately 1 in every 800 births (Bull 2020). In the USA, there are approximately 5500 births annually (12.6 per 10,000) (De Graaf et al. 2021). Within a European context, it was estimated that between 2011 and 2015, there were 8031 births (10.1 per 10,000) (De Graaf et al. 2021). Prevalence rates for Down syndrome in the UK have been estimated at 6.3 per 10,000 (Alexander et al. 2016). The incidence in Ireland is estimated to be 1 in 546 births, with approximately 7000 people with Down syndrome living in Ireland (Caples et al. 2018).

Diagnosis of Down Syndrome

Down syndrome is diagnosed during the prenatal or postnatal stages of pregnancy. In some instances, it is identified during a routine ultrasound. The expectant mother may also be offered non-invasive prenatal screening for chromosomal abnormalities, such as the Panorama test or Harmony test. If these tests give a positive result,

diagnostic tests are then undertaken to confirm the results including amniocentesis or chorionic villus sampling (CVS).

A baby may be diagnosed with Down syndrome based on the appearance of the baby. Specific characteristics, including epicanthal folds and upslanting palpebral fissures, leading to an upward slant to the eyes, Brushfield spots in the iris of the eye, hypotonia, a single palmer crease and a flat nasal bridge, may also be evident. Chromosomal analysis is undertaken using karyotyping (Fig. 8.1).

Features and Health Conditions of Children and Adults with Down Syndrome

Children and adults with Down syndrome are unique individuals with a diverse range of abilities and support needs. Like all individuals, people with Down syndrome and their families will face challenges in life, but despite these challenges, the QoL of people with Down syndrome has improved over time (Antonarakis et al. 2020). The QoL and the life expectancy of people with Down syndrome can be negatively impacted by the burden of medical conditions they may experience such as cardiac and respiratory conditions (Burke et al. 2014; Haddad et al. 2018). However, with appropriate supports, people with Down syndrome and their families lead full and productive lives, despite the challenges they face (Caples et al. 2018). The features and co-morbid health conditions associated with Down syndrome can impact across the lifespan and are identified in Table 8.3.

Table 8.3 Features and health conditions associated with Down syndrome

Conditions	Overview
Neurodevelopmental, neurological and psychiatric	• Intellectual disability • Language disorders • Cerebellar hypoplasia • Alzheimer's disease • Epilepsy • Anxiety and depression • Behaviours that challenge
Craniofacial	• Small, low set ears • Epicanthic folds • Flat nasal bridge • Flat occiput • Small mouth • Upslanting palpebral fissures
Cardiovascular	• Congenital heart defects • Pulmonary hypertension
Musculoskeletal	• Atlantoaxial instability • Small stature • Short fingers • Hypotonia
Sensory	• Conductive and sensorineural hearing loss • Refractive errors, cataracts, keratoconus and amblyopia
Respiratory	• Obstructive sleep apnoea • Respiratory tract infections • Aspiration pneumonia
Autoimmune	• Thyroid disease • Coeliac disease • Alopecia • Type 1 diabetes mellitus • Psoriasis
Other	• Haematological disorders • Immune dysfunction • Obesity • Dysphagia • Bowel dysfunction • Gastrointestinal structural defects • Leukaemia • Male infertility

Developed from Antonarakis et al. (2020); Bull (2020) and the Global Down Syndrome Foundation (2020)

Management of Health Conditions Associated with Down Syndrome

Ongoing management of the co-morbid health conditions experienced by people with Down syndrome is required. Areas of specific focus include congenital heart defects (CHD), atlanto-axial instability, thyroid dysfunction, epilepsy and respiratory conditions including sleep apnoea and Alzheimer's disease, although this is not an exhaustive list.

Cardiovascular Conditions: A cardiology examination to identify CHD should be carried out at birth and when the infant is a month old. The treatment of CHD in children with Down syndrome is the same as for all children and surgical repair is recommended. Infants may develop pulmonary-artery hypertension later in life, so ongoing surveillance is required. Individuals with Down syndrome should have annual screening for acquired valve disease and heart failure (Antonarakis et al. 2020; Bull 2020; Bunt and Bunt 2022).

Atlantoaxial Instability: Where diagnosed, ongoing surveillance is required. Participation in sports may increase the risk of spinal injury. Symptoms such as neck pain and weakness, issues with gait, spasticity and hyperflexion should be observed and managed, and spinal X-rays undertaken routinely, where recommended (Antonarakis et al. 2020; Bunt and Bunt 2022).

Thyroid Dysfunction: Congenital hypothyroidism can be an issue for children and adults. There is an increased risk of developing the condition across the lifespan and measurements of thyroid-stimulating hormone (TSH) should be undertaken. The Global Down Syndrome Foundation (2020) recommends screening adults for hypothyroidism every 1–2 years from the age of 21.

Respiratory Conditions: Both children and adults are prone to respiratory conditions, which have been identified as one of the most frequent causes of hospitalisation in people with an intellectual disability (Doody et al. 2021). Vigilance is required in recognising and treating these conditions. Obstructive sleep apnoea is also an issue, and symptoms such as snoring, sleepiness during the day, restlessness at night and heavy breathing should be observed. A range of approaches can be used to manage this condition including continuous positive airway pressure (CPAP) (Antonarakis et al. 2020).

Epilepsy: Children and adults with Down syndrome have a higher prevalence of epilepsy in comparison to the general population. Infantile spasms and West syndrome can occur in children, and an electroencephalogram should occur promptly when seizures are detected, as early treatment leads to improved outcomes (Lopes et al. 2018). Late-onset myoclonic epilepsy in Down syndrome (LOMEDS) is a significant issue in those diagnosed with Alzheimer's dementia, negatively impacting quality of life. Anti-epileptic medication should be used in the management of epilepsy, under the guidance of a neurologist (Altuna et al. 2021).

Alzheimer's Disease: Increases in longevity mean that people with Down syndrome are experiencing many of the health conditions common in older adults. The risk of developing Alzheimer's increased from 25% in those over 50 years to 80% in those aged 65 and over (Mccarron et al. 2017). A baseline assessment of cognitive and adaptive functioning should be undertaken in those over 30, to ensure early detection of the symptoms of this condition (Antonarakis et al. 2020).

Quality of Life and Down Syndrome

The quality of life of people with Down syndrome can be negatively impacted by health-related issues, hence the importance of proactive screening and early intervention programmes that can mitigate the impact of these co-morbid health conditions. However, the quality of life of people with Down syndrome is also impacted by a broader range of factors linked to social inclusion such as friendship (Haddad et al. 2018), employment (Kumin and Schoenbrodt 2016), leisure activities (Poelke et al. 2016) autonomy and living independently (Santoro et al. 2022). These issues must also be addressed to ensure that peo-

ple with Down syndrome have the best possible quality of life with access to appropriate supports, in a timely manner, reflective of a right-based approach to service provision.

Exploring Cerebral Palsy

Cerebral palsy is a group of disorders defined as 'any non-progressive central motor deficit linked to events in the prenatal, perinatal or postnatal period that resulted in damage to or dysfunction of the central nervous system' (Axton and Fugate 2009, p. 244). Cerebral palsy impacts an individual's movement, posture and balance, and the impact of these disorders varies from person to person (CDC 2022). The various types of cerebral palsy are outlined in Table 8.4.

Table 8.4 Types of cerebral palsy

Types of cerebral palsy	Overview

Spastic cerebral palsy	• Most common form of cerebral palsy (80%)
	• Increased muscle tone: Muscles are tight and contract strongly with attempted movement or stretching and movements can be awkward
	• Spastic cerebral palsy is frequently identified by the parts of the body affected:
	  – Monoplegia: One limb is affected
	  – Diplegia: Both limbs are affected (mainly the legs are affected. People have difficulty walking as their legs pull together and turn inward)
	  – Triplegia: Three limbs are affected
	  – Quadriplegia: All limbs are affected (most severe form as the limbs, trunk and face are affected. People cannot walk and often have a number of co-morbid health conditions) intellectual disability, seizures or problems with vision, hearing or speech
	  – Hemiplegia: Both limbs on the same side of the body are affected (usually the arm is more affected than the leg)
	  – Paraplegia: Both legs are affected due to damage to spinal cord

Types of cerebral palsy	Overview
Dyskinetic cerebral palsy	• Includes athetoid, choreoathetoid and dystonic cerebral palsies • Uncontrolled movements that are slow and writhing or rapid and jerking • Involuntary movements such as twitches or spasms • Movements can affect any part of the body, including the face, mouth and tongue making sucking difficult
Ataxic cerebral palsy	• Difficulty coordinating muscle groups and problems with balance, coordination, walking, etc. • Gait is probably unsteady if the person can walk • Difficulty with movements that are quick or require a great deal of control such as writing or when reaching for something
Mixed	Features of more than one form of cerebral palsy are present, most commonly a combination of spastic-dyskinetic cerebral palsy

Causes of Cerebral Palsy

Cerebral palsy is caused by the abnormal development of or damage to the developing brain, and this can occur prior to, during or after the birth of a child. The majority of cases of cerebral palsy occur during the perinatal phase (O'Callaghan et al. 2011; CDC 2022). Perinatal risk factors include congenital developmental deformities, preterm births, low birth rate, multiple births and brain haemorrhage. Perinatal infections including **t**oxoplasmosis, **o**thers (e.g. hepatitis B, syphillis, chickenpox, HIV), **r**ubella, **c**ytomegalovirus and **h**erpes simplex virus (**TORCH**) are also linked to cerebral palsy. Birth injuries account for a small percentage of cases of cerebral palsy and are linked to birth asphyxia, placenta abruption and cord prolapse. After birth, factors including infections such as meningitis, accidental injuries following a road traffic accident or near drowning and non-accidental injuries such as shaken baby syndrome (Vitrikas et al. 2020;Upadhyay et al. 2020; CDC 2022) can lead to cerebral palsy.

Table 8.5 Assessment tools

Name of tool	Purpose
Gross Motor Function Classification System Movement Disorder—Childhood Rating Scale Gillette Mobility Scale	Functional ability focused on mobility, posture and balance
Burke–Fahn–Marsden Dystonia Rating Scale Barry Albright Dystonia Scale Unified Dystonia Rating Scale Dyskinesia Rating Scale Dyskinesia Impairment Scale Kinematic Dystonia Measures	Dystonia
Hypertonia Assessment Scale Ashworth Scale	Hypertonia
Manual Ability Classification System Quality of Upper Extremity Skills Test Assisting Hand Assessment	Upper limb function

Prevalence of Cerebral Palsy

Cerebral palsy is the most common physical disability of childhood (Vitrikas et al. 2020). Prevalence rates vary, but a number of population-based studies have identified prevalence rates varying from 1 to 4 per 1000 live births (Maenner et al. 2016; Surveillance of Cerebral Palsy in Europe 2000). While rates of cerebral palsy have remained relatively stable over time, research suggests that rates are declining (Sellier et al. 2016).

Assessment of Cerebral Palsy

Children and adults with cerebral palsy are unique individuals with a diverse range of abilities and support needs. Like all individuals, people with cerebral palsy and their families will face challenges in life. Children and adults with cerebral palsy will need to have comprehensive assessments undertaken for health-related issues linked to this condition and co-morbid healthy conditions that may occur. Having been diagnosed with cerebral palsy, a variety of assessment approaches can be utilised to establish the level of cerebral palsy and its impact. An overview of some of these scales is available in Table 8.5.

In conjunction with these, an assessment for fixed contractures may need to be undertaken in some circumstances. Issues with eating and swallowing can also impact on up to 80% of people with cerebral palsy (Edvinsson and Lundqvist 2016). Children and adults with cerebral palsy may experience a range of co-morbid health conditions including pain (75%), intellectual disability (50%), unable to walk (33%), hip displacement (33%), nonverbal (25%), epilepsy (25%), behavioural issues (25%), bladder control (25%), sleep disorder (25%), dribbling (20%), blind (10%) and deaf (4%) (Novak et al. 2012). These co-morbid conditions also need to be assessed and monitored, on an ongoing basis.

Quality of Life (QoL)

The QoL of people with cerebral palsy has been shown to be negatively impacted by health-related issues, hence the importance of appropriate assessment strategies, early intervention programmes and the continued evolution of supports across the lifespan. However, the QoL of people with cerebral palsy has also been shown to be impacted by a broader range of factors linked to issues including access to further education, employment opportunities, meaningful relationships and ability to live independently (Reddihough et al. 2013). People with cerebral palsy and their families have shown that with determination, the development of competencies, typical parental expectations and support, access to further education, acceptance and involvement in school life and strategies for addressing bullying (Gaskin et al. 2021), their QoL can be improved.

Exploring Autism Spectrum Disorder (ASD)

Signs, Symptoms and General Diagnostic Issues

ASD is a neurodevelopmental disorder characterised by deficits in social communication and the presence of restricted and repetitive interests or activities and sensory anomalies, beginning in the early developmental period (APA 2013). The Centres for Disease Control and Prevention (CDC) described an autism prevalence of 1 in 44 children with a male-to-female ratio of 4.5 to 1. In 2013, the *Diagnostic and Statistical Manual of Mental Disorders*, fifth ed. (DSM-5) created the umbrella diagnosis of ASD, consolidating four previously separate disorders: autistic disorder, Asperger syndrome, childhood disintegrative disorder and pervasive developmental disorder not otherwise specified (APA 2013). This evolution in diagnostic classification may explain the increase of ASD that previously had been unrecognised in some children (Zylstra et al. 2014; Sanchack and Thomas 2016).

Although individuals with ASD are very different from one another, the disorder is characterised by core features in two areas—social communication and restricted, repetitive sensory–motor behaviours—irrespective of culture, race, ethnicity or socioeconomic group. ASD results from early altered brain development and neural reorganisation. However, because there are no reliable biomarkers, the diagnosis must be made based on behaviour (Sanchack and Thomas 2016; Lord et al. 2018).

Screening Tools and Standardised Diagnostic Instruments

Since signs of ASD can be detected early, routine developmental screening is suggested at 9-, 18- and 24- or 30-month well-child visits. Targeted screening for ASD with a validated screening tool at 18 and 24 months of age is recommended by paediatricians for early identification. The Modified Checklist for Autism in Toddlers (M-CHAT) is widely used (Hyman et al. 2020). Assessment of children's symptoms can be obtained from a variety of scales, such as the Childhood Autism Rating Scale, Social Responsiveness Scale and Social Communication Questionnaire. The most frequently used screening instruments vary from observational measures (e.g. Autism Diagnostic Observation Schedule (ADOS)) (Lord et al. 2012) to caregiver interviews (e.g. Autism Diagnostic Interview Revised) (Lord et al. 1994). The most robust observational measure for ASD diagnosis in adulthood is the ADOS (module 4) (Lord et al. 2000). Adaptive scales are also used as measures of everyday functioning. Obtaining information about receptive and expressive language level, general behavioural difficulties and motor skills, including an estimate of cognitive functioning or IQ, is considered standard practice (Hyman et al. 2020). A diagnosis of ASD requires a multidisciplinary assessment by an interdisciplinary team. Symptoms can manifest and be interpreted differently depending on the environmental context. Thus, evaluation of symptomatology in different environments (home, school, community, in addition to the clinic) is recommended.

Sensory Processing Issues in ASD

Atypical sensory processing is a central aspect of ASD. Difficulties in registration of meaningful sensory input are often one of the most disabling and commonly observed aspects in children with ASD. Inability to cope with sensation can also lead to 'overload' and 'shutdown', which interferes with the person's ability to process incoming input that produces an appearance of lack of registration (Dellapiazza et al. 2019). People with autism can demonstrate a great deal of variability in their abilities and reactions. Behaviours like gravitational insecurity or having the head tilted backward or moving across uneven surfaces can create significant feelings of anxiety and fear. In response these children commonly show both sensory-seeking and sensory avoidance behaviours in relation to movement (Kuhaneck and Watling 2010). Movement seeking frequently takes the form of rocking or rhythmic motions (usually considered to be calming or organising to the child) or twirling and swinging motions (usually consider it to be alerting and activating). Professionals often categorise these behaviours as 'self-stimulatory' and 'non-purposeful' (Sefen et al. 2020).

People with ASD experience tactile sensitivity and have difficulty reading environmental cues that normally help an individual know what to expect next, leading to feelings of anxiety and discomfort (Normansell-Mossa et al. 2021). Auditory processing problems are also evident in children with ASD. At times they give the impression of being deaf or hard of hearing, yet some children experience certain sounds as painful and are unable to tune out irrelevant noises. Celebrations such as birthday parties can be particularly troublesome, because of the quality of spontaneous noise (balloons popping, children singing). Participation in the community such as walking through a shopping mall, attending school assembly, watching a movie or attending a sporting event can be irritating, due in part to the levels and quality of sounds (Schafer et al. 2020).

Praxis is another challenge that people with ASD experience with other sensory processing disorders. The term praxis has been approached from different perspectives and although it is associated with the ability to plan a motor action, this term incorporates cognitive elements, such as the conceptualisation of the actions (ideation) necessary for the organisation, sequencing and execution of a motor plan.

Of note is a common difficulty in ideation (Serrada-Tejeda et al. 2021). Ideation and planning of action are essential in all novel activities. The difficulty that people with ASD routinely have with these functions makes new or novel activities confusing and anxiety producing. This leaves people with ASD with a tendency to favour sameness and routines.

Co-occurring Psychiatric Conditions in ASD

In addition to ASD, co-morbid conditions such as intellectual disability and language and motor difficulties can also be evident. Attention-deficit hyperactivity disorder (ADHD) is the most common comorbidity in individuals with ASD and significantly impacts outcomes in children with ASD who have average intelligence or intellectual disability. The impact of ADHD on children and adults changes over time in terms of interactions with executive functioning, peer relationships and depression and should be monitored.

Anxiety in various forms including social anxiety, generalised anxiety, separation anxiety in younger children and phobias also affect many children with ASD. Anxiety and depression are more common, or at least more prominent, in language-proficient individuals and increase in adolescence in girls, while they also occur in a substantial minority of boys. Irritability and aggression are more common (25%) in ASD than in other developmental disorders, although they take many different forms, from mild physical aggression in very young children to verbal aggression in adults.

Management of ASD

There are a variety of intervention models specific to ASD, whose methods follow certain theoretical and methodological constructs (see Table 8.6). Intervention and support should be individualised, multidimensional and interdisciplinary. The goals are to maximise an individual's functional independence and quality of life through development and learning, improvements in social skills and communication, reductions in disability and comorbidity, promotion of independence and provision of support to families. Additionally, individuals should be helped to fulfil their potential in areas of strength (Hyman et al. 2020).

Quality of Life (QoL) in ASD

Diagnostic severity and IQ levels are the best predictors of the future individual functioning of people with ASD. Most adults with ASD with intellectual disability can communicate verbally,

Table 8.6 Classification of the intervention models in autism

Biologically based interventions
• Medication
• Complementary and alternative medicine
Psychodynamic interventions
Educational interventions
• Behavioural interventions
– Early intensive behavioural intervention (EIBI)
– Contemporary applied behaviour analysis
Pivotal response training (PRT)
Natural language paradigm (NLP)
Incidental teaching
• Developmental interventions
– Floortime (DIR)
– Responsive teaching
– Relationship development intervention (RDI)
• Therapy-based interventions
– Communication-focused interventions
Visual strategies and visually cued instruction
Manual signing
The picture exchange communication system (PECS)
Social stories
Speech-generating devices
Facilitated communication
Functional communication training
– Sensory–motor interventions
Auditory integration training (AIT)
– Sensory integration
• Combined interventions
– The SCERTS model
– Treatment and education of autistic and related communication handicapped children (TEACCH)
– Learning Experiences: An Alternative Programme for Preschoolers and Parents (LEAP)
• Family-based interventions
– Family-centred positive behaviour support (PBS) programmes
– The Hanen programme

Adapted from Ros Cervera et al. (2011)

can take care of basic needs and have the ability to work but need daily support. Marriage and long-term intimate relationships can be rare for adults with ASD, and it can be difficult for them to find suitable jobs and services. Improvements in QoL are not only related to the development and improvement of the services for these people but also ensuring that an early diagnosis occurs.

Early intervention in special education can improve developmental trajectories of children with ASD. Research shows that increasing daytime recreational activities and community inclusion improves the person-environment fit, resulting in higher levels of satisfaction for the person with ASD (Sanchack and Thomas 2016). Given existing healthcare systems, there is a clear and ongoing need for coordination among health, education and other services (e.g. intensive support for challenging behaviours and planning of housing and employment programmes for adults with ASD). Working with families, schools and community agencies, the multidisciplinary team can transform the lives of individual children and adults by providing accurate and realistic information, support and hope.

Case Study

The following case study explores the impact of a potential diagnosis of autism on Gabriel and her family:

Case study		
Background	Gabriel is 3 years old and is the youngest of three siblings. Her parents Luke and Sarah have brought her to see their GP; they have concerns about how she is meeting some of her developmental milestones. In the past 6 months, Gabriel has reached some milestones, at quite an early age. For example, she found toilet training easy, although she occasionally has 'accidents' when absorbed in playing with her favourite toy. Gabriel can become distressed if she does not have access to this toy	
	Gabriel has some words or approximation of words, which her parents and siblings understand. Her main focus is to get access to objects and things, but she is picking up words more quickly. Her parents are concerned that Gabriel shows little interest in engaging with them and her siblings. She does not turn and look at them when they come into the room and does not respond when they call her name. Gabriel had a hearing test done and no issues were identified	
	Her siblings play together, but Gabriel rarely joins them unless her brothers Luke and Eoghan are playing with their trains. She lines up the trains one after the other and becomes upset if the boys change anything. The other area of concern is how Gabriel responds to different textures and sounds in her environment. Gabriel does not like any material that is scratchy, such as wool, and does not like buttons. She becomes upset if her drinks are too cold, so a lot of time is spent trying to ensure these issues are addressed. Sarah and Luke are quite concerned about Gabriel's overall development and are unsure how to proceed and have attended their GP for support	
Support structures	History	• Not meeting all her developmental milestones • No medical conditions • Reviewed by audiologist – no issues identified
	Family support	• Parents resident in the family home • Parents work with childcare provided by the wider family network • Grandparents live nearby and support the family
	Community services	• Public health nurse • General practitioner
Suspected diagnosis	Autism spectrum disorder because: • Deficits in social communication (speech acquisition is delayed/not engaging with siblings/peers) • Presence of restricted and repetitive interests or activities and unusual play patterns (Gabriel likes to line up the trains one after the other) • Change in routine is a significant challenge (Gabriel becomes upset if the boys change anything around) • Sensory processing issues (hyperreactive to touch)	

Family concerns	For Gabriel's family, behaviours that challenge are a major barrier to inclusive education, community participation and opportunities to develop friendship with peers. Gabriel's family report that such behaviour negatively affects many elements of their lifestyle including relationships between siblings, relationships with extended family members, participation in religious activities and the quality of home routines (e.g. feeding, bath)
	Gabriel demonstrates problems in processing tactile information, reacting defensively to tactile information leads to discomfort during self-care tasks such as toothbrushing, hair washing and combing, dressing and eating
	Economic stressors are also a concern for Gabriel's parents because they are afraid of missing time at work or one of the parents having to give up work to support Gabriel. The cost of medical care/behavioural interventions for Gabriel is something that also concerns them
	The impairments in reciprocal social interaction, communication and imagination, symbolic play and peer interaction are also a source of concern
	If Gabriel does not have access to early intervention service with a multidisciplinary team, her ASD characteristics may worsen and the family may, at some point, stop engaging in the public activities and routines which Gabriel can find difficult (e.g. shopping, attending religious services, eating out, going to the park). Therefore, Gabriel's behaviour has the potential to disrupt meals, vacations and family outings, negatively impacting both on the quality of life of Gabriel and her family
	Gabriel's family feels it is imperative that she finds a nursery place so that she can interact and have normative role models with her peers and family in all activities of daily life. It is important to support the development of Gabriel's communicative abilities with different partners in varied social contexts and expand Gabriel's initiated communication and focus of attention
Management	The family, and Gabriel, must be fully involved in the provision of holistic care and support, in conjunction with professional support services
	Gabriel must be referred to an early intervention service, which is a family-centred and built around how Gabriel interacts with her family, and her family interacts with her, and how Gabriel and her family are embedded within and engage with their local community
	There are two goals in providing family-centred supports: One goal is to support family members as the primary and most constant care providers in Gabriel's life. In doing so, an intervention programme should provide support to Gabriel's family system so that issues that may stress the family unit (including social, financial, physical, psychological issues) and thus affect family's ability to support Gabriel are mitigated as much as possible
	The second goal of family-centred intervention is to support the family in strengthening their ability to influence Gabriel's development and well-being. The provision of family-centred intervention that includes positive behavioural support is important for children with ASD who have behaviours that challenge, for three reasons
	First, the impact of these behaviours on family life can be highly disruptive and pervasive, affecting all family members, including Gabriel and the family lifestyle. Second, a highly effective approach to changing persistent behaviours that is challenging is to use a communication-based approach to teaching new patterns of communication and social interaction. Finally, effective behavioural support is enhanced by the development of partnerships with the people who are most intimately involved with Gabriel
	The implementation of comprehensive, positive behavioural support (within the natural routines of family life) provides a process for developing interventions that focus on Gabriel's communication skill development, challenging behaviour reduction and family support
	Those engaging with Gabriel must also respond to echolalia or unconventional communication specific to the functions that it serves for Gabriel and model/teach more conventional means. Always monitor Gabriel's emotion regulation and make the necessary accommodations or modifications to support emotion regulation, attention and learning
	Visual supports must be used by all partners in every context because information using visual aids such as individual or sequences of objects, photographs, logos or picture symbols will enhance Gabriel's active participation and understanding.
	As Gabriel is tactile defensive, the professional team and family must be aware of limited development of hand skills in the child because tolerating a variety of tactile experiences in play and craft activities are significant experiences in the typical progression of manual dexterity. Additionally, because tactile processing is an important aspect in connecting to others on an emotional level and participating in social situations, the social withdrawal that can occur in Gabriel could have a tactile component

Subsequent investigations	Multidisciplinary team assessment Griffiths III tool Schedule of growing skills II tool Sensory profile	
Roles and interventions	Intellectual disability nurse	– Engage with the family as part of the early intervention team – Undertake childhood assessments – Provide support and education to the family – Link the family to support groups
	Psychologist	– Parental guidance (development of parent's capacities in dealing with Gabriel) – Group therapy (the psychologist leading the sessions offers guided programmes as the group works through the issues together) – Support groups (for parents, siblings, etc., explore thoughts and feelings of having a child with ASD)
	Occupational therapist	Sensory and motor modulation and integration (e.g. games and activities to improve sensory modulation and integration include start-stop activities, running and changing direction); perceptual motor challenges (e.g. activities to sharpen perceptual motor skills include looking and playing games and activities involving destinations such as throwing and catching; reaching for a desired object moving on a string to the left, right and across midline); visuospatial processing activities (e.g. completing obstacle courses or playing hide-and-seek); tactile discrimination (e.g. finding objects hidden in materials of different textures, paints or shaving cream); peer play (e.g. once a child is fully engaged, she should begin to play with another peer) Motor planning and sequencing, including the capacity to sequence actions, behaviours and symbols (e.g. thoughts, words, visual images, spatial concepts) promoting autonomy in activities during Gabriel's daily life
	Speech and language therapist (SLT)	Development of pragmatics and strategies of communication based on Gabriel's communication abilities as well as learning strengths and needs. Gabriel will become a competent communicator when she is able to demonstrate a balance in socio-communicative skills including initiating, maintaining and responding to communicative partners. SLT will implement augmentative communication support to enhance Gabriel's communication and expressive language (i.e. non-speech communication system, e.g. gestures, signs, objects, pictures, photographs, picture symbols). Augmentative communication will support Gabriel to enhance her understanding of language, expression and understanding of emotion and to enhance Gabriel's emotional regulation
	Dentist	Early intervention is important in order to invest in prevention and early diagnosis of oral diseases and in the implementation of healthy routines from an early age. It is important to instruct Gabriel's caregivers on the care to be taken with oral health, in order to avoid more complex and costly dental treatments
	Dietitian	Screening for gastrointestinal disorders. Ensure that Gabriel's sensory processing characteristics will not negatively impact on her diet and nutrition. The dietitian must assess Gabriel's nutritional status, identify her support needs and intervene with an appropriate diet, reflective of her likes and dislikes

Conclusion

This chapter aimed to describe the characteristics and conditions of Down syndrome, cerebral palsy and ASD. The assessment and intervention approaches vary according to each condition and the needs of the person and the family. The provision of services is a complex undertaking governed by governmental laws, funded by multiple sources and structured and administered in different ways, but it is a given that the family is an essential member of the team and that the team includes practitioners from multiple disciplines as needed. The role of the multidisciplinary teams should be to maximise an individual's functional independence and quality of life through development and learning, improvements in social skills and communication, enhancing functional ability, addressing comorbidities, promotion of independence and provision of support to families.

Key Concepts Discussed

- People with intellectual disabilities may experience a wide range of neurodevelopmental condition that impact on them from a biopsychosocial perspective and can impact their quality of life.
- The causes of these neurodevelopmental conditions are diverse and the manner in which they impact the person and the co-morbid conditions associated with them can have a significant impact on the health and quality of life of people with an intellectual disability.
- Early intervention and appropriate person-centred supports and services are paramount in ensuring that people with an intellectual disability and their families can mitigate the impact of these conditions on the quality of life of the individuals involved.

References

Alexander M, Ding Y, Foskett N, Petri H, Wandel C, Khwaja O (2016) Population prevalence of Down's syndrome in the United Kingdom. J Intellect Disabil Res 60:874–878

Altuna M, Gimenez S, Fortrea J (2021) Epilepsy in down syndrome: a highly prevalent comorbidity. J Clin Med 10

Antonarakis SE, Skotko BG, Rafii MS, Strydom A, Pape SE, Bianchi DW, Sherman SL, Reeves RH (2020) Down syndrome. Nat Rev Dis Primers 6:9

APA (2013) Diagnostic and statistical manual of mental disorders (DSM-5). American Psychiatric Association, Washington, DC

Axton S, Fugate T (2009) Pediatric nursing care plans for the hospitalized child. Pearson Education, Upper Saddle River, NJ

Bull MJ (2020) Down syndrome. N Engl J Med 382:2344–2352

Bunt CW, Bunt SK (2022) Medical care for adults with down syndrome: Guidelines from the global down syndrome foundation. Am Fam Physician 105:436–437

Burke E, McCarron M, McCallion P (eds) (2014) Advancing years, different challenges: wave 2: IDS-TILDA. Findings of the ageing of people with an intellectual disability. School of Nursing and Midwifery, University of Dublin, Dublin

Caples M, Martin A-M, Dalton C, Marsh L, Savage E, Knafl G, Van Riper M (2018) Adaptation and resilience in families of individuals with down syndrome living in Ireland. Br J Learn Disabil 46:1–9

CDC (2022) Center for Disease Control and Prevention. https://www.cdc.gov/

De Graaf G, Buckley F, Skotko BG (2021) Estimation of the number of people with down syndrome in Europe. Eur J Hum Genet 29:402–410

Dellapiazza F, Michelon C, Oreve MJ, Robel L, Schoenberger M, Chatel C, Vesperini S, Maffre T, Schmidt R, Blanc N, Vernhet C, Picot MC, Baghdadli A (2019) The impact of atypical sensory processing on adaptive functioning and maladaptive behaviors in autism Spectrum disorder during childhood: results from the ELENA cohort. J Autism Dev Disord 50:2142–2152

Doody O, Bailey ME, Hennessy T (2021) Nature and extent of intellectual disability nursing research in Ireland: a scoping review to inform health and health service research. BMJ Open 11:e051858

Edvinsson SE, Lundqvist LO (2016) Prevalence of orofacial dysfunction in cerebral palsy and its association with gross motor function and manual ability. Dev Med Child Neurol 58:385–394

Gaskin C, Imms C, Dagley GR, Msall ME, Reddihough D (2021) Successfully negotiating life challenges: learnings from adults with cerebral palsy. Qual Health Res 31(12):2176–2193

Global Down Syndrome Foundation (2020) Global medical care guidelines for adults with down syndrome checklist. https://www.globaldown-syndrome.org/wp-content/uploads/2020/10/Global-Down-Syndrome-Foundation-Medical-Care-Guidelines-for-Adults-with-Down-Syndrome-Checklist-v.1-10-20-2020

Haddad, F., Bourke,J., Wong, K. & Leonard H. (2018) An investigation of the determinants of quality of life in adolescents and young adults with down syndrome. PLoS One, 13(6), e0197394. https://doi.org/10.1371/journal.pone.0197394

HSE (2020) Down syndrome. https://www.hse.ie/eng/health/az/d/down's-syndrome/complications-of-down's-syndrome.html

Hyman, S. L., Levy, S. E., Myers, S. M., & Behavioral, P. Council on Children With Disabilities, Section on Developmental and Behavioral Pediatrics. (2020) Identification, evaluation, and management of children with autism spectrum disorder. Pediatrics, 145: e20193447

Kuhaneck HM, Watling R (2010) Autism: a comprehensive occupational therapy approach. AOTA Press, Bethesda, MD

Kumin L, Schoenbrodt L (2016) Employment in adults with down syndrome in the United States: results from a National Survey. J Appl Res Intellect Disabil 29:330–345

Lopes J, Miziara I, Kahani D, Lazzari R, Guerreiro L, Moura R, Cordeiro L, Naves E, Conway B, Oliveira C (2018) P 115—Brain activity after transcranial stimulation combined with virtual reality training in children with down syndrome: case report. Gait Posture 66:426–437

Lord C, Rutter M, Le Couteur A (1994) Autism diagnostic interview-revised: a revised version of a diagnostic interview for caregivers of individuals with possible pervasive developmental disorders. J Autism Dev Disord 24:659–685

Lord C, Risi S, Lambrecht L, Cook EH Jr, Leventhal BL, Dilavore PC, Pickles A, Rutter M (2000) The autism diagnostic observation schedule-generic: a standard measure of social and communication deficits associated with the spectrum of autism. J Autism Dev Disord 30:205–223

Lord C, Rutter M, Dilavore P, Risi S, Gotham K, Bishop S (2012) Autism diagnostic observation schedule–2nd edition (ADOS-2). Western Psychological Corporation, Los Angeles, CA

Lord C, Elsabbagh M, Baird G, Veenstra-Vanderweele J (2018) Autism spectrum disorder. Lancet 392:508–520

Maenner MJ, Blumberg SJ, Kogan MD, Christensen D, Yeargin-Allsopp M, Schieve LA (2016) Prevalence of cerebral palsy and intellectual disability among children identified in two U.S. National Surveys, 2011-2013. Ann Epidemiol 26:222–226

Mccarron M, Mccallion P, Reilly E, Dunne P, Carroll R, Mulryan N (2017) A prospective 20-year longitudinal follow-up of dementia in persons with down syndrome. J Intellect Disabil Res 61:843–852

Normansell-Mossa KM, Top DN Jr, Russell N, Freeston M, Rodgers J, South M (2021) Sensory sensitivity and intolerance of uncertainty influence anxiety in autistic adults. Front Psychol 12:731753

Novak I, Hines M, Goldsmith S, Barclay R (2012) Clinical prognostic messages from a systematic review on cerebral palsy. Pediatrics 130:e1285–e1312

O'Callaghan ME, Maclennan AH, Gibson CS, Mcmichael GL, Haan EA, Broadbent JL, Goldwater PN, Dekker GA, Australian Collaborative Cerebral Palsy Research, G (2011) Epidemiologic associations with cerebral palsy. Obstet Gynecol 118:576–582

Poelke G, Ventura MI, Byers AL, Yaffe K, Sudore R, Barnes DE (2016) Leisure activities and depressive symptoms in older adults with cognitive complaints. Int Psychogeriatr 28:63–69

Reddihough DS, Jiang B, Lanigan A, Reid SM, Walstab JE, Davis E (2013) Social outcomes of young adults with cerebral palsy. J Intellect Develop Disabil 38(3):215–222. https://doi.org/10.3109/13668250.2013.788690

Ros G, Milla Romero MG, Abad L, Mulas F (2011) Intervention models in children with autism Spectrum disorders. In: Williams T (ed) Autism spectrum disorders. InTech. https://doi.org/10.5772/18512

Sanchack KE, Thomas CA (2016) Autism Spectrum disorder: primary care principles. Am Fam Physician 94:972–979

Santoro SL, Hendrix J, White N, Chandan P (2022) Caregivers evaluate independence in individuals with down syndrome. Am J Med Genet A 188:1526–1537

Schafer EC, Mathews L, Gopal K, Canale E, Creech A, Manning J, Kaiser K (2020) Behavioral auditory processing in children and young adults with autism spectrum disorder. J Am Acad Audiol 31:680–689

Sefen JAN, Al-Salmi S, Shaikh Z, Almulhem JT, Rajab E, Fredericks S (2020) Beneficial use and potential effectiveness of physical activity in managing autism Spectrum disorder. Front Behav Neurosci 14:587560

Sellier E, Platt MJ, Andersen GL, Krageloh-Mann I, De La Cruz J, Cans C, Surveillance Of Cerebral Palsy, N (2016) Decreasing prevalence in cerebral palsy: a multi-site European population-based study, 1980 to 2003. Dev Med Child Neurol 58:85–92

Serrada-Tejeda S, Santos-Del-Riego S, May-Benson TA, Perez-De-Heredia-Torres M (2021) Influence of ideational praxis on the development of play and adaptive behavior of children with autism spectrum disorder: a comparative analysis. Int J Environ Res Public Health 18:5704

Surveillance Of Cerebral Palsy In Europe (2000) Surveillance of cerebral palsy in Europe: a collaboration of cerebral palsy surveys and registers. Surveillance of cerebral palsy in Europe (SCPE). Dev Med Child Neurol 42:816–824

Upadhyay J, Tiwari N, Ansari MN (2020) Cerebral palsy: aetiology, pathophysiology and therapeutic interventions. Clin Exp Pharmacol Physiol 47:1891–1901

Vitrikas K, Dalton H, Breish D (2020) Cerebral palsy: an overview. Am Fam Physician 101:213–220

Zylstra RG, Prater CD, Walthour AE, Aponte AF (2014) Autism: why the rise in rates? J Fam Pract 63:316–320

Part III

From Adulthood to Older Age

Chronic Health Among Those with an Intellectual Disability

9

Eilish Burke, Máire O'Dwyer,
Dederieke Maes-Festen, and Alyt Oppewal

Chapter Topics

- This chapter considers the most prevalent chronic health conditions experienced by people with intellectual disabilities:
- Epilepsy
- Musculoskeletal conditions focusing on osteoporosis
- Cardiovascular disease
- Respiratory disease
- Gastrointestinal disease
- Sensory impairment
- The contributing factors to chronic health conditions are also explored.
- Factors to consider in addressing chronic health conditions are also identified.

E. Burke (✉) · M. O'Dwyer
Trinity College Dublin, Dublin, Ireland
e-mail: eburke7@tcd.ie; modwyer6@tcd.ie

D. Maes-Festen · A. Oppewa
Erasmus Medical Centre, Rotterdam, Netherlands
e-mail: d.maes-festen@erasmusmc.nl;
a.oppewal@erasumumc.nl

Introduction

For many individuals with intellectual disability, their physical health profile is complex and poses challenges throughout their lifetime. How one ages impacts on physical health; however, ageing is a lifelong process, and as there is no definitive age when one is said to be old, promoting and considering physical health across the lifespan is prudent. As noted by Forty (2021) for the general population, early childhood experiences, particularly adverse events, can impact on outcomes in later years. Similarly, the health a person with intellectual disability experiences in childhood, as well as the contribution of genetics, psychological issues, behavioural problems and poorer health experiences, culminates in a myriad of challenges and possible negative outcomes that can manifest in adulthood (Gerber 2012). So, for example, bone mineral density increases steadily from birth and reaches its peak in early adulthood, the greatest increase occurring within the pubescent years at which time the peak bone mass is reached. Any insult experienced during this period, such as the impact of lifelong medications for epilepsy, something common among people with intellectual disability, can impact bone health in later years, resulting in an increased risk of osteoporosis developing (Walsh et al. 2009). Therefore, one can con-

© The Author(s), under exclusive license to Springer Nature Switzerland AG 2023
F. Sheerin, C. Doyle (eds.), *Intellectual Disabilities: Health and Social Care Across the Lifespan*,
https://doi.org/10.1007/978-3-031-27496-1_9

clude that health experiences and health habits built through the early years of life impact later in life and, as people with intellectual disability are living longer, health challenges are to be expected.

Globally the prevalence of intellectual disability is estimated between 0.05% and 1.55% based on a recent meta-analysis finding (McKenzie et al. 2016). The population of adults with intellectual disability has grown over the last number of decades with life expectancy increasing across almost all Western societies; however, these trends are not seen to a great extent among developing countries (Dolan et al. 2019). Estimates from Ireland, the UK and the USA show significant improvement in life expectancy, with an average age of 65 years (McBride et al. 2021). However, these trends decrease with increasing severity of intellectual disability (Doyle et al. 2021). Generally, this increase has been attributed to better healthcare, improved living conditions and better education. However, despite these trends people with intellectual disability continue to die on average 20 years earlier than their peers without intellectual disability (McCarron et al. 2015; Doyle et al. 2021). Increased attention to health and health disparity is evident within the literature, emphasising the difficulties people experience (Burke et al. 2014; Burke et al. 2017). Overall, however, as a group, adults with intellectual disability are at higher risk of chronic disease. Multimorbidity and disease patterns for people with intellectual disability differ greatly from those in the general population with mental health, neurological disease, eye disease gastrointestinal and bone disease being among the most common, as opposed to the dominance of cardiovascular disease seen among the general population (McCarron et al. 2013; Kinnear et al. 2018). This chapter will explore some of the most prevalent chronic health conditions, the contributing factors and challenges and propose lifestyle behavioural changes that can improve health and quality of life for adults with intellectual disability.

Chronic Health Conditions

Epilepsy

Epilepsy is a chronic neurological disorder whereby brain activity becomes abnormal causing seizures. It is defined as having two or more seizures which are characterised by episodes of involuntary movement involving part or all the body, sometimes accompanied by loss of consciousness (Sarmast et al. 2020). Fundamentally, epilepsy is an organic condition that can begin at any age; however, it predominantly begins in childhood. Characteristics of epilepsy vary, and the International League Against Epilepsy classify them as *focal*, which can be with or without loss of consciousness, and *generalised* seizures including absence, tonic, atonic, clonic, myoclonic and tonic-clonic forms (Sarmast et al. 2020). With no identifiable cause in about half of those with epilepsy, contributing factors include brain trauma such as stroke or head injury, environmental factors such as drug abuse and infections such as meningitis. It is commonly associated with specific syndromes among those with intellectual disability, such as tuberous sclerosis complex (TSC), or Down syndrome and dementia (Franz et al. 2010; Altuna et al. 2021; Yang et al. 2021). Epilepsy is one of the most common neurological conditions worldwide with around 1% of the global population having epilepsy. However, for people with intellectual disability, the picture is vastly different. The prevalence of epilepsy among those with intellectual disability has been estimated between 22% and 28% (Haveman et al. 2011; Robertson et al. 2015). In an Irish longitudinal study, the prevalence demonstrated an increase from 30.5% to 35.7% between 2011 and 2017 in adults over the age of 40 years, with epilepsy identified as the most common non-cardiovascular condition (Burke et al. 2017). Comparing this to the non-disabled population, epilepsy prevalence is approximately 20–30 times higher, with seizure activity often reported as poorly controlled or resistant to drug treatment which is especially true for those with a more severe to profound intellectual disability particularly those with complex

Table 9.1 Overview of epilepsy investigations

Investigations	Rationale
Electroencephalography (EEG)	Helps in identifying the location of the epileptic focus
Neuroimaging including computed tomography (CT scanning)	Can provide information on potential epileptogenic lesions or tumours
Magnetic resonance imaging (MRI)	Similar to CT scanning, MRI is more precise; however, the person requires careful preparation and desensitising for success
Electrocardiogram (ECG)	Conducted to exclude cardiac conditions that could resemble epilepsy such as cardiac arrhythmia

multimorbidity (Matthews et al. 2008). Those with epilepsy are more likely to have a more severe level of intellectual disability, live with greater comorbid conditions and experience greater deficits in their activities of daily living. It is widely accepted that epilepsy contributes to poorer physical health and well-being; impacts on the persons psychological, social and mental health overall; and leads to a lower life expectancy for persons with intellectual disability and epilepsy (Varley et al. 2010). Investigations to diagnose epilepsy can be challenging among those with intellectual disability, and diagnosis is frequently based on clinical presentation; however, this should not be a single seizure or occurrence. The National Institute for Health and Care Excellence (NICE) guidelines recommend where possible further investigations and referral to a specialist should be considered, which will particularly avoid differential diagnosis (NICE 2012); see Table 9.1 for an overview of investigations.

Epidemiological studies have shown greater morbidities for those with epilepsy than those without; for example, Weatherburn et al. (2017) identified over 30% of those with epilepsy to have three or more comorbidities compared to those without epilepsy at 15% particularly those with lower socioeconomic circumstance. For people with intellectual disability, epilepsy has been associated with stroke, gastrointestinal disease and joint disease (Burke et al. 2014), blindness, speech impairment, motor difficulties and bone loss

(Robertson et al. 2015; Burke et al. 2017). Along with this, seizure occurrence may be unpredictable and increase the risk of falls, fractures and, ultimately, hospitalisation and mortality. Mental and psychological problems are also associated with epilepsy with Turky et al. (2011) noting a seven-fold increase in psychopathology in people with epilepsy and intellectual disability compared to those with intellectual disability without epilepsy; however, these findings have been challenged with Arshad et al. (2011) reporting no association and more recently Brizard et al. (2021) noting the results of their systematic review and meta-analysis as inconclusive. A correlation between epilepsy and behaviour of concern has also been suggested; however, the evidence is indeterminate. Some studies demonstrate increase in self-injurious behaviour and higher aggression rates in those with epilepsy and intellectual disability compared to the non-epileptic group; however, the authors of this meta-analysis do caution the interpretation of the results due to the small effect size (0.16) (Blickwedel et al. 2019; Deb et al. 2020a). Nevertheless, rates and patterns of comorbid mental health conditions, particularly depression, are seen at greater rates among those with epilepsy. Consequently, emerging evidence points to epilepsy contributing to higher levels of morbidity and also higher levels of premature mortality among those with intellectual disability (Kiani et al. 2014). People with intellectual disability are at risk of dying earlier than their non-disabled counterparts; however, this risk is increased in the presence of epilepsy. In a systematic review by Robertson et al. (2015), those having regular seizures, once or more a week, were 16.8 times at greater risk of death than the general population. Liao et al. (2022) found that in the cases of those who died with epilepsy and intellectual disability, almost 33% experienced a potentially avoidable death. These avoidable deaths are associated with environmental challenges, communication difficulties and poorer health surveillance, much of which can be accounted for as difficulties for the person with intellectual disability during health encounters. However, there is a paucity of evidence of the risk factors that contribute to death among those with epilepsy and intellectual disability.

Use of antiepileptic medicines (AED) is common among adults with intellectual disability, for both epilepsy and mood-stabilising indications in the treatment of psychiatric conditions. Epilepsy in adults with intellectual disability is more likely to require polypharmacy, and there are challenges associated with detection of side effects and seizure control. Seizures may be resistant to single-drug treatment (Amiet et al. 2008). A cross-sectional study from a nationally representative cohort of older adults with intellectual disability in Ireland found that 50% of those with epilepsy were taking two or more antiepileptic medicines, yet four in ten still experienced monthly seizures (O'Dwyer et al. 2018). There are few high-quality observational/intervention studies of the treatment of epilepsy in people with intellectual disability. A Cochrane review examining pharmacological interventions for epilepsy in people with intellectual disability concluded the quality of studies to be low to moderate (Jackson et al. 2015). Polypharmacy, which is commonplace for people with intellectual disability, increases the risk of drug-drug interactions, and exposure to sedative and anticholinergic medicines contributes to additional adverse effects on cognitive function for adults with intellectual disability who have epilepsy. In addition, certain psychotropic medicines, for example, the antipsychotic clozapine, may also be pro-convulsive, which may worsen seizure control (Mula 2017; Monaghan et al. 2021). In a cross-sectional study of 190 older adults with intellectual disability who had epilepsy in Ireland, 30.5% were exposed to a medicine classified as moderate/high risk of decreasing the seizure threshold (Monaghan et al. 2021). Enzyme-inducing AEDs may also lower the plasma levels of other psychotropic medicines taken concurrently, therefore reducing the efficacy of the psychotropic medicine (Ruiz-Giménez et al. 2010).

Epilepsy and seizure activity is a feature for those with Down syndrome. The seizure activity is said to have a bimodal distribution whereby the first occurrence may happen within the first 2 years of life and the second during the fifth or sixth decade of life (Altuna et al. 2021). For people with Down syndrome, late development of epilepsy is particularly associated with the development of Alzheimer's disease (AD), a condition shown to be dominant in those with Down syndrome as they age (McCarron et al. 2017a). The combination of the triplication of chromosome 21 contributing to the overproduction and accumulation of amyloid-B plaques that ultimately induce synaptic degeneration and potentially contribute to increased cortical irritability induces an epileptic effect (Lott et al. 2012). The seizure presentation in those with Down syndrome and AD is quite specific and, due to its presentation and late onset, has a specific name, late-onset myoclonic epilepsy (LOME). As people with Down syndrome are now living to middle and late age, their risk of presenting with AD and ergo LOME has increased (Altuna et al. 2021). This increase has also been demonstrated by the Intellectual Disability Supplement to the Irish Longitudinal Study on Ageing (IDS-TILDA), whereby an increase of almost 20% was seen over a 10-year period (McCarron et al. 2017b). Other syndrome-specific presentations that increase the risk of epilepsy include TSC in which epilepsy is a common feature. TSC is a genetic disorder with a global prevalence of approximately 1:6000. Epilepsy can present in 80–90% of individuals with neuropsychological disorders including intellectual disability common in about 85% and almost half presenting with ASD (de Vries et al. 2018).

The consequences of epilepsy are both clinical—increased risk of hospitalisation and mortality—and functional—impacting on the individuals' abilities to conduct their activities of daily living. Therefore, management is key and pharmacological treatment is the treatment of choice. However, AED contributes to gastrointestinal adverse effects, which in turn can impact negatively on the efficacy of the AED treatment. Appropriate diagnosis includes robust history taking, health screening and classification to avoid differential diagnosis and ensure appropriate management and care can be planned in a person-centred way. The WHO recognises epilepsy as a major health concern for those with intellectual disability; however, those with intellectual disability and epilepsy are very much underrepresented in research (Shankar et al. 2018). To improve quality of care and provide an

Table 9.2 Key concepts discussed

- Epilepsy is one of the most common neurological conditions worldwide
- Prevalence among people with intellectual disability is 20–30 times higher than the general population
- Higher prevalence of epilepsy is present under certain circumstances, e.g. people with Down syndrome as they age
- Epilepsy increases the risk of death among those with intellectual disability
- Epilepsy is difficult to treat for people with intellectual disability and may require polypharmacy
- Appropriate diagnosis and management are essential to promote optimal health

evidence base for care delivery, there is a need for increased research in this relatively neglected group (see Table 9.2 for summary).

Musculoskeletal Health and Osteoporosis

Musculoskeletal health is where there is an absence of disease in any part of the musculoskeletal system encompassing the muscles, bones, joints, tendons and ligaments. Essential for functioning, the musculoskeletal system gives the body structure, enables movement and provides a protective function for the body's internal organs (Peate 2018). Whilst many musculoskeletal conditions such as arthritis or osteoporosis are associated with ageing, there is evidence to suggest that functional decline in later years can be deterred if individuals act during critical times in their lives to build up biological reserve. So, for example, bone mass is laid down early in life, emphasising the importance of considering musculoskeletal health across the lifespan. Musculoskeletal conditions include osteoarthritis, rheumatoid arthritis, spondyloarthritis, gout, osteoporosis, osteopenia, associated fragility fractures, sarcopenia and inflammatory diseases of the connective tissue. The WHO has attributed musculoskeletal conditions as the leading contributors to years lived with disability worldwide, and whilst the majority of people will age well, there is a substantial number who will present with clinical problems due to musculoskeletal deterioration as they age (Briggs et al. 2016). These conditions interfere with the

ability to carry out normal functioning and activities of daily living, increase the risk of living with chronic pain and increase the risk of falls and subsequent fractures, frailty and loss of independence. As the population of people with intellectual disability age, musculoskeletal conditions will contribute to significantly poorer health (Burke et al. 2019). This increase in poorer health places a burden on the individual, their carer and the health system. The WHO has noted that the extent of the problem of musculoskeletal conditions is not fully understood or appreciated and that, overall, there is a lack of knowledge of these conditions as well as a lack of information (WHO 2003).

Bone is a living organ that is in a continual state of remodelling, whereby new bone cells are replacing older or damaged cells on a continuous basis (Peate 2018). Specific conditions such as diabetes, arthritis, thyroid disease and gastrointestinal disease all contribute to poor bone health, and when it is considered that over 71% of people with intellectual disability are classed as multimorbid, that is, the presence of two or more chronic conditions (McCarron et al. 2013), maintaining a healthy bone status, preventing bone fatigue and ensuring bone resorption does not outpace bone formation as the bone regenerates are challenging endeavours.

Osteoporosis occurs due to the deterioration of the microarchitectural structures within the bone, which increases the susceptibility to fracture due to increased bone fragility. Osteoporosis is insidious, often going undiagnosed until the first clinical fracture. The WHO based their definition of osteoporosis on bone mineral density (BMD) measured by dual-emission X-ray absorptiometry (DXA) scanning. The DXA measure provides a t-score which classifies the results into three categories (see Table 9.3). The WHO notes that if BMD is 2.5 SD or more below the average value for a young healthy female, osteoporosis is present. However,

Table 9.3 World Health Organization BMD cut-offs

BMD category	T-score
Normal	−1 or above
Osteopenia	−1.1 to −2.4
Osteoporosis	−2.5 and below

this definition has its flaws, and that although there is a connection between low t-score and fracture risk, the risk is ongoing, that is, fractures also occur within the osteopenia range, so if the cut-off for osteoporosis is only considered, then there is a risk of disregarding treatment for those with osteopenia (Kanis et al. 2013); therefore, using t-scores as the bases of identifying osteoporosis and treatment is fraught with difficulty.

This dependence on DXA measurement directly influences the known prevalence of osteoporosis, and it is noted that within society there are quite a number of undiagnosed cases, the Irish Osteoporosis Society estimates there are over 300,000 people undiagnosed in Ireland (HSE 2008), and the probability is that this is replicated worldwide. For people with intellectual disability, the prevalence has been reported as low as 8% (McCarron et al. 2011). However, there is a variance noted within the literature with Lin et al. (2015) reporting 21% among residences with intellectual disabilities in Taiwan and Leslie et al. (2009) reporting a 78.5% prevalence in a Canadian residential setting. In the IDS-TILDA study, the doctor's diagnosis of osteoporosis has depicted a steady increase over the first 10 years of this longitudinal study from 8% to 21% by 2017 (Burke et al. 2017). However, these rates varied significantly to those objectively measured within the study whereby using quantitative ultrasound the prevalence of 41% osteoporosis and 33% osteopenia was identified (Burke et al. 2019). The challenges that exist for those with intellectual disability are diagnostic screening and the dependence on DXA. People with intellectual disability may have anxiety or non-compliance issues with DXA and may have access or mobility issues and frequently report lack of reasonable adjustment when it comes to health screening (Moloney et al. 2021); therefore, with a paucity of diagnostic screening, measurement of risk is compromised, and the prevalence is possibly higher than reported. Alternate approaches and the consideration of risk factors ought to be taken into account. The classical risk factors include smoking, increased alcohol consumption, family history, female gender, imbalanced diet, sedentary behaviour, lack of sunlight exposure and glucocorticoids (WHO 2003;

Kanis et al. 2013). However, people with intellectual disability have unique and differing issues predisposing them to greater risk. The high prevalence of epilepsy resulting in an increased AED exposure across their lifespan directly impacts on bone tissue. Those who are already at risk for poor bone health may be further adversely impacted by enzyme-inducing AEDs, for example, phenytoin, which may increase bone turnover (Ruiz-Giménez et al. 2010; Watkins et al. 2019). Mobility challenges and comorbid conditions such as scoliosis increase osteoporosis risk. Some factors are negligible such as smoking or increased alcohol consumption which are reported as low among those with intellectual disability (McCarron et al. 2011). However, some factors whilst they apply may mean others are overlooked. Take, for example, gender, among those with intellectual disability; it has been noted risks with behavioural lifestyle, level of intellectual disability and AED medications are emerging strongly (Burke et al. 2021).

It is known that behavioural lifestyle as a modifiable factor can make substantial improvements when addressed; however, overweight and obesity levels are substantial among those with intellectual disability (Ryan et al. 2021) and sedentary behaviour is considerable (Lynch et al. 2021), all contributing negatively to bone health. In addition, people with intellectual disability have great difficulty engaging in health promotion, may have compliance issues in the presence of behaviours of concern or autism, have challenges expressing their health needs and frequently have their health neglected due to a lack of reasonable adjustments (Ali et al. 2013), resulting in challenges in maintaining their own health; for full overview of increased burden of risk, see Table 9.4.

An investment in musculoskeletal health is required for those with intellectual disability, and more attention is needed to be placed on overall musculoskeletal health. Good bone health provides stability, promotes strength and coordination and enables independent pain-free activities as one ages; therefore, maintaining a healthy musculoskeletal system across the lifespan by optimising bone health arrests decline and promotes an active healthier life (see Table 9.5 for summary).

Table 9.4 Increased burden of risk for people with intellectual disability

Modifiable factors	Non-modifiable factors
• Lifestyle behaviours including inactivity and sedentary behaviour, poor nutrition, low vitamin D and calcium, obesity indicative of poor diet and vitamin D deficiency • Barriers impacting on healthcare access including poor reasonable adjustments, individuals' communication difficulties, fragmentation of service provision, lack of specifically designed health promotion • An inadequately built environment impeding individuals' access to screening and health promotion • Impairing attitudes and carers' lack of knowledge	• Sex • Increased age • Family history • Caucasian • Previous history of fracture • Late menarche • Early menopause • Low endogenous oestrogen • Hypogonadism in males • Syndrome-specific risk such as Down syndrome and Prader-Willi syndrome • Antiepileptic medicines • Antipsychotic medicines • Proton-pump inhibitors

Table 9.5 Key concepts discussed

• Bone is a living tissue that needs to be stimulated to maintain optimal health
• Bone mass is laid down in the early years
• Taking care of your bone health across the lifespan, particularly as crucial junctures such as adolescence, is essential to minimise deterioration in later years
• Osteoporosis is an insidious condition, and many people with intellectual disability go undiagnosed, making them more susceptible to fracture
• Lack of diagnostic screening exists for those with intellectual disability
• Modifiable factors can be addressed to arrest the deterioration of bone health

Cardiovascular Disease

According to the WHO cardiovascular disease (CVD) is one of the leading causes of death worldwide with an annual estimate of 17.8 million lives lost globally mainly attributed to heart attacks and strokes (Roth et al. 2018). CVD is an umbrella term used to describe conditions that

Table 9.6 Risk factors for atherosclerotic cardiovascular disease in people with intellectual disability

Higher prevalence compared to the general population
Obesity (BMI) in women
Diabetes mellitus
Peripheral arterial disease
Similar prevalence compared to the general population
Hypertension
Metabolic syndrome
Obesity (men)
Intellectual disability-specific issues, associated with increased risk
Use of antipsychotics
Sedentary lifestyle, low physical fitness
Genetic syndromes, such as Bardet-Biedl and Prader-Willi syndrome, sex chromosomal abnormalities, Werner's syndrome, mitochondrial defects and congenital rubella syndrome

affect the heart and circulation and are usually associated with a build-up of fatty deposits over time. A high concentration of these fatty deposits, otherwise known as hypercholesterolaemia, which is an accumulation of low-density-lipoprotein cholesterol within the arteries, contributes to atherosclerosis (Gidding and Allen 2019). As atherosclerosis progresses the arteries narrow, reducing or occluding blood flow, contributing to a number of CVD, most commonly heart attack and stroke. In addition, lifestyle behaviour, smoking, alcohol overuse, obesity, diabetes, family history and hypertension have been identified as some of the risk factors for the presence of CVD, with hypertension as one of the greatest contributors (Gidding et al. 2016); see Table 9.6 for specific issues associated with increased risk for those with intellectual disability.

Cardiovascular epidemiological investigation among those with intellectual disability is not extensive; however, CVD risk factors are reported as high with a marked difference observed between sexes. Women in the main have been reported to be at greater risk (McCarron et al. 2011, 2017b; Burke et al. 2014). Conversely with objective measurement, prevalence has been identified as higher among men than women with intellectual disability although not significantly

(O'Brien et al. 2021). Similarly, the health ageing and intellectual disability (HA-ID) study reported high prevalence and demonstrated that hypertension, diabetes, hypercholesterolaemia and metabolic syndrome in older adults with intellectual disability over the age of 50 years were not diagnosed in 50, 45, 46 and 94%, respectively, prior to participation in the study (de Winter et al. 2012). Depending on the specific condition, prevalence rates vary, for example, the Irish Longitudinal Study on Ageing reported heart attack and heart failure as the highest CVD among the general older population compared to IDS-TILDA who reported heart murmur, abnormal heart rhythm and congestive heart failure as the most common CVD among those with intellectual disability, with heart attack five times lower in people with intellectual disability compared to the general population (Barrett et al. 2011; McCarron et al. 2011; Burke et al. 2014). For people with intellectual disability, the prevalence of CVD overall has been estimated between 4% and 26% with frequent rates of specific CVD reported lower than the general population (Wallace and Schluter 2008; de Winter et al. 2016). However, some of these particular studies are chart reviews; therefore, the likelihood of undiagnosed cases going unreported is high. The possibility of underdiagnosed cases is proposed in a Dutch longitudinal study, HA-ID, due to individuals' atypical presentation or absent complaints (deWinter et al. 2012; de Winter and Evenhuis 2014). Nevertheless, CVD is a feature for people with intellectual disability due to increased risk factors, longevity and frequently missed diagnoses. For example, for people with intellectual disability, there is evidence that peripheral arterial disease develops as they age; in fact de Winter et al. (2013) identified that people with intellectual disability have a significantly higher prevalence than an aged-matched cohort without intellectual disability. The presence of peripheral arterial disease can be an indicator of atherosclerosis which contributes to heart attack and stroke.

CVD among those with intellectual disability in some instances is associated with genetic causes of intellectual disability. It is estimated that nearly 50% of those born with Down syndrome present with some form of cardiovascular anomaly (Versacci et al. 2018). Congenital heart defects are common among people with intellectual disability particularly those with Down syndrome compared to the general population (Van Den Akker et al. 2006). Early detection and corrective surgery are standard practice for those born with Down syndrome; however, this has only been in vogue since the 1980s (Tsou et al. 2020). Therefore, this implies there may be a cohort of adults with Down syndrome and undiagnosed congenital heart defect. This of course has implications for pulmonary hypertension and other cardiovascular complications as they age (Vis et al. 2010). Investigating cardiac defects among adults with Down syndrome, Vis et al. (2010) identified 17% of those with Down syndrome with undiagnosed congenital heart defect with a further 77% with unknown cardiac regurgitation, and whilst this study was conducted in the Netherlands, the possibility of similar circumstance of undiagnosed defects is highly likely in other countries.

One major risk factor for CVD is hypertension as it causes structural changes to the walls of the arteries, making them more susceptible to atherosclerosis. People with intellectual disability present with two major risks for hypertension, overweight/obesity and sedentary lifestyle (Lynch et al. 2021; Ryan et al. 2021). These factors combined with the predisposition of poorer health associated with intellectual disability increase their vulnerability for hypertension. Unfortunately, there have been contradictory results among studies of the prevalence of hypertension among those with intellectual disability with reports of lower, higher or similar rates among those with intellectual disability compared to the general population (de Winter et al. 2012; Stevens et al. 2014; Axmon et al. 2017). This is mainly due to limited sample sizes; bias of selected samples, for example, from residential services only; differences in definitions for hypertension used; too high cut-off points; or reliance on self-report rather than objective measurement. However, Schroeder et al. (2020) screened a large cohort (33,122) of individuals with intellectual disability over the age of

18 years and identified a similar prevalence to the general population at 48% with higher levels reported for men versus women (50.7% v 43.1%, respectively). What was interesting was the identification of an increase in prevalence associated with age, obesity and low or no physical activity. Nevertheless, it is reported that those who present with hypertension respond well to treatment. O'Brien et al. (2021) report that comparing the treatment of those with and without intellectual disability, those with intellectual disability are more likely to be detected and be in receipt of antihypertensive treatment and the treatment is effective in controlling hypertension. However, what was notable in this study was the lack of awareness and treatment in those with more severe to profound level of intellectual disability, a fact previously highlighted by Van de Louw et al. (2009) when they noted the difficulty in preforming measurement in this group due to resistance or repetitive movement. Despite this, internationally the attention on hypertension among those with intellectual disability is poor, and considering the challenges in identifying prevalence and developing a state of the science picture of hypertension among those with intellectual disability, it is safe to say there are hidden undiagnosed cases. Therefore, more stringent detection and treatment needs to be instigated, particularly among those with more severe levels of intellectual disability.

Another connection to CVD has been identified between behaviours of concern and metabolic syndrome, a leading risk for CVD. Exploring this issue, Smith et al. (2022) note that antipsychotic use demonstrated significant weight gain among those with intellectual disability. In their systematic review and meta-analysis, they describe how most studies identified these trends among children and young adults with intellectual disability, noting that this trend predisposes an already vulnerable population to lifetime health adversity particularly CVD. Many individuals with intellectual disability are treated with antipsychotic medications, which contribute to the adverse effects of weight gain and metabolic syndrome (O'Dwyer et al. 2017; Carli et al.

2021). The use of antipsychotic medicines among those with intellectual disability is increasing their risk of CVD; therefore, metabolic monitoring along with the efficacy and efficiency of using antipsychotic medicines ought to be included in individuals' healthcare plan and medicine reviews.

CVD for people with intellectual disability, apart from congenital heart disease, are becoming some of the greatest contributors to death with most CVD related to poor lifestyle behaviours (de Winter et al. 2016). However, it is known that angina pectoris, peripheral arterial disease and myocardial infarction may be missed or diagnosed at a later stage (Jansen et al. 2013). Underdiagnosis and undertreatment may result in health inequity. Therefore, the diagnosis of cardiovascular disease should be considered when the individual presents with atypical symptoms, such as behavioural changes (de Winter and Evenhuis 2014). Diagnosis and treatment of cardiovascular diseases occur according to the guidelines for the general population. In clinical practice, it appears that invasive cardiac surgery is rarely performed in this group, which leaves questions regarding supposed feasibility of these treatments (Jansen et al. 2013). Undertreatment of CVD in this population should be considered an undesirable health inequity. By managing specific risk factors for CVD, the increased risk of morbidity and mortality among those with intellectual disability can be managed. So, for example, managing hypertension is one aspect to address, considering that those who are treated respond well (O'Brien et al. 2021). It is expected as people with intellectual disability age and become more independent in community settings, morbidity and mortality due to CVD will increase (Van Den Akker et al. 2006); therefore, there is an urgent need to focus attention on these aspects of healthcare. Despite the ageing trajectory of those with intellectual disability, the fact remains that longevity in recent years has plateaued and people with intellectual disability continue to die earlier than their non-disabled peers (Doyle et al. 2021). It is possible that many of these deaths could be attributed to undiagnosed CVD (see Table 9.7 for summary).

Table 9.7 Key concepts discussed

- CVD prevalence is high among people with intellectual disability however often undiagnosed
- Undertreatment of CVD is common and ought to be considered an undesirable health inequity
- People with intellectual disability can present atypically
- Proactive screening for CVD is essential for people with intellectual disability

Respiratory Disease

Respiratory disease includes asthma, pneumonia, upper respiratory tract infection, chronic obstructive pulmonary disease (COPD) and lung cancer. In Ireland one in five deaths are attributed to respiratory disease with similar figures reported for the UK (O'Connor et al. 2018; Truesdale et al. 2021). Respiratory disease accounts for over 14% of inpatient hospitalisations and over 18% of emergency admissions (O'Connor et al. 2018). For people with intellectual disability, higher rates of respiratory disease have been reported as all too often individual's respiratory system is compromised due to, for example, dysphagia (Truesdale et al. 2021). Prevalence range differs according to the condition; however, a prevalence of between 8% and 27% has been reported with higher levels noted among those with a more profound level of intellectual disability (Van Timmeren et al. 2017). Whilst the diagnosis of COPD is less common among those with intellectual disability, the prevalence of asthma has been reported as higher than the general population. Gale et al. (2009) report the prevalence of asthma among those with intellectual disability at 12%, which was double that of the general population and was associated with obesity and smoking risk factors. Considering that obesity rates have been identified at almost 80% (Burke et al. 2017; Ryan et al. 2021), this does not bode well for respiratory function among those with intellectual disability especially as they age. The presence of intellectual disability is directly related to outcomes as often those with intellectual disability are inefficient when using their inhalers (Davis et al. 2016). When examining data on death as a result of asthma, it is noted that

those who died were more likely to have an intellectual disability, which has led the British Thoracic Society (BTS) to include intellectual disability as a risk factor in their guidelines on fatal asthma (BTS 2018).

The Mencap report 'Death by Indifference' highlights the disparity and inequities in the healthcare of those with intellectual disability with many deaths potentially preventable (Heslop et al. 2013). One of the leading causes of death among those with intellectual disability is respiratory disease (Brameld et al. 2018; Oppewal et al. 2018; O'Leary et al. 2018a, b; Truesdale et al. 2021). Brameld et al. (2018) note that whilst people with intellectual disability are admitted to hospital less often than their non-disabled peers, their most frequent admissions were associated with respiratory conditions such as pneumonia, asthma and vaccine-preventable respiratory disease. Similarly, Truesdale et al. (2021) report respiratory mortality at almost 11 times higher than the general population with pneumonia as one of the major contributors. Dysphagia, which can lead to aspiration and subsequently chest infection or pneumonia, is an important factor to consider in relation to respiratory conditions. For those whose positioning is compromised, who have scoliosis or have swallowing issues due to comorbidities such as cerebral palsy, the negative impact on their respiratory function can lead to the occurrence of respiratory disease. Dysphagia is frequently associated with individuals with intellectual disability, particularly those with more complex needs, syndromic implications or multimorbidity. So, for example, those with a more profound intellectual disability, Prader-Willi syndrome, cerebral palsy or Alzheimer's dementia are at greater risk as neurological damage often impairs gag reflexes or inappropriate eating, packing the mouth with food, and subsequently the person can either choke or aspirate (Manduchi et al. 2021). The prevalence of dysphagia is unknown; however, it is estimated that most individuals with intellectual disability can present with dysphagia, and it has been reported that up to 85% of people with cerebral palsy experience episodes of dysphagia (Benfer et al. 2013) and approximately 74% of children with

Down syndrome exhibit dysphagia (O'Neill and Richter 2013). In the HA-ID study, a prevalence of 43.8% was found in a near-representative sample of adults aged 50 years and over (Maes-Festen et al. IN PRESS). Therefore, it is important to raise awareness on the possibility of dysphagia and the potential consequences for both carers and individuals with intellectual disability. Individual health assessment ought to include a swallowing baseline assessment particularly if the individuals are within these at-risk groups. What is challenging for carers is the fact that aspiration can often be silent and can go unnoticed, leading to the progression of disease and causes of respiratory infections going unrecognised. Recurrent chest infections are high among those with intellectual disability, specifically due to dysphagia (Truesdale et al. 2021). Dysphagia as a prelude to adverse respiratory conditions is a concern, not least for its association with mortality (Robertson et al. 2018a). Improved educational packages for carers and individuals with intellectual disability should include recognition and management of dysphagia which should be incorporated into care plans to reduce the possibility of respiratory conditions such as aspiration pneumonia.

Choking episodes have serious and potentially fatal consequences as well as respiratory disease implications for those with intellectual disability. Choking is also frequently under-recognised or sometimes missed altogether by carers when coughing episodes are not recognised or not reported as choking episodes particularly at mealtimes (Guthrie et al. 2015). For individuals with intellectual disability, choking is directly related to a number of factors associated with having an intellectual disability including poor oral status, presenting with behaviours of concern, using antipsychotic medications as well as other common comorbidities such as epilepsy or cerebral palsy. It is known that people with intellectual disability have a higher edentulous status than the general population (Mac Giolla Phadraig et al. 2015) and the levels of antipsychotic prescriptions (O'Dwyer et al. 2017) among those with epilepsy are up to 30 times higher than the general population (Matthews et al. 2008). Oral

Table 9.8 Key concepts discussed

- High prevalence of respiratory disease, dysphagia and choking among those with intellectual disability
- Respiratory mortality is almost 11 times higher among those with intellectual disability than the general population
- Dysphagia is common and leads to aspiration and consequent respiratory infection
- Recognition in people with intellectual disability is difficult and screening is recommended
- Early recognition and management of dysphagia reduces the risk of severe associated health problems
- Educational packages for carers and individuals with intellectual disability should include recognition and management of dysphagia, choking and their associated factors

health needs to be methodically monitored to promote good oral and dental hygiene. Postural and mealtime supports and liaison with speech and language therapist as well as physiotherapy to assess and monitor the individual promote good posture and ultimately good lung function. The use of accessible easy-read information should be prioritised for people at risk, again to support their respiratory health. Practical sessions on the use of inhalers and the use of spacers and other adaptations should be taught to people with intellectual disability in an effort to improve skill and overall improve respiratory health (see Table 9.8 for summary).

Gastrointestinal Disease

Patterns and prevalence of chronic disease are much different and the burden much greater for those with intellectual disability across their lifespan. There is evidence that there is a continual increase in chronic conditions as individuals age, none more so than gastrointestinal [GI] disease (Burke et al. 2017). Individuals with intellectual disability are at risk across their lifespan where some genetic disorders such as Down syndrome or Edwards syndrome predispose individuals to GI congenital abnormalities such as duodenal stenosis or oesophageal atresia (Prasher and Janicki 2018). GI disease involves disorders of the digestive tract including the oesophagus, stomach, small and large intestine and rectum.

Some of the main GI diseases that impact on those with intellectual disability include gastro-oesophageal reflux disease (GERD), coeliac disease and constipation with infection with *Helicobacter pylori* reported as higher in children with intellectual disability than the general population particularly those who live in congregated settings. Unfortunately, *Helicobacter pylori* is not routinely screened within the healthcare clinics (Somerville et al. 2008).

GERD is highly prevalent among those with intellectual disability with reports of prevalence as high as 50% and over 70% of those who present with reflux oesophagitis (Böhmer et al. 2000). Factors contributing to these high levels among those with intellectual disability may include, for example, neurological factors such as dysfunction of the chemoreceptor trigger zone for emesis, which may cause abnormal gastric motility and vomiting, instigating GERD (Dellon et al. 2018; Curtis et al. 2021). Often individuals with intellectual disability present with additional factors such as medication irritation, infections or allergies that exacerbate GERD, causing increased pain and discomfort. Frequently the pain associated with GERD can present as agitation, spasm, persistent cough and sleep disorders, and children are often difficult to pacify and may display self-aggressive behaviour, malnourishment, rumination, regurgitation and hematemesis often being a feature (Gössler et al. 2007). It is therefore possible that GERD and its sequelae, Barrett's oesophagus and gastritis, contribute further to the presence of peptic ulceration and the possibility of oesophageal adenocarcinoma (de Castilho et al. 2020). Early recognition of GERD is the basis of addressing the issue; however, this can be challenging. Factors that may identify the presence of GERD have been reported by Swender et al. (2006) when they recounted that hand mouthing was exhibited to a greater extent among those who were diagnosed with GERD, noting that this behaviour ought to alert healthcare staff to the possible presence of GERD and the importance of baseline functional assessment (Swender et al. 2006). What is concerning is the frequent use of proton-pump inhibitors (PPI) among those with intellectual disability, with almost a quarter of adults over the age of 40 years reporting use for more than a year particularly among women and frequently without a confirmed diagnosis (Al Mutairi et al. 2018). Interestingly, Al Mutairi et al. (2018) noted that PPI use was similar to that within the older general population, seen predominantly among those over the age of 50 years and mostly among those with a more severe to profound level of intellectual disability. The trouble with this type of use is that it contributes to polypharmacy and increases the potential for drug interactions (Wedemeyer and Blume 2014), and PPIs have been identified as harmful to bone health among those with intellectual disability (Burke et al. 2021).

Coeliac disease appears to be on the increase with between 1% and 3% prevalence among the general population; however, it is estimated that people with Down syndrome are at greater risk for coeliac disease with a prevalence estimated to be over six times higher than the general population (Sharr et al. 2016). Coeliac disease is highly associated with autoimmune disease, and as those with Down syndrome have an impaired immune response and present with abnormalities of their immune system, their risk is increased (Pavlovic et al. 2017). It is often not identified among individuals with intellectual disability as they may present atypically, and for children with Down syndrome, common signs and symptoms can be typical without coeliac disease being present. Growth impairment, intermittent diarrhoea with constipation and anaemia are often identified among children and adolescents with Down syndrome, making diagnosis of coeliac disease challenging; therefore, clinical vigilance to increase awareness must be exercised for the screening and diagnosis of coeliac disease among those with Down syndrome (Sharr et al. 2016).

Of significant concern are the rates of constipation among those with intellectual disability, a modifiable but life-threatening condition. Constipation is an issue across the life course for those with intellectual disability with rates reported as significant at all ages (Veugelers et al. 2010; Leader et al. 2018; Robertson et al. 2018b). Chaidez et al. (2014) report that children with intellectual disability can be five times more likely to present with constipation than their non-disabled peers. Evidence suggests that damage to the central nervous system is a significant factor for the presence of constipation which implies that any disruption of the neural modulation of colonic motility contributes to its presence; in other words peristalsis if interrupted slows the passing of matter through the bowel, resulting in constipation (Sarna 2010; Veugelers et al. 2010). Overall rates of between 33% and 57% are reported in the literature with identified contributing factors including medications such as anticholinergic use, tube feeding, cerebral palsy, mobility issues or severe to profound level of intellectual disability (Veugelers et al. 2010; Robertson et al. 2018b; Maslen et al. 2022). The IDS-TILDA study has recorded substantial increases in the prevalence of constipation over time. Its prevalence has escalated from 17.3% in 2011 to 43.5% in 2017 with greater prevalence among women particularly older women (65 years+) at 54.3% (McCarron et al. 2011; Burke et al. 2017). Similar to other reports levels of constipation increase with severity of intellectual disability, and of particular concern is that many older adults (37.6%) reported never having a normal bowel motion without the use of laxatives (Burke et al. 2017). Additionally, a sizable proportion of individuals remain constipated despite the use of laxatives, and frequently laxatives were used inappropriately (Robertson et al. 2018b; Al Mutairi et al. 2020). Individualised prescription management is essential to ensure evidence-based guidelines are recommended and instigated so that medicine use is optimised; this is particularly pertinent when considering laxative use as there appears to be an unstructured approach to its management. Unfortunately, constipation is commonly ignored and often not reported on time and is associated with death. Sumida and colleagues whilst investigating constipation and cardiovascular disease report that those presenting with constipation have a higher risk of all-cause mortality (Sumida et al. 2019). Gross failures of care of individuals with intellectual disability have been reported, resulting in the unnecessary death of individuals from constipation (Hill 2018). This report highlights serious concerns that being constipated is

Table 9.9 Key concepts discussed

- Gastrointestinal disease is highly prevalent among those with intellectual disability with specific syndromes such as Down syndrome increasing risk
- Prevalence of GERD has been recognised as high as 70% with the possibility of contributing to other GI conditions such as oesophagitis
- Coeliac disease is almost six times higher among those with Down syndrome than the general population
- Constipation, a life-threatening condition, is highly prevalent across all ages and specifically those with a more severe intellectual disability
- There is a frequent use of PPI often without a confirmed diagnosis
- Medication management appears highly prevalent, and often inappropriate laxative prescribing is noted
- Delay in diagnosis can be a feature due to complexities such as individuals' communication difficulties of expressing their own needs
- Addressing lifestyle behaviours is required to promote good gut health

not something that ought to be ignored and many individuals with intellectual disability require support and assistance in recognising its occurrence and addressing their own toilet hygiene.

It is important to note that the assessment and diagnosis of GERD and other GI conditions is challenging among people with intellectual disability most often in relation to impaired communication or complex behaviours of concern which may be difficult to understand. Often the person's complexities and multimorbidities contribute to a delay in identifying the condition or missing the diagnosis altogether and symptoms or behaviour being attributed to their intellectual disability, resulting in diagnostic overshadowing. It is therefore imperative that a multidisciplinary team approach to care is taken as this collaborative approach will support the identification of issues for the person as a whole, lend to more person-centred care and inspire improved health outcomes for the individual overall (see Table 9.9 for summary).

Sensory Impairment

Sight and hearing are key elements to support communication, navigate our environment and help make sense of the world around us.

Unfortunately, sensory impairments are common among individuals with intellectual disability, contributing substantially to challenges in everyday life (Dijkhuizen et al. 2016; Fellinger 2022). Anatomical anomalies, for example, keratoconus or narrow ear canals, which implies a lifelong risk of sensory impairment, are a feature for those with Down syndrome. Cataracts are also frequently part of the life for those with Down syndrome and often go untreated which is in part disempowering and impairs the rights of the individual to be independent, a fact that needs to be addressed and highlighted with healthcare practitioners. In the IDS-TILDA study, self-reported eye disease rose by over 4–19.5% in a 10-year period with cataracts as the most prevalent condition identified among those with Down syndrome across all age groups (Burke et al. 2017). In total over 21% of individuals with intellectual disability reported their eyesight as poor with an increase of over 5% in the same period; what is concerning is that the previous work identified eye disease as the most common condition among this cohort at 51% (McCarron et al. 2013); however, screening does appear to be ongoing with only 61% of the IDS-TILDA cohort reporting they had an eye exam in the last year (Burke et al. 2017). However, this would leave one to wonder the vigilance or the suitability of these eye exams; is there a need for reasonable adjustments for screening to improve detection of poor eye health? Similarly, poorer hearing health was noted within the IDS-TILDA study with the uptake of hearing assessment low. In total 39% reported not having a hearing assessment within the previous 3 years, the majority stating they felt there was no need for it (Burke et al. 2017). However, when one considers that most individuals depend on support to identify their health needs, there is a need for further education among healthcare workers specifically targeting the sensory health needs of those for whom they care. Across the life course sensory impairments impact on language development, social engagement, cognitive development, education as well as physical health and well-being. Despite this sensory impairment frequently goes underdiagnosed and under-recognised

Table 9.10 Key concepts discussed

- Sensory impairment is highly prevalent among those with intellectual disability
- Often sensory impairment goes unrecognised and underdiagnosed
- Those with Down syndrome are at specific risk
- Improved educational packages for carers and individuals with intellectual disability are required

among individuals with intellectual disability (Evenhuis et al. 2009; Kiani and Miller 2010). The estimated prevalence differs depending on the level of intellectual disability, syndrome and comorbidities (Van Naarden Braun et al. 2015; Rydzewska et al. 2019); however, what is agreed is that the level of undiagnosed impairment is substantial with Van Splunder et al. (2006) reporting levels of over 40%. Often the person's intellectual disability is the overshadowing aspect with staff attributing lower levels of function to their cognitive ability (Fellinger 2022). Health for those with intellectual disability is complex, and healthcare practitioners need to be aware that the fact that they have an intellectual disability increases their chances of sensory impairment; therefore, vigilance, robust screening and specifically educated carers with the ability to make reasonable adjustments are essential (see Table 9.10 for summary).

Contributing Factors to Poor Health Outcomes

Due to greater health challenges and a cascade of disparities, such as lack of health education, communication difficulties and lack of reasonable adjustment in health provision or health promotion, people with intellectual disability experience significant health disparities globally (Krahn and Fox 2014). Often health promotion is inaccessible with scant regards to reasonable adjustment for this population. A healthy lifestyle is key for good health and healthy ageing. However, research has consistently shown that adults with intellectual disability often have unhealthy lifestyles. Apart from non-modifiable factors, such as syndrome-specific challenges,

Fig. 9.1 Modifiable factors increasing the burden of disease

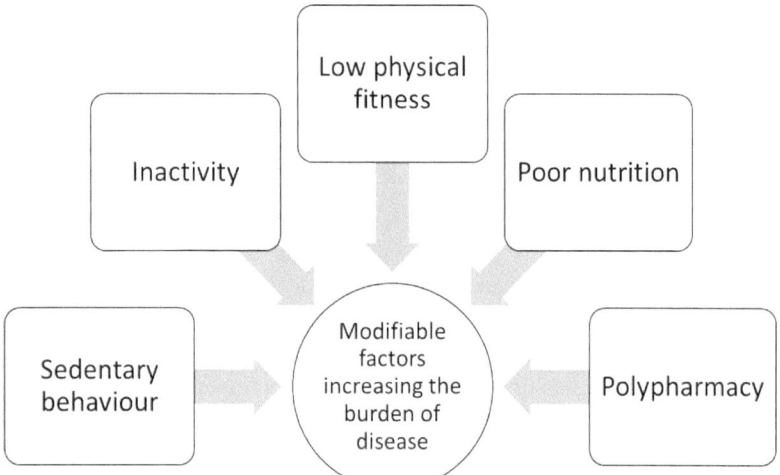

the relationship between Down syndrome and dementia or uncontrolled epilepsy among those with intellectual disability, there are modifiable factors like low physical activity, lack of physical fitness, poor nutrition and polypharmacy that contribute to poorer health outcomes (see Fig. 9.1).

Physical Activity and Fitness

The physical activity levels of adults with intellectual disability are low, and often well under the recommended daily activity levels (Lynch et al. 2021). Although the number of adults with intellectual disability not meeting the physical activity guidelines differs per study, Dairo et al. (2016) showed in a systematic review that only 9% of the adults with intellectual disability worldwide achieved the minimum physical activity guidelines. Similarly, Melville et al. (2017), in another review, demonstrated that besides these low physical activity levels, sedentary behaviour levels are also high. They reported that objectively assessed sedentary time ranged from 8.7 to 10.7 h per day. Low physical activity levels have consistently been demonstrated to be associated with poor health outcomes, putting people at a higher risk for cardiovascular diseases, hypertension, type 2 diabetes mellitus, metabolic syndrome, obesity, certain types of cancer, mental

health problems and premature mortality (American College of Sports Medicine (ACSM) 2021). Apart from that, sedentary behaviour is also independently associated with higher risks for diabetes, cardiovascular diseases, cancers and premature mortality (ACSM 2022). Ultimately, this low physical activity and high sedentary behaviour levels are concerning and put adults with intellectual disability at an unnecessary risk for adverse health outcomes. It has also been identified that adults with intellectual disability are often less fit than adults of the general population. This may partly be explained by their inactive lifestyles. In the HA-ID study those within the 50 years age group were only as fit as individuals within a 70–80-year age group in the general population (Hilgenkamp et al. 2012). These low physical fitness levels were associated with a higher risk for premature mortality and a decline in mobility and the ability to perform daily activities (Oppewal et al. 2014, 2015; Oppewal and Hilgenkamp 2019). Low fitness levels therefore increase the risk for unnecessary adverse health outcomes for these individuals. Because even small improvements in physical fitness levels are expected to result in major improvements in health (Oppewal et al. 2020), improving physical fitness is an important target area to improve the overall health of adults with intellectual disability and work towards healthy ageing within this population.

Nutrition

Besides being active and fit, healthy nutrition is also an important aspect of a healthy lifestyle and a key determinant of overall health across the life course. The HA-ID study previously illustrated that adults with intellectual disability have inadequate dietary intake. None of the 287 participants met all Dutch recommendations for a healthy dietary intake or recommended daily allowance (RDA). The dietary intake was too low in calories in 68.6% of the participants, too low in protein in 30.2%, too low in fibre in 98.2% and too high in saturated fat in 89.5% (de Leeuw et al. 2022). This finding is supported in other studies, for example, it was found that adults with intellectual disability tend to have diets with sugar, salt and saturated fat intake above the recommendations and hardly met the recommendations for fruit, vegetables, fibre and micronutrient intake (Bossink et al. 2017; Dean et al. 2021; Harper et al. 2021). Similarly, in the IDS-TILDA study, dietary consumption did not meet the RDA with fruit and vegetable intake the lowest in terms of the food pyramid [1] and over 28% reporting they ate takeaway fast food at least once a week (Burke et al. 2014). Mostly, people with intellectual disability rely on others for support with their grocery shopping or this is provided, and others make the choice (O'Donovan et al. 2020). There is a plethora of evidence noting that paid support workers do not always make healthy food choices (Adolfsson et al. 2012; O'Leary et al. 2018b), which leaves individuals with intellectual disability exposed to less favourable options.

Poor dietary habits contribute to malnutrition and particularly states of overweight and obesity. With levels of obesity reaching epidemic levels, for example, nearly 80% objectively measured as overweight/obese (Ryan et al. 2021), improving nutrition is a key factor in alleviating poor health outcomes. Whilst individuals have the right to choose their own food, a right that has to be respected, they may not always know the implications of the choice, or they may lack the ability to understand the consequences of their choices (Kolset et al. 2018). Therefore, the need for lifelong support, education and policy to include individuals with intellectual disability is a requirement (Dean et al. 2021; Røstad-Tollefsen et al. 2021). Supporting people with intellectual disability to improve their lifestyle can help this group to become healthier and to age with better health.

Polypharmacy

Polypharmacy (the use of multiple medicines) can be beneficial and improve health outcomes, quality of life and disease management. However, inappropriate polypharmacy carries extra risk in adults and older adults with intellectual disability. People with intellectual disability may not be able to communicate the side effects associated with polypharmacy, there is a limited evidence base of the safety of polypharmacy in adults with intellectual disability who have multimorbidity, and people with intellectual disability may have increased sensitivity to adverse effects associated with medicines (Taylor et al. 2015). People with intellectual disability have been described as one of the most medicated groups in society (Straetmans et al. 2007). Numerous studies have shown rates of polypharmacy that far exceed rates in the general population (Häßler et al. 2015; Peklar et al. 2017). A cross-sectional study in Ireland of 753 adults over 40 years of age found that 35% reported taking 5–9 medicines (polypharmacy) and 21% ten or more medicines (excessive polypharmacy) (O'Dwyer et al. 2016). In addition, in this study, the most commonly reported medication classes implicated in polypharmacy differed compared to the older population reflecting different disease patterns: with antipsychotics being most commonly reported by 43%, followed by antiepileptics (39%) and laxa-

---

[1] *'The Food Pyramid is a visual representation of how different foods and drinks contribute towards a healthy balanced diet. The Food Pyramid allows individuals the flexibility to choose foods and drinks from each shelf depending on their food preferences. It organises foods and drinks into 5 main shelves, starting from the most important shelf on the bottom'* (Department of Health 2020).

Table 9.11 Ways to optimise polypharmacy in adults with intellectual disability

- Holistic multidisciplinary regular review of medicines
- Use of a structured tool for review, e.g. Scottish NHS seven-step medication review (National Health Service Scotland 2022)
- Focus on medicines associated with adverse cognitive and physical adverse effects, for example, anticholinergic medicines, through the use of structured tool to measure anticholinergic burden such as an anticholinergic cognitive burden scale (ACB scale) (Campbell et al. 2013)
- Development of national policy and guidance around optimising polypharmacy specifically for adults with intellectual disability
- Patient-centred approach with people with intellectual disability and carers about experiences of polypharmacy and its benefits and side effects

Table 9.12 Key concepts discussed

- Physical inactivity is reported at over 70%
- Sedentary behaviour is highly prevalent with some studies reporting up to 10 h of sitting per person
- Fitness among those with intellectual disability is poor with those in younger age groups identifying as having fitness equivalent to much older aged categories
- Inactivity, sedentary behaviour and low fitness contribute to unnecessary adverse health
- Nutrition has been identified as poor among those with intellectual disability with the overall nutrient values of individual's diets identified as not meeting RDA
- Being overweight or obese is common among those with intellectual disability
- Polypharmacy is frequently observed, and whilst sometimes this is necessary, the rates far exceed those observed among the general population
- Inappropriate polypharmacy increases risk of poorer health outcomes
- Medication optimisation and deprescribing interventions ought to be considered across the broad spectrum of medication management

tives (38%). This is in contrast to the older adult population, where gastrointestinal medicines, cardiac therapies and analgesics are more frequently reported. Several factors have been associated in the literature with polypharmacy in adults with intellectual disability: living in congregated settings and having multimorbidity, mental health conditions and epilepsy (Haider et al. 2014; O'Dwyer et al. 2016). In the general population, there has been increasing focus on deprescribing to reduce inappropriate polypharmacy. Many deprescribing interventions to date in the population with intellectual disability have focused on reducing use of antipsychotics (Shankar et al. 2019; Deb et al. 2020b). Medication optimisation ought to be the approach taken (Table 9.11).

In response to reports published in England highlighting inappropriate use of antipsychotics and psychotropics, particularly in institutional settings, the NHS England began the 'stopping over medication of people with a learning disability, autism or both (STOMP)' project (Branford et al. 2018). The STOMP pledge was signed by different healthcare professions in the UK, including NHS England, the Royal College of Psychiatrists and the Royal Pharmaceutical Society. There has been no coordinated national response to polypharmacy and inappropriate psychotropic use in Ireland or many other European countries. Specific validated prescribing criteria need to be developed for people with intellectual disabil-

ity to guide identification of inappropriate polypharmacy to optimise medicine use and improve safety and health outcomes for people with intellectual disability (see Table 9.12 for summary).

What Can Be Done to Improve Health Among Those with Intellectual Disability?

People with intellectual disability have higher health needs, appear to present with older age conditions much earlier than the general population and often have atypical presentation of these conditions. Individuals frequently have communication difficulties and may find it challenging to express or interpret their own health needs. This imposes greater responsibility on healthcare professionals and those who support their care. The need for reasonable adjustment is clear, and further education is required for both individuals themselves, those who support them and indeed primary healthcare professionals who, heretofore, may never have supported individuals with intellectual disability (Doherty et al. 2020). Nevertheless, there are a number of aspects that are important and can be addressed (see Table 9.13).

Table 9.13 Factors that support addressing health issues among people with intellectual disability

- Being proactive in improving education for individuals with intellectual disability and their carers
- Underpinning policy with core indicators; see, for example, 'Positive Ageing Indicators for People with an Intellectual Disability' (McGlinchey et al. 2019)
- Addressing disparities in health promotion with the introduction of reasonable adjustments such as easy read
- Enhancing health surveillance and ensuring a proactive approach to screening and interventions to address behavioural issues identified
- Annual health assessment to include all domains of health: social, emotional, psychological, environmental, physical and mental
- Recognising the importance of specialist knowledge and having multidisciplinary and interdisciplinary collaboration
- Medication review on an annual basis
- Emphasis being placed on the importance of lifestyle and working towards healthier lifestyle behaviours

Working Towards a Healthier Lifestyle

Improving the lifestyles of people with intellectual disability is an important area for health improvement. However, this is not an easy task, because of the heterogeneity of this population and their often-complex surroundings. We have to take into account the variety in cognitive and physical capabilities, the often-complex coexisting and intertwined health conditions and the dependency of people with intellectual disability on others to become active and eat healthy. Besides that, often experienced barriers, such as lack of education or inaccessible health promotion, have a big influence on the opportunities people with intellectual disability have for a healthier lifestyle. Lack of transport and finances, lack of support and limited accessible opportunities to become active are all too frequent barriers (Bossink et al. 2017). Therefore, to support people with intellectual disability towards a healthier lifestyle, it is crucial that the methods are personalised, include reasonable adjustments to support their inclusion, promote person-centred care and include the whole system surrounding the person with intellectual disability (McLeroy et al. 1988; Sallis et al. 2006). Social-ecological models are helpful to get insight into the complex dynamic interrelations among individual, interpersonal and environmental factors of health promotion; see Fig. 9.2 for an example of the rainbow model (Dahlgren and Whitehead 2021). Applying this model to care delivery encourages healthcare professionals to think beyond the immediate medical needs and consider the wider social, educational, lifestyle and environmental determinants of health. For each level, different techniques are helpful, such as specifically designed activities for the person with intellectual disability at an individual level (van Schijndel-Speet et al. 2017), behavioural change techniques at the interpersonal level (Michie et al. 2011; Willems et al. 2017), tools to get insight into the assets in the environment for a healthy lifestyle (Vlot-van Anrooij et al. 2020) and the plan-do-check-act cycle for implementation and maintenance of lifestyle approaches and policies (Steenbergen et al. n.d.) at an environmental level. This will hopefully facilitate the development of more appropriate person-centred management strategies for this vulnerable group with the ultimate aim of improving their quality of life.

The Main Determinants of Health

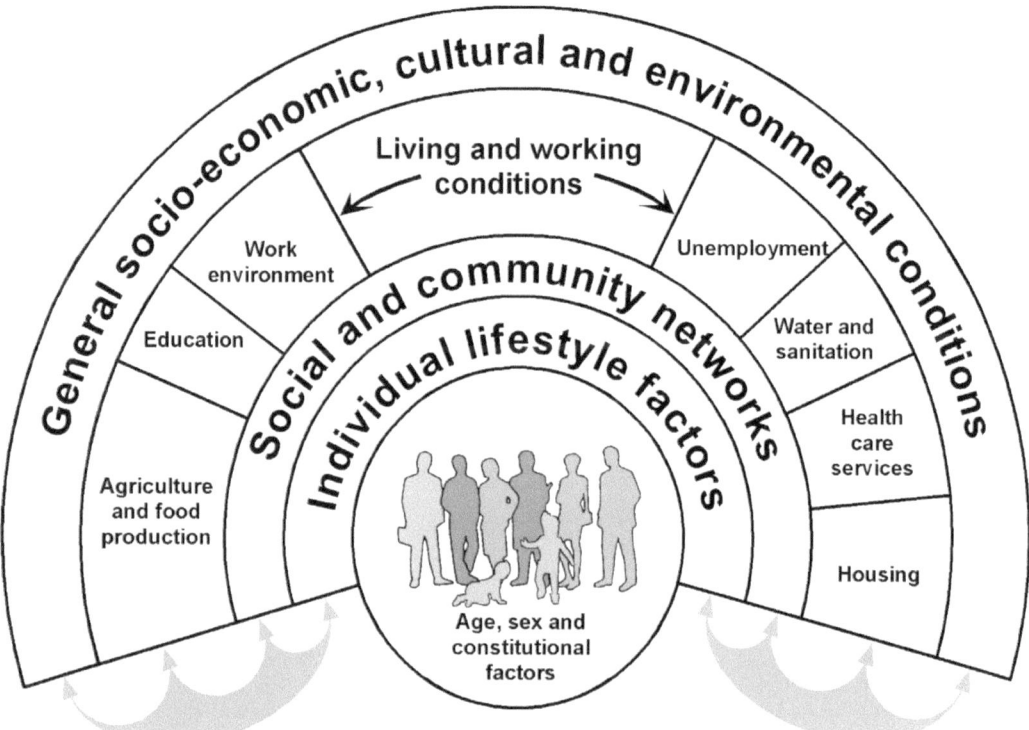

Fig. 9.2   The rainbow model (Adapted from Dahlgren and Whitehead 1993)

Conclusion

Chronic health conditions and particularly multi-morbidity are features in the lives of many individuals with intellectual disability. This chapter explored the most prevalent chronic health conditions across their lifespan. Conditions such as epilepsy, osteoporosis, cardiovascular disease, respiratory disease, gastrointestinal disease and sensory impairment are among the most prevalent conditions and pose some of the greatest challenges to the promotion of a healthy life for those with intellectual disability across all ages and all levels of intellectual disability. Throughout the chapter the reader is reminded of the health disparity experienced by individuals across their life course. There is a diversity of care across the world for those with intellectual disability, what is available in one health services may not or is not available in another and this is particularly relevant in developing countries. Nevertheless, there is a need to increase awareness of the disparities in health experienced by individuals with intellectual disability, and support carers and healthcare professionals recognise the potential increased disease loading for these individuals. There is a need for more proactive action to address health disparity among those with intellectual disability, the risk being that without action disparity will remain and people with intellectual disability will continue to experience poorer health. Policy makers and healthcare professionals alike need to focus on supporting healthcare practice, identifying the specific need for those with intellectual disability and instigating healthcare change in the form of improved education for all and standards for health assessment as well as addressing the environmental challenges to mitigate disparity in an effort to avoid extra burden and disability being placed on this already marginalised group.

Key Concepts Discussed

- This chapter considered the most prevalent chronic health conditions experienced by people with intellectual disabilities:
  Epilepsy
  Musculoskeletal conditions focusing on osteoporosis
  Cardiovascular disease
  Respiratory disease
  Gastrointestinal disease
  Sensory impairment
- The contributing factors to chronic health conditions were also explored.
- Factors to consider in addressing chronic health conditions were identified.

Reader Activity

Chronic health is highly prevalent among those with intellectual disability across their lifespan; with consideration to the content of the chapter and what you have learned, identify key aspects that would influence your provision of care to those with an intellectual disability.

Useful Resources to Promote Better Physical Health

- Positive ageing indicators for people with intellectual disability—chrome-extension://efaidnbmnnnibpca-jpcglclefindmkaj/ https://assets.gov.ie/9674/abcd-feef1474423b983e531d2bde645d.pdf
- Get wise about your health—https://www.getwiseid.eu/#/
- People with intellectual disability as physical activity leaders [PPALs]—https://www.tcd.ie/tcaid/research/Project5.php
- Get fit and keep fit with modifiable exercise—https://www.tcd.ie/tcaid/research/ppalsvideos.php
- Healthy Ageing and Intellectual Disability [HA-ID]—https://bmjopen.bmj.com/content/12/2/e053499
- Intellectual Disability Supplement to the Irish Longitudinal Study on Ageing [IDS-TILDA]—https://idstilda.tcd.ie/
- Trinity Centre for Ageing and Intellectual Disability [TCAID]—https://www.tcd.ie/tcaid/

References

Adolfsson P, Fjellström C, Lewin B, Mattsson Sydner Y (2012) Foodwork among people with intellectual disabilities and dietary implications depending on staff involvement. Scand J Disabil Res 14(1):40–55

Al Mutairi H, O'Dwyer M, McCarron M, McCallion P, Henman MC (2018) The use of proton pump inhibitors among older adults with intellectual disability: a cross sectional observational study. Saudi Pharmac J 26(7):1012–1021

Al Mutairi H, O'Dwyer M, Burke E, McCarron M, McCallion P, Henman MC (2020) Laxative use among older adults with intellectual disability: a cross-sectional observational study. Int J Clin Pharm 42(1):89–99

Ali A, Scior K, Ratti V, Strydom A, King M, Hassiotis A (2013) Discrimination and other barriers to accessing health care: perspectives of patients with mild and moderate intellectual disability and their carers. PLoS One 8(8):e70855

Altuna M, Giménez S, Fortea J (2021) Epilepsy in down syndrome: A highly prevalent comorbidity. J Clin Med 10(13):2776

American College of Sports Medicine (2021) ACSM's guidelines for exercise testing and prescription, 11th edn. Lippincott Williams & Wilkins, Philadelphia, PA

American College of Sports Medicine (2022) ACSM's Guidelines for Exercise Testing and Prescription. 11th ed. Lippincott Williams & Wilkins, Philadelphia, PA

Amiet C, Gourfinkel-An I, Bouzamondo A, Tordjman S, Baulac M, Lechat P, Mottron L, Cohen D (2008) Epilepsy in autism is associated with intellectual disability and gender: evidence from a meta-analysis. Biol Psychiatry 64(7):577–582

Arshad S, Winterhalder R, Underwood L, Kelesidi K, Chaplin E, Kravariti E, Anagnostopoulos D, Bouras N, McCarthy J, Tsakanikos E (2011) Epilepsy and intellectual disability: does epilepsy increase the likelihood of co-morbid psychopathology? Res Dev Disabil 32(1):353–357

Axmon A, Ahlström G, Höglund P (2017) Prevalence and treatment of diabetes mellitus and hypertension among older adults with intellectual disability in comparison with the general population. BMC Geriatr 17(1):1–12

Barrett A, Burke H, Cronin H, Hickey A, Kamiya Y, Kenny RA, Layte R, Maty S, McGee H, Morgan K, Mosca I (2011) Fifty plus in Ireland 2011: first results from the Irish longitudinal study on ageing (TILDA), vol 10. Trinity College Dublin, Dublin, pp 2011–2000

Benfer KA, Weir KA, Bell KL, Ware RS, Davies PS, Boyd RN (2013) Oropharyngeal dysphagia and gross motor skills in children with cerebral palsy. Pediatrics 131(5):e1553–e1562

Blickwedel J, Ali A, Hassiotis A (2019) Epilepsy and challenging behaviour in adults with intellectual disability: a systematic review. J Intellect Develop Disabil 44(2):219–231

Böhmer CJM, Klinkenberg-Knol EC, Niezen-de Boer MC, Meuwissen SGM (2000) Gastroesophageal reflux disease in intellectually disabled individuals: how often, how serious, how manageable? Am J Gastroenterol 95(8):1868–1872

Bossink LW, van der Putten AA, Vlaskamp C (2017) Understanding low levels of physical activity in people with intellectual disabilities: A systematic review to identify barriers and facilitators. Res Dev Disabil 68:95–110

Brameld K, Spilsbury K, Rosenwax L, Leonard H, Semmens J (2018) Use of health services in the last year of life and cause of death in people with intellectual disability: a retrospective matched cohort study. BMJ Open 8(2):e020268

Branford D, Gerrard D, Saleem N, Shaw C, Webster A (2018) Stopping over-medication of people with intellectual disability, autism or both (STOMP) in England part 1–history and background of STOMP. Adv Mental Health Intellect Disabil 13(1):31–40

Briggs AM, Cross MJ, Hoy DG, Sanchez-Riera L, Blyth FM, Woolf AD, March L (2016) Musculoskeletal health conditions represent a global threat to healthy aging: a report for the 2015 World Health Organization world report on ageing and health. The Gerontologist 56(suppl_2):S243–S255

British Thoracic Society (2018) British Guideline on the Management of Asthma. British Thoracic Society, Scottish Intercollegiate Guidelines Network. Thorax 63(Suppl 4).: iv1–121

Brizard BA, Limbu B, Baeza-Velasco C, Deb S (2021) Association between epilepsy and psychiatric disorders in adults with intellectual disabilities: systematic review and meta-analysis. BJPsych open 7(3):e95

Burke EA, McCallion P, McCarron M (2014) Advancing years, different challenges: wave 2 IDS-TILDA: findings on the ageing of people with an intellectual disability: an intellectual disability supplement to the Irish longitudinal study on ageing. Dublin: Trinity College Dublin

Burke EA, McGlinchey E, O'Dwyer M, Foran S, Mac Giolla Phadraig C, O'Connell J, Yan J, McCallion P, McCarron M (2017) Physical health IN: Health, Wellbeing and Social Inclusion: Ageing with an Intellectual Disability in Ireland Evidence from the First Ten Years of The Intellectual Disability Supplement to The Irish Longitudinal Study on Ageing (IDS-TILDA). Trinity College Dublin, Dublin

Burke EA, Carroll R, O'Dwyer M, Walsh JB, McCallion P, McCarron M (2019) Quantitative examination of the bone health status of older adults with intellectual and developmental disability in Ireland: a cross-sectional nationwide study. BMJ Open 9(4):e026939

Burke EA, Carroll R, Ding AW, Yaman M, Walsh JB, McCallion P, McCarron M (2021) Men's bones matter too, a cross sectional study examining bone health among men with intellectual disability in Ireland. OBM Geriatr 5(4):1–1

Campbell NL, Maidment I, Fox C, Khan B, Boustani M (2013) The 2012 update to the anticholinergic cognitive burden scale. J Am Geriatr Soc 61(S1):S142–S143

Carli M, Kolachalam S, Longoni B, Pintaudi A, Baldini M, Aringhieri S, Fasciani I, Annibale P, Maggio R, Scarselli M (2021) Atypical antipsychotics and metabolic syndrome: from molecular mechanisms to clinical differences. Pharmaceuticals 14(3):238

Chaidez V, Hansen RL, Hertz-Picciotto I (2014) Gastrointestinal problems in children with autism, developmental delays or typical development. J Autism Dev Disord 44(5):1117–1127

Curtis JS, Kennedy SE, Attarha B, Edwards L, Jacob R (2021) Upper gastrointestinal disorders in adult patients with intellectual and developmental disabilities. Cureus 13(6):e15384

Dahlgren G, Whitehead M (1993) Tackling inequalities in health: what can we learn from what has been tried? Working paper, London: King's Fund, accessible in: Dahlgren G, Whitehead M. (2007) European strategies for tackling social inequities in health: Levelling up Part 2. WHO Regional office for Europe, Copenhagen. http://www.euro.who.int/__data/assets/pdf_file/0018/103824/E89384.pdf

Dahlgren G, Whitehead M (2021) The Dahlgren-Whitehead model of health determinants: 30 years on and still chasing rainbows. Public Health 199:20–24

Dairo YM, Collett J, Dawes H, Oskrochi GR (2016) Physical activity levels in adults with intellectual disabilities: A systematic review. Prev Med Rep 4:209–219

Davis S, Durvasula S, Merhi D, Young P, Traini D, Bosnic-Anticevich S (2016) The ability of people with intellectual disability to use inhalers–an exploratory mixed methods study. J Asthma 53(1):86–93

de Castilho LS, de Menezes Rampi C, Cruz AJS, Lages FS, Leão DM, Abreu MHNG (2020) Gastroesophageal reflux disease in patients with developmental disabilities. Extensio 17(36):22–32

de Leeuw MJ, Oppewal A, Elbers RG, Knulst MW, van Maurik MC, van Bruggen MC, Hilgenkamp TI, Bindels PJ, Maes-Festen DA (2022) Healthy ageing and intellectual disability study: summary of findings and the protocol for the 10-year follow-up study. BMJ Open 12(2):e053499

de Vries PJ, Belousova E, Benedik MP, Carter T, Cottin V, Curatolo P, Dahlin M, D'Amato L, d'Augères GB, Ferreira JC, Feucht M (2018) TSC-associated neuropsychiatric disorders (TAND): findings from the TOSCA natural history study. Orphanet J Rare Dis 13(1):1–13

de Winter CF, Evenhuis HM (2014) Cardiovascular disease risks in people with an intellectual disability: causes and interventions. Ned Tijdschr Geneeskd 158:A8002–A8002

de Winter CF, Bastiaanse LP, Hilgenkamp TIM, Evenhuis HM, Echteld MA (2012) Cardiovascular risk factors (diabetes, hypertension, hypercholesterolemia and metabolic syndrome) in older people with intellectual disability: results of the HA-ID study. Res Dev Disabil 33(6):1722–1731

de Winter CF, Bastiaanse LP, Kranendonk SE, Hilgenkamp TIM, Evenhuis HM, Echteld MA (2013) Peripheral arterial disease in older people with intellectual disability in The Netherlands using the ankle-brachial index: results of the HA-ID study. Res Dev Disabil 34(5):1663–1668

de Winter CF, Van den Berge APJ, Schoufour JD, Oppewal A, Evenhuis HM (2016) A 3-year follow-up study on cardiovascular disease and mortality in older people with intellectual disabilities. Res Dev Disabil 53:115–126

Dean S, Marshall J, Whelan E, Watson J, Zorbas C, Cameron AJ (2021) A systematic review of health promotion programs to improve nutrition for people with intellectual disability. Curr Nutrit Rep 10(4):255–266

Deb S, Brizard BA, Limbu B (2020a) Association between epilepsy and challenging behaviour in adults with intellectual disabilities: systematic review and meta-analysis. BJPsych Open 6(5):e114

Deb S, Nancarrow T, Limbu B, Sheehan R, Wilcock M, Branford D, Courtenay K, Perera B, Shankar R (2020b) UK psychiatrists' experience of withdrawal of antipsychotics prescribed for challenging behaviours in adults with intellectual disabilities and/or autism. BJPsych open 6(5):e112

Dellon ES, Liacouras CA, Molina-Infante J, Furuta GT, Spergel JM, Zevit N, Spechler SJ, Attwood SE, Straumann A, Aceves SS, Alexander JA (2018) Updated international consensus diagnostic criteria for eosinophilic esophagitis: proceedings of the AGREE conference. Gastroenterology 155(4):1022–1033

Department of Health (2020) Healthy Ireland, Healthy Eating Guidelines. Government of Ireland. https://www.gov.ie/en/publication/70a2e4-the-food-pyramid/

Dijkhuizen A, Hilgenkamp TI, Krijnen WP, van der Schans CP, Waninge A (2016) The impact of visual impairment on the ability to perform activities of daily living for persons with severe/profound intellectual disability. Res Dev Disabil 48:35–42

Doherty AJ, Atherton H, Boland P, Hastings R, Hives L, Hood K, James-Jenkinson L, Leavey R, Randell E, Reed J, Taggart L (2020) Barriers and facilitators to primary health care for people with intellectual disabilities and/or autism: an integrative review. BJGP open 4(3):bjgpopen20X101030

Dolan E, Lane J, Hillis G, Delanty N (2019) Changing trends in life expectancy in intellectual disability over time. Ir Med J 112(9):1006

Doyle A, O'Sullivan M, Craig S, McConkey R (2021) People with intellectual disability in Ireland are still dying young. J Appl Res Intellect Disabil 34(4):1057–1065

Evenhuis HM, Sjoukes L, Koot HM, Kooijman AC (2009) Does visual impairment lead to additional disability in adults with intellectual disabilities? J Intellect Disabil Res 53(1):19–28

Fellinger J (2022) Intellectual disability and sensory impairment. In Textbook of psychiatry for intellectual disability and autism Spectrum disorder. Springer, Cham, pp 849–867

Forty L (2021) How early childhood events impact upon adult health. In A prescription for healthy living. Academic Press, Elsevier, UK, pp 17–29. https://doi.org/10.1016/B978-0-12-821573-9.00002-3

Franz DN, Bissler JJ, McCormack FX (2010) Tuberous sclerosis complex: neurological, renal and pulmonary manifestations. Neuropediatrics 41(05):199–208

Gale L, Naqvi H, Russ L (2009) Asthma, smoking and BMI in adults with intellectual disabilities: a community-based survey. J Intellect Disabil Res 53(9):787–796

Gerber PJ (2012) The impact of learning disabilities on adulthood: A review of the evidenced-based literature for research and practice in adult education. J Learn Disabil 45(1):31–46

Gidding SS, Allen NB (2019) Cholesterol and atherosclerotic cardiovascular disease: a lifelong problem. J Am Heart Assoc 8(11):e012924

Gidding SS, Rana JS, Prendergast C, McGill H, Carr JJ, Liu K, Colangelo LA, Loria CM, Lima J, Terry JG, Reis JP (2016) Pathobiological determinants of atherosclerosis in youth (PDAY) risk score in young adults predicts coronary artery and abdominal aorta calcium in middle age: the CARDIA study. Circulation 133(2):139–146

Gössler A, Schalamon J, Huber-Zeyringer A, Höllwarth ME (2007) Gastroesophageal reflux and behavior in neurologically impaired children. J Pediatr Surg 42(9):1486–1490

Guthrie S, Lecko C, Roddam H (2015) Care staff perceptions of choking incidents: what details are reported? J Appl Res Intellect Disabil 28(2):121–132

Haider SI, Ansari Z, Vaughan L, Matters H, Emerson E (2014) Prevalence and factors associated with polypharmacy in Victorian adults with intellectual disability. Res Dev Disabil 35(11):3071–3080

Harper L, Ooms A, Tuffrey Wijne I (2021) The impact of nutrition on sleep in people with an intellectual disability: An integrative literature review. J Appl Res Intellect Disabil 34(6):1393–1407

Haveman M, Perry J, Salvador-Carulla L, Walsh PN, Kerr M, van Schrojenstein Lantman-de Valk H, Van Hove G, Berger DM, Azema B, Buono S, Cara AC (2011) Ageing and health status in adults with intellectual disabilities: results of the European POMONA II study. J Intellect Dev Disabil 36(1):49–60

Häßler F, Thome J, Reis O (2015) Polypharmacy in the treatment of subjects with intellectual disability. J Neural Transm 122(1):93–100

Health Service Executive (2008) Strategy to Prevent Falls and Fractures in Ireland's Ageing Population. Report of the National Steering Group on the Prevention of Falls in Older People and the Prevention and Management of Osteoporosis throughout Life. In: Strategic Health Planning. Dr Steeven's Hospital, Dublin 8

Heslop P, Blair P, Fleming P, Hoghton M, Marriott A, Russ L (2013) Confidential inquiry into premature deaths of people with learning disabilities (CIPOLD). Norah Fry Research Centre, Bristol

Hilgenkamp TI, van Wijck R, Evenhuis HM (2012) Low physical fitness levels in older adults with ID: results of the HA-ID study. Res Dev Disabil 33(4):1048–1058

Hill A (2018) 'Gross failure' in man's care led to death from constipation. The Guardian online https://www.theguardian.com/uk-news/2018/feb/08/gross-failure-in-mans-care-led-to-death-from-constipation

Jackson CF, Makin SM, Marson AG, Kerr M (2015) Pharmacological interventions for epilepsy in people with intellectual disabilities. Cochrane Database Syst Rev 2015(9):CD005399

Jansen J, Rozeboom W, Penning C, Evenhuis HM (2013) Prevalence and incidence of myocardial infarction and cerebrovascular accident in ageing persons with intellectual disability. J Intellect Disabil Res 57(7): 681–685

Kanis JA, McCloskey EV, Johansson H, Cooper C, Rizzoli R, Reginster JY (2013) European guidance for the diagnosis and management of osteoporosis in postmenopausal women. Osteoporos Int 24(1):23–57

Kiani R, Miller H (2010) Sensory impairment and intellectual disability. Adv Psychiatr Treat 16(3):228–235

Kiani R, Tyrer F, Jesu A, Bhaumik S, Gangavati S, Walker G, Kazmi S, Barrett M (2014) Mortality from sudden unexpected death in epilepsy (SUDEP) in a cohort of adults with intellectual disability. J Intellect Disabil Res 58(6):508–520

Kinnear D, Morrison J, Allan L, Henderson A, Smiley E, Cooper SA (2018) Prevalence of physical conditions and multimorbidity in a cohort of adults with intellectual disabilities with and without down syndrome: cross-sectional study. BMJ Open 8(2):e018292

Kolset SO, Nordstrøm M, Hope S, Retterstøl K, Iversen PO (2018) Securing rights and nutritional health for persons with intellectual disabilities–a pressing challenge. Food Nutr Res 62. https://doi.org/10.29219/fnr.v62.1268

Krahn GL, Fox MH (2014) Health disparities of adults with intellectual disabilities: what do we know? What do we do? J Appl Res Intellect Disabil 27(5): 431–446

Leader G, Francis K, Mannion A, Chen J (2018) Toileting problems in children and adolescents with parent-reported diagnoses of autism spectrum disorder. J Dev Phys Disabil 30(3):307–327

Leslie WD, Pahlavan PS, Roe EB, Dittberner K (2009) Bone density and fragility fractures in patients with developmental disabilities. Osteoporos Int 20(3): 379–383

Liao P, Vajdic CM, Reppermund S, Cvejic RC, Srasuebkul P, Trollor JN (2022) Mortality rate, risk factors, and causes of death in people with epilepsy and intellectual disability. Seizure 101:75–82

Lin LP, Hsu SW, Yao CH, Lai WJ, Hsu PJ, Wu JL, Chu CM, Lin JD (2015) Risk for osteopenia and osteoporosis in institution-dwelling individuals with intellectual and/or developmental disabilities. Res Dev Disabil 36:108–113

Lott IT, Doran E, Nguyen VQ, Tournay A, Movsesyan N, Gillen DL (2012) Down syndrome and dementia: seizures and cognitive decline. J Alzheimers Dis 29(1):177–185

Lynch L, McCarron M, McCallion P, Burke E (2021) Sedentary behaviour levels in adults with an intellectual disability: a systematic review and meta-analysis. HRB Open Res 3:57

Mac Giolla Phadraig C, McCallion P, Cleary E, McGlinchey E, Burke E, McCarron M, Nunn J (2015) Total tooth loss and complete denture use in older adults with intellectual disabilities in Ireland. J Public Health Dent 75(2):101–108

Manduchi B, Walshe M, Burke É, Carroll R, McCallion P, McCarron M (2021) Prevalence and risk factors of choking in older adults with intellectual disability: results from a national cross-sectional study. J Intellect Develop Disabil 46(2):126–137

Maslen C, Hodge R, Tie K, Lagharne R, Lamb K, Shankar R (2022) Constipation in autistic people and people with learning disabilities. Br J Gen Pract 72(720):348–351

Matthews T, Weston N, Baxter H, Felce D, Kerr M (2008) A general practice-based prevalence study of epilepsy among adults with intellectual disabilities and of its association with psychiatric disorder, behaviour disturbance and carer stress. J Intellect Disabil Res 52(2):163–173

McBride O, Heslop P, Glover G, Taggart T, Hanna-Trainor L, Shevlin M, Murphy J (2021) Prevalence estimation of intellectual disability using national administrative and household survey data: the importance of survey question specificity. Int J Popul Data Sci 6(1):1342

Burke, EA., McCallion, P., Carroll, R., Walsh, J.B. and McCarron, M. (2017) An exploration of the bone health of older adults with an intellectual disability in Ireland. J Intellect Disabil Res, 61(2), pp.99–114

McCarron M, Swinburne J, Burke E, McGlinchey E, Andrews V, Mulryan N, Foran S, McCallion P (2011) Growing older with an intellectual disability in Ireland: first results from the intellectual disability supplement to the Irish longitudinal study on ageing (IDS-TILDA). School of Nursing and Midwifery, Trinity College Dublin, Dublin

McCarron M, Swinburne J, Burke E, McGlinchey E, Carroll R, McCallion P (2013) Patterns of multimorbidity in an older population of persons with an intellectual disability: results from the intellectual disability supplement to the Irish longitudinal study on aging (IDS-TILDA). Res Dev Disabil 34(1):521–527

McCarron M, Carroll R, Kelly C, McCallion P (2015) Mortality rates in the general Irish population compared to those with an intellectual disability from 2003 to 2012. J Appl Res Intellect Disabil 28(5):406–413

McCarron M, McCallion P, Reilly E, Dunne P, Carroll R, Mulryan N (2017a) A prospective 20-year longitudinal follow-up of dementia in persons with down syndrome. J Intellect Disabil Res 61(9):843–852

McCarron M, Haigh M, McCallion P, McCallion P, Carroll R, Burke E, McGlinchey E, O'Donovan MA, McCausland D, Sheerin F, O'Dwyer M (2017b) Health, well-being and social inclusion: ageing with an intellectual disability in Ireland. Evidence from the first ten years of The Intellectual Disability Supplement to The Irish Longitudinal Study on Ageing (IDS-TILDA). https://www.tcd.ie/tcaid/assets/pdf/wave3report.pdf

McGlinchey E, McCallion P, McDermott S, Foley M, Burke EA, O'Donovan M-A, McCausland D, Gibney S, McCarron M (2019) Positive ageing indicators for people with an intellectual disability 2018. Trinity Centre for Ageing and Intellectual Disability, Dublin

McKenzie K, Milton M, Smith G, Ouellette-Kuntz H (2016) Systematic review of the prevalence and incidence of intellectual disabilities: current trends and issues. Curr Dev Disord Rep 3(2):104–115

McLeroy KR, Bibeau D, Steckler A, Glanz K (1988) An ecological perspective on health promotion programs. Health Educ Q 15(4):351–377

Melville CA, Oppewal A, Elinder LS, Freiberger E, Guerra-Balic M, Hilgenkamp TI, Einarsson I, Izquierdo-Gomez RH, Sansano-Nadal O, Rintala P, Cuesta-Vargas A (2017) Definitions, measurement and prevalence of sedentary behaviour in adults with intellectual disabilities—A systematic review. Prev Med 97:62–71

Michie S, Ashford S, Sniehotta FF, Dombrowski SU, Bishop A, French DP (2011) A refined taxonomy of behaviour change techniques to help people change their physical activity and healthy eating behaviours: the CALO-RE taxonomy. Psychol Health 26(11):1479–1498

Moloney M, Hennessy T, Doody O (2021) Reasonable adjustments for people with intellectual disability in acute care: a scoping review of the evidence. BMJ Open 11(2):e039647

Monaghan R, O'Dwyer M, Luus R, Mulryan N, McCallion P, McCarron M, Henman MC (2021) Antiepileptics, psychotropic drugs and seizures in adults with epilepsy and intellectual disability. J Appl Res Intellect Disabil 34(5):1316–1317. 111 Hoboken, NJ : Wiley

Mula M (2017) Epilepsy and psychiatric comorbidities: drug selection. Curr Treat Options Neurol 19(12): 1–11

National Health Service Scotland (2022) The 7-Steps medication review. https://managemeds.scot.nhs.uk/for-healthcare-professionals/principles/the-7-steps-medication-review/. Accessed 21 Nov 2022

NICE (2012) The epilepsies: the diagnosis and management of the epilepsies in adults and children in primary and secondary care. NICE clinical guideline 137 guidance.nice.org.uk/cg137

O'Brien F, McCallion P, Carroll R, O'Dwyer M, Burke E, McCarron M (2021) The prevalence, awareness, treatment, and control of hypertension in older adults with an intellectual disability in Ireland: a cross sectional study. Eur J Cardiovasc Nurs 20(4):315–323

O'Connor M, Hurley E, O'Connor T (2018) Respiratory health of the nation. Irish Thoracic Society. https://tinyurl.com/2p88b43e

O'Donovan MA, McCallion P, McCausland D, McCarron M (2020) Choice as people age with intellectual disability: An Irish perspective. In Choice, preference, and disability. Springer, Cham, pp 303–315

O'Neill AC, Richter GT (2013) Pharyngeal dysphagia in children with down syndrome. Otolaryngol Head Neck Surg 149(1):146–150

O'Dwyer M, Peklar J, McCallion P, McCarron M, Henman MC (2016) Factors associated with polypharmacy and excessive polypharmacy in older people with intellectual disability differ from the general population: a cross-sectional observational nationwide study. BMJ Open 6(4):e010505

O'Dwyer M, Peklar J, Mulryan N, McCallion P, McCarron M, Henman MC (2017) Prevalence, patterns and factors associated with psychotropic use in older adults with intellectual disabilities in Ireland. J Intellect Disabil Res 61(10):969–983

O'Dwyer M, Peklar J, Mulryan N, McCallion P, McCarron M, Henman MC (2018) Prevalence and patterns of anti-epileptic medication prescribing in the treatment of epilepsy in older adults with intellectual disabilities. J Intellect Disabil Res 62(3):245–261

O'Leary L, Cooper SA, Hughes-McCormack L (2018a) Early death and causes of death of people with intellectual disabilities: a systematic review. J Appl Res Intellect Disabil 31(3):325–342

O'Leary L, Taggart L, Cousins W (2018b) Healthy lifestyle behaviours for people with intellectual disabilities: An exploration of organizational barriers and enablers. J Appl Res Intellect Disabil 31:122–135

Oppewal A, Hilgenkamp TI (2019) Physical fitness is predictive for 5-year survival in older adults with intellectual disabilities. J Appl Res Intellect Disabil 32(4):958–966

Oppewal A, Hilgenkamp TI, van Wijck R, Schoufour JD, Evenhuis HM (2014) Physical fitness is predictive for a decline in daily functioning in older adults with intellectual disabilities: results of the HA-ID study. Res Dev Disabil 35(10):2299–2315

Oppewal A, Hilgenkamp TI, van Wijck R, Schoufour JD, Evenhuis HM (2015) Physical fitness is predictive for a decline in the ability to perform instrumental activities of daily living in older adults with intellectual disabilities: results of the HA-ID study. Res Dev Disabil 41:76–85

Oppewal A, Schoufour JD, van der Maarl HJ, Evenhuis HM, Hilgenkamp TI, Festen DA (2018) Causes of mortality in older people with intellectual disability: results from the HA-ID study. Am J Intellect Dev Disabil 123(1):61–71

Oppewal A, Maes-Festen D, Hilgenkamp TIM (2020) Small steps in fitness, major leaps in health for adults with intellectual disabilities. Exerc Sport Sci Rev 48(2):92–97

Pavlovic M, Berenji K, Bukurov M (2017) Screening of celiac disease in down syndrome-old and new dilemmas. World J Clin Cases 5(7):264

Peate I (2018) Anatomy and physiology, 5. The musculoskeletal system. Br J Healthcare Assist 12(1):6–9

Peklar J, Kos M, O'Dwyer M, McCarron M, McCallion P, Kenny RA, Henman MC (2017) Medication and supplement use in older people with and without intellectual disability: an observational, cross-sectional study. PLoS One 12(9):e0184390

Prasher VP, Janicki MP (eds) (2018) Physical health of adults with intellectual and developmental disabilities. Springer, New York

Robertson J, Hatton C, Emerson E, Baines S (2015) Prevalence of epilepsy among people with intellectual disabilities: a systematic review. Seizure 29:46–62

Robertson J, Chadwick D, Baines S, Emerson E, Hatton C (2018a) People with intellectual disabilities and dysphagia. Disabil Rehabil 40(11):1345–1360

Robertson J, Baines S, Emerson E, Hatton C (2018b) Prevalence of constipation in people with intellectual disability: A systematic review. J Intellect Develop Disabil 43(4):392–406

Røstad-Tollefsen HK, Kolset SO, Retterstøl K, Hesselberg H, Nordstrøm M (2021) Factors influencing the opportunities of supporting staff to promote a healthy diet in adults with intellectual disabilities. J Appl Res Intellect Disabil 34(3):733–741

Roth GA, Abate D, Abate KH, Abay SM, Abbafati C, Abbasi N, Abbastabar H, Abd-Allah F, Abdela J, Abdelalim A, Abdollahpour I (2018) Global, regional, and national age-sex-specific mortality for 282 causes of death in 195 countries and territories, 1980–2017: a systematic analysis for the global burden of disease study 2017. Lancet 392(10159):1736–1788

Ruiz-Giménez J, Sánchez-Alvarez JC, Cañadillas-Hidalgo F, Serrano-Castro PJ (2010) Antiepileptic treatment in patients with epilepsy and other comorbidities. Seizure 19(7):375–382

Ryan J, McCallion P, McCarron M, Luus R, Burke EA (2021) Overweight/obesity and chronic health conditions in older people with intellectual disability in Ireland. J Intellect Disabil Res 65(12):1097–1109

Rydzewska E, Hughes-McCormack LA, Gillberg C, Henderson A, MacIntyre C, Rintoul J, Cooper SA (2019) Prevalence of sensory impairments, physical and intellectual disabilities, and mental health in children and young people with self/proxy-reported autism: observational study of a whole country population. Autism 23(5):1201–1209

Sallis JF, Cervero RB, Ascher W, Henderson KA, Kraft MK, Kerr J (2006) An ecological approach to creating active living communities. Annu Rev Public Health 27:297–322

Sarmast ST, Abdullahi AM, Jahan N (2020) Current classification of seizures and epilepsies: scope, limitations and recommendations for future action. Cureus 12(9):e10549

Sarna SK (2010) Colonic motility in health. In Colonic Motility: From Bench Side to Bedside. Morgan & Claypool Life Sciences, San Rafael, CA

Schroeder EC, DuBois L, Sadowsky M, Hilgenkamp TI (2020) Hypertension in adults with intellectual disability: prevalence and risk factors. Am J Prev Med 58(5):630–637

Service Scotland (2022) https://managemeds.scot.nhs.uk/for-healthcare-professionals/principles/the-7-steps-medicationreview/

Shankar R, Rowe C, Van Hoorn A, Henley W, Laugharne R, Cox D, Pande R, Roy A, Sander JW (2018) Under representation of people with epilepsy and intellectual disability in research. PLoS One 13(6):e0198261

Shankar R, Wilcock M, Oak K, McGowan P, Sheehan R (2019) Stopping, rationalising or optimising antipsychotic drug treatment in people with intellectual disability and/or autism. Drug Ther Bull 57(1):10–13

Sharr C, Lavigne J, Elsharkawi IM, Ozonoff A, Baumer N, Brasington C, Cannon S, Crissman B, Davidson E, Florez JC, Kishnani P (2016) Detecting celiac disease in patients with down syndrome. Am J Med Genet A 170(12):3098–3105

Smith E, Stogios N, Au E, Maksyutynska K, De R, Ji A, Sørensen ME, John LS, Lin HY, Desarkar P, Lunsky Y (2022) The metabolic adverse effects of antipsychotic use in individuals with intellectual and/or developmental disability (IDD): A systematic review and meta-analysis. Acta Psychiatrica Scand 146(3):201–214

Somerville H, Tzannes G, Wood J, Shun A, Hill C, Arrowsmith F, Slater A, O'Loughlin EV (2008) Gastrointestinal and nutritional problems in severe developmental disability. Dev Med Child Neurol 50(9):712–716

Steenbergen HA, Waninge A, van Wijck R, de Jong J, van der Schans CP (n.d.) Maintenance and quality assurance of a healthy lifestyle in an organization for people with intellectual disability

Stevens A, Courtney-Long E, Gillespie C, Armour BS (2014) Peer reviewed: hypertension among US adults by disability status and type, national health and nutrition examination survey, 2001–2010. Prev Chronic Dis 11:E139

Straetmans JM, van Schrojenstein Lantman-de HM, Schellevis FG, Dinant GJ (2007) Health problems of people with intellectual disabilities: the impact for general practice. Br J Gen Pract 57(534):64–66

Sumida K, Molnar MZ, Potukuchi PK, Thomas F, Lu JL, Yamagata K, Kalantar-Zadeh K, Kovesdy CP (2019) Constipation and risk of death and cardiovascular events. Atherosclerosis 281:114–120

Swender SL, Matson JL, Mayville SB, Gonzalez ML, McDowell D (2006) A functional assessment of handmouthing among persons with severe and profound intellectual disability. J Intellect Dev Disabil 31(2):95–100

Taylor D, Paton C, Kapur S (2015) The Maudsley prescribing guidelines in psychiatry. John Wiley and sons Ltd., Chichester

Truesdale M, Melville C, Barlow F, Dunn K, Henderson A, Hughes-McCormack LA, McGarty A, Rydzewska E, Smith GS, Symonds J, Jani B (2021) Respiratory-associated deaths in people with intellectual disabilities: a systematic review and meta-analysis. BMJ Open 11(7):e043658

Tsou AY, Bulova P, Capone G, Chicoine B, Gelaro B, Harville TO, Martin BA, McGuire DE, McKelvey KD, Peterson M, Tyler C (2020) Medical care of adults with down syndrome: A clinical guideline. JAMA 324(15):1543–1556

Turky A, Felce D, Jones G, Kerr M (2011) A prospective case control study of psychiatric disorders in adults with epilepsy and intellectual disability. Epilepsia 52(7):1223–1230

Van De Louw J, Vorstenbosch R, Vinck L, Penning C, Evenhuis H (2009) Prevalence of hypertension in adults with intellectual disability in The Netherlands. J Intellect Disabil Res 53(1):78–84

Van Den Akker M, Maaskant MA, Van der Meijden RJM (2006) Cardiac diseases in people with intellectual disability. J Intellect Disabil Res 50(7): 515–522

Van Naarden Braun K, Christensen D, Doernberg N, Schieve L, Rice C, Wiggins L, Schendel D, Yeargin-Allsopp M (2015) Trends in the prevalence of autism spectrum disorder, cerebral palsy, hearing loss, intellectual disability, and vision impairment, metropolitan Atlanta, 1991–2010. PLoS One 10(4):e0124120

van Schijndel-Speet M, Evenhuis HM, van Wijck R, Van Montfort KCAGM, Echteld MA (2017) A structured physical activity and fitness programme for older adults with intellectual disabilities: results of a cluster-randomised clinical trial. J Intellect Disabil Res 61(1):16–29

Van Splunder JANG, Stilma JS, Bernsen RM, Evenhuis HM (2006) Prevalence of visual impairment in adults with intellectual disabilities in The Netherlands: cross-sectional study. Eye 20(9):1004–1010

Van Timmeren EA, Van der Schans CP, Van der Putten AAJ, Krijnen WP, Steenbergen HA, van Schrojenstein Lantman-de Valk HMJ, Waninge A (2017) Physical health issues in adults with severe or profound intellectual and motor disabilities: a systematic review of cross-sectional studies. J Intellect Disabil Res 61(1):30–49

Varley J, Delanty N, Normand C, Coyne I, McQuaid L, Collins C, Boland M, Grimson J, Fitzsimons M (2010) Epilepsy in Ireland: towards the primary–tertiary care continuum. Seizure 19(1):47–52

Versacci P, Di Carlo D, Digilio MC, Marino B (2018) Cardiovascular disease in down syndrome. Curr Opin Pediatr 30(5):616–622

Veugelers R, Benninga MA, Calis EA, Willemsen SP, Evenhuis H, Tibboel D, Penning C (2010) Prevalence and clinical presentation of constipation in children with severe generalized cerebral palsy. Dev Med Child Neurol 52(9):e216–e221

Vis JC, de Bruin-Bon RH, Bouma BJ, Huisman SA, Imschoot L, van den Brink K, Mulder BJ (2010) Congenital heart defects are under-recognised in adult patients with Down's syndrome. Heart 96(18): 1480–1484

Vlot-van Anrooij K, Hilgenkamp TI, Leusink GL, van der Cruijsen A, Jansen H, Naaldenberg J, van der Velden K (2020) Improving environmental capacities for health promotion in support settings for people with intellectual disabilities: inclusive design of the DIHASID tool. Int J Environ Res Public Health 17(3):794

Wallace RA, Schluter P (2008) Audit of cardiovascular disease risk factors among supported adults with intellectual disability attending an ageing clinic. J Intellect Dev Disabil 33(1):48–58

Walsh J, Henry Y, Fatayerji D, Eastell R (2009) Lumbar spine peak bone mass and bone turnover in men and women: a longitudinal study. Osteoporos Int 20: 355–362

Watkins L, O'Dwyer M, Shankar R (2019) New anti-seizure medication for elderly epileptic patients. Expert Opin Pharmacother 20(13):1601–1608

Weatherburn CJ, Heath CA, Mercer SW, Guthrie B (2017) Physical and mental health comorbidities of epilepsy: population-based cross-sectional analysis of 1.5 million people in Scotland. Seizure 45:125–131

Wedemeyer RS, Blume H (2014) Pharmacokinetic drug interaction profiles of proton pump inhibitors: an update. Drug Saf 37(4):201–211

WHO Scientific Group on Prevention, Management of Osteoporosis and World Health Organization (2003) Prevention and management of osteoporosis: report of a WHO scientific group (No. 921). World Health Organization, Geneva

Willems M, Hilgenkamp TI, Havik E, Waninge A, Melville CA (2017) Use of behaviour change techniques in lifestyle change interventions for people with intellectual disabilities: A systematic review. Res Dev Disabil 60:256–268

Yang L, Wang Y, Chen X, Zhang C, Chen J, Cheng H, Zhang L (2021) Risk Factors for Epilepsy: A National Cross-Sectional Study from National Health and Nutrition Examination Survey 2013 to 2018. Int Gen Med 14:4405

Ageing and Intellectual Disability

10

Philip McCallion and Mary McCarron

Chapter Topics

Growth in the ageing population of people with intellectual disability is well established as are increasing concerns about health, changes in function and the potential for loneliness and isolation and often unwanted transitions to other settings, which may be justified as better able to address increasing needs.

- This chapter acknowledges such concerns but also addresses what it means to grow older successfully, to age in place and to continue to exercise self-determination.
- Drawing on international and interdisciplinary perspectives as well as longitudinal data on the ageing of this population, the emphasis will be on prevention, health promotion and supports rather than "treatment" of ageing.
- The chapter will also highlight major challenges to be addressed, how services are changing and the need to shift to recognising a greater likelihood of ageing independently and with family rather than in out-of-home and provider-based care.

- The specific issues related to ageing and intellectual disabilities to include healthy ageing, dementia and palliative care will be explored.
- New and continuing needs for family caregiver support, training for staff, the holistic provision of end-of-life care and continuing needs for policy change will also be addressed.

Introduction

The efforts of families, providers, communities, professionals and people themselves have improved the lives of people with intellectual disability and they are now ageing in greater numbers. All older adults need good management of age-related chronic conditions, housing that accommodates their changing abilities with age, adequate nutrition, timely and appropriate health care and opportunities for positive social engagement. However, older adults with intellectual disability also have unique needs and life experiences compared with age peers in the general population that must be considered including high levels of avoidable or treatable causes of premature death (Heslop et al. 2014) and less opportunities for self-determination in their ageing lives (McCallion and Ferretti 2017). It also appears that comparatively, health became progressively poorer as people with intellectual disability age beyond 45 years (McCallion et al. 2021). Problems with definitions, timeframes and

P. McCallion
Temple University, Philadelphia, PA, USA
e-mail: philip.mccallion@temple.edu

M. McCarron (✉)
Trinity College Dublin, Dublin, Ireland
e-mail: mccarrm@tcd.ie

© The Author(s), under exclusive license to Springer Nature Switzerland AG 2023
F. Sheerin, C. Doyle (eds.), *Intellectual Disabilities: Health and Social Care Across the Lifespan*,
https://doi.org/10.1007/978-3-031-27496-1_10

sources of data notwithstanding in the studies available, there appears to be a greater prevalence among ageing adults with intellectual disability, as compared to the general population and their own younger years, of epilepsy, sensory impairments, dental disease, osteoporosis, dementia, gastrointestinal disorders, respiratory disorders (such as pneumonia), mental illness and behavioural challenges (McCarron et al. 2011). Ageing people with intellectual disability have also been shown to become high and frequent users of primary healthcare services given different patterns and combinations of morbidities and are less likely to receive preventive interventions, with utilisation data particularly suggesting a lack of preparedness for ageing people with intellectual disability in general population health delivery (McCarron et al. 2013; McCallion et al. 2019). A lack of surveillance, inequalities in access to health services and little training in the typical health and functioning issues in older adults with intellectual disability may increase the potential for under-reporting of conditions (McCallion et al. 2017a). The higher and different comorbidity, and poorer management of health conditions, may also mean greater and significant physical health-related burdens fall upon caregivers and older persons with intellectual disabilities themselves (McCarron et al. 2013).

Ageing with Disadvantages

Data available does suggest that people with intellectual disabilities enter the ageing process from a particularly disadvantaged position with long-standing health concerns and greater risk of adverse outcomes (McCallion et al. 2017b). In childhood and younger adulthood, they are more likely to have lived in poverty, experienced poorer physical and mental health and lived unhealthy and sedentary lifestyles than the general population. The lives of adults with intellectual disabilities have featured economic, educational and social exclusion. The low rates of employment (Bigby et al. 2014) people with intellectual disabilities experience mean limited opportunities to accumulate wealth, and there is a heavy reliance on government income support schemes that are frequently close to or below poverty lines. There is little access to private health and social care systems, often features of best health and longer lives in the general population; and they are instead dependent on underfunded public health and welfare systems. People with intellectual disabilities also experience social exclusion even when living in "community" and this results in their having small and deficient informal networks to offer instrumental support, social participation and emotional well-being. More recent advances in offering individual advocacy have helped but are more likely targeted to younger adults, and despite individualised, person-centred and participant-directed planning strategies, there is little history of individualised negotiation of formal services.

Premature Ageing

Research on premature ageing among people with intellectual disabilities has reflected unique patterns of ageing, particularly in people with Down syndrome, where features appear earlier such as dementia symptoms (McCarron et al. 2014). This has encouraged efforts to have mainstream services re-examine ages 60 and 65 years as eligibility cut-offs for ageing-focused services. However, it has also obscured middle age for people with intellectual disabilities with many regarding people in their 40s or 50s as old (Bigby et al. 2014). This is a disservice to the individuals themselves and encourages neglect of the middle-age stage of life in people with intellectual disabilities including attention to the opportunities in that stage of life for screening and health promotion to prepare for ageing years. Given an ever-extending old age in the general population, we now see efforts to differentiate between young, middle and old-old (McCallion et al. 2021). Attention to a healthy and extended older age for people with intellectual disabilities requires similar attention.

Evenhuis et al. (2012) in the Netherlands have challenged the notion of premature ageing, believing that if people with intellectual disabilities have a pattern of age-related health vulnerabilities different from the general population, this results from frailty and high vulnerability to adverse health conditions, rather than ageing itself. They confirmed that people with intellectual disabilities at age 50–64 had prevalence levels of frailty (11%) similar to that of the general population aged at 65 years and older (7–9%), but argued that such frailty among people with intellectual disabilities was associated with preventable and reversible low levels of physical activity, social relationships and community participation (Hilgenkamp et al. 2012; Schoufour et al. 2012). Such findings have important implications for the design of services and encourage investment in prevention and health promotion approaches rather than the more expensive treatment and care management approaches our service system tends to favour (Kaneda 2006).

Nevertheless, these findings of health impairments at an earlier age for people with intellectual disabilities encourage attention to physical and mental health issues. Similarly, findings on social isolation and lack of engagement suggest that remediation of these issues should be a primary target for staff supporting people with intellectual disabilities.

Table 10.1 Physical and mental health concerns and differences

- Higher rates of unhealthy lifestyles, with highest rates of unhealthy weight gain, obesity, cardiovascular disease (CVD) and CVD-related mortality among those living independently
- Higher levels of medication use and excess polypharmacy
- Poorer dental hygiene with elevated levels of missing teeth but poor rates of replacement, e.g. with dentures
- Higher rates of females having poorer health than males as they age
- Rates of sedentary lifestyles meaning they are less likely than the general population to achieve levels of physical activity that would positively affect health
- Higher rates of chronic conditions
- Earlier onset of menopause for women with intellectual disability with implications for dementia and early mortality
- Increased pain levels, sarcopenia, osteoporosis and arthritis
- Rates of mental health concerns range from 20% to 40% of assessed older people with intellectual disability with rates increasing as they age
- Great levels of side effects of medications as they may metabolise these differently from others
- Higher rates of sensory impairments that increase communication difficulties
- Rates of ageing-specific disorders (such as Alzheimer's disease) that may increase predisposition of persons with intellectual disability to depression and anxiety, as may poorly understood life events such as bereavements and abuse

Ageing: The Impact on Physical and Mental Health

Using both administrative datasets and population surveys, ageing persons with intellectual disabilities (as compared with older adults in the general population) have been found to have a range of different health needs and experiences (see Table 10.1, and for a more comprehensive review, see McCallion et al. 2019).

van Schrojenstein Lantman-De Valk et al. (2000) found, compared with others, that 318 people with intellectual disabilities, receiving health care within a general practice had 2.5 times the health problems of those without such lifelong disabilities. Haveman et al. (2009) agreed that this state was highly influenced by a lack of information, lack of exercise, poor mobility, poor

eating habits and medication use. Other findings are that epilepsy, unaddressed pain, comorbidity, life events and the consequences of polypharmacy appear of most concern (McCallion 2014). Longer life in people with intellectual disabilities (McCallion et al. 2019) is also the greatest known risk factor for dementia. Prevalence of dementia in people with Down syndrome, for example, has been reported to double every 5 years from 9% between the ages of 45 and 49 years to 18% between ages 50 and 54 years and 32% between ages 55 and 59 years (Coppus et al. 2008), with an estimated cumulative risk of 90% by age 65 (McCarron et al. 2017).

As noted by McCallion and McCarron (2015) the type of care and surveillance offered is also of concern:

- People with intellectual disabilities are more likely (compared to general population peers) to lead unhealthy lifestyles, not accessing health promotion and health screening services, all of which contribute to physical ailments in later life.
- Health problems of persons with intellectual disabilities are less likely to be recognised, and the reliance for their health management on decisions by proxy (family members and care staff) increases access barriers including that health needs identified at screening are not subsequently met.
- People with intellectual disabilities as compared to peers without identified disability have higher levels of obesity, have a more sedentary lifestyle, participate less in physical activity and are more likely to consume high-fat diets, prepared by staff and family members with their own challenges in these areas.
- Health promotion programmes themselves are seldom targeted at people with intellectual disabilities, yet they have been shown to increase disease prevention and case finding.
- There is a lack of specialist knowledge and training among multidisciplinary team members such as therapists, social workers and psychologists.

Given ageing presents increased health needs, opportunities for community living and quality lives must also be addressed, as they too promote better health. For the general population, independent, successful ageing and retirement is supported by pensions and other financial resources, good health and health care, social networks and family supports (McCallion et al. 2013); these resources are not always available to people with intellectual disabilities. The absence of their own children and spouses and of accrued retirement income means that for people with intellectual disabilities, community maintenance and participation in older age will be more difficult. In addition, as the family caregivers of adults with intellectual disabilities themselves age and move perhaps beyond their caring capacity, additional formal supervised living arrangements may need to be developed, but there are questions by societies about their affordability (Bigby et al. 2014). Even in countries with well-developed residential networks, such as Ireland, the USA and the UK, the increased longevity among those already living there means that fewer places are becoming freed up over time, leaving many to wonder how additional ageing lives will be supported (McCallion and McCarron 2015). An equally critical issue is where is the voice of people with intellectual disabilities themselves as decisions are made about their ageing lives.

Approaches to Care in Ageing

People are often stigmatised when they have dementia, other chronic disease and intellectual disability (McCarron et al. 2022). Person-centred approaches to care that empower the individual and improve their quality of life often counteract perceptions that individuality is lessened (Kitwood 1997) by disease, particularly if the approach by staff addresses comfort, attachment, inclusion, occupation and identity.

Relationship-Based Care

A relationship-based approach to care emphasises how relationships impact quality of life and how care is given meaning by those relationships. The care triad (Adams and Grieder 2005) involves the person with an intellectual disability, family and paid caregivers and is nested within larger care networks and broader health systems that impact upon the individual and caregivers, for example: by making available resources such as respite care.

In intellectual disability care settings this is particularly important where relationships with staff carers have developed over long periods of time (McCarron et al. 2017) and emotional connection to people whom the individual knows, and loves remains intact as a disease such as dementia progresses. Decades of knowing and working with someone and the authenticity of relationships become the cornerstone of good person-centred care. The promotion of person-based and relationship-based approaches to care must be combined with a strengths-based approach, emphasising the character strengths and values (such as kindness, honesty) (Niemiec et al. 2017) of both the person and of caregivers such as families and staff. In older age there is also an opportunity for staff-based services to reach out to and include families (both previously connected and previously distant or separated), as later years for all are often a time to rekindle connections and address losses. Older age is a time that benefits from planning.

Advance Care Planning

Issues such as guardianship and advance care planning should be addressed early in the ageing process. A health crisis and imminent death is not the moment to address nutrition and hydration concerns, pain management, seizure control, resuscitation or place of death as decisions are often charged by high emotions resulting in great distress for everyone involved (McCarron et al. 2017). Individuals with intellectual disability present with different needs and varying levels of ability and willingness to engage in decision-making regarding their end-of-life care. As noted by the International Summit on Intellectual Disability and Dementia, advance care planning is recommended prior to extensive progression of dementia, and specialist training is required for staff who work in more generalised intellectual disability, palliative, hospice or dementia services (McCallion et al. 2017b). A proactive approach to decision-making with regard to end-of-life care was emphasised. There are previously documented concerns that staff often lack training in talking about death with people with intellectual disabilities and may even fear discussing death (Tuffrey-Wijne et al. 2017). This is likely to be also true for caring families. There are educational materials on end-of-life preparations available for carers as well as materials for persons with intellectual disability and their peers (Weise 2022). Care is also best supported when underpinned by person-centred, relationship-based and family-focused strategies (Kirkendall et al. 2012).

People with mild to moderate intellectual disabilities are often able to articulate their wishes with regard to advanced illness and end-of-life decision-making (Stancliffe et al. 2017). In a study of four people with intellectual disabilities, advance care planning was positively influenced by a pacing and process of planning where they felt supported in making their own choices, there was open and honest communication, and there was confidence that there would be continued support in their current lifestyle and associated plans (McKenzie et al. 2017). Facilitating such processes is increasingly the role of staff supporting people with intellectual disabilities.

Social Networks and Supports

Community living and the support of social networks for people with intellectual disabilities are relatively new phenomena given that institutional approaches have previously dominated service delivery. The continuing influence of normalisation (Nirje 1969) and later, social role valorisation (Wolfensberger 1985) has moved people from institutional, congregated settings into the community and increased commitment to the community maintenance of those living in family care (Lightfoot and McCallion 2016). Yet, there are reports of people with intellectual disabilities moving to institutional settings as they age (Bigby et al. 2014).

The issue is further complicated by questioning by some, of the absolute value of community living. There are arguments that the data actually highlights that community presence is easier to achieve than community integration, and although movement of people with intellectual disabilities into the community has successfully occurred, achieving actual integration has not (Verdonschot et al. 2009). But such questions rather than permitting a return to institutions instead challenge whether the community-based system of care for adults with intellectual disability is fit for purpose when it comes to ageing.

The concept of continuing community integration of adults with intellectual disabilities is poorly understood and deserves to be considered in a manner similar to that of ageing in the general population. Placing value on relationships with families and peers, developing and supporting friendships and further exploring of the "sense of community" for people with intellectual disabilities as they age are warranted (McCausland et al. 2020).

In addition, the prevalent negative perceptions of ageing services for the general population held by disability providers and advocates and outright ageism are actually producing protective attitudes among staff towards ageing persons with intellectual disabilities and perhaps supporting self-serving desires to continue to maintain these individuals within intellectual disabilities services. An openness to new types of supports, engagement with service provision for other older adults and a shared view of the attributes of successful ageing (Rowe and Kahn 1998) are needed. This approach would have the additional benefit of potentially supporting improved cross-system responses and more affordable support. Nevertheless, the disadvantages for health and well-being in ageing of the well-documented smaller social networks and absence for many of meaningful family and friend relationships must be acknowledged (McCausland et al. 2020).

Family Caregiving

Changing family demographics—declines in birth rates and family sizes, economic concerns and rural to urban transitions—have been straining family caring (Jackson et al. 2011). Popular conceptions are that caregiving families are likely to include children, persons with less severe levels of intellectual disability and persons with less significant health and care issues. But families are coping with care needs at least as pressing and demanding as those in group home facilities (Lightfoot and McCallion 2015). When parents die, siblings or more distant relatives often assume care and there have been suggestions they are less ready to replace the "caring for" primary care role (Bigby 1997). However, siblings are stepping in and assuming such care in very large

numbers (Zendell 2011; Fujiura 2012). There are new challenges for caregivers given the increased ageing of people with intellectual disabilities.

Siblings have always played a role in the care of their family members with intellectual disabilities (McCallion and Toseland 1993). Zendell (2011), in a national survey sample, found a full range of caregiving experiences for siblings regardless of gender. Traditionally, women were the primary caregivers but gender patterns are now changing. An important concern for care workers and nurses is not to stereotype families. Male caregivers, in particular, have reported feeling isolated and judged in the role (McCallion and Kolomer 2003; Fujiura 2012). Where families will need help is in exploring continued maintenance in their existing home; accessing of services for both the individual with intellectual disabilities and themselves; involvement of other family members, neighbours and friends in "circles of support" (O'Brien and O'Brien 1998); and how to purchase services from a range of providers (Hewitt et al. 2010; Bigby et al. 2014; McCallion and McCarron 2015).

There are increasing questions as to how nations will afford expanding formal systems of old age supports. The care of ageing persons with intellectual disabilities and support for caregivers have remained largely with disabilities service providers. This is now changing, for example, in the USA, the Administration on Aging/Administration on Community Living has included family caregivers of people with intellectual disabilities as a targeted population for agencies that traditionally serve older adults (McCallion and McCarron 2015). Such programs represent an area where expertise in intellectual disabilities needs to be embedded.

Ageing in the Community as Opposed to Ageing in Community-Based Services

There has been a long-standing concern that the organisation of services for persons with intellectual disabilities has been focused upon those not living independently or with family. A view of ageing as illness and decline has encouraged maintenance of people in group homes and residential settings and delivery of professionally led services or in some cases transfer to nursing home settings (McCallion et al. 2017b). Yet success in moving people with intellectual disabilities to more community-based options and the avoidance of placement in out-of-family and independent home settings mean an increasing number of independent and family-based living situations. This has created a need for new types of service options such as participant-directed services and individualised budget, disability-sensitive and informed health and hospital services, greater supports of family caregivers, both parent and sibling, future planning initiatives and home modification and other supports so that living independently or with family continues to meet personal desires and not become increasingly restrictive (Lightfoot and McCallion 2015; McCarron et al. 2018). Success in achieving supports for continued living will require more of a household rather than individual focus (everyone in the home, caregiver and peers as well as the person with an intellectual disability) by staff and by service packages (Lightfoot and McCallion 2015). There is also an on-going need to redesign social care and nursing roles including embedding intellectual disabilities expertise in hospital and other community-based service providers currently only equipped to support others in the general population (Sheerin et al. 2021).

"Services" should not be seen only in terms of placement and day programs. Attention to quality health care, physical activity and social connection/participation earlier in life may positively influence both the nature and severity of issues that otherwise would impair the later life of people with intellectual disabilities. Person-centred, flexible, individualised support available during adulthood may reduce the challenge of adapting support to meet changed needs as people age. Finally, if the focus of remaining in the community was less on building group homes and intellectual disability-specific formal programs and instead was focused on supporting people where they have always lived, there will likely be a greater range of alternatives and greater integration with other ageing-related resources. The reorientation of workforces to support this is critical (McCarron et al. 2018).

A growing interest in such maintenance of independence and community living of ageing persons with intellectual disabilities is being informed by consideration of self-determination principles.

Self-Determination

Much attention in ageing for the general population is on self-determination and the relationship between autonomy and competence. Autonomy is experiencing choice in one's behaviours as opposed to pressure or coercion, believing one's own actions will improve their situation (health or otherwise) and the perception of having competence (the skills, knowledge and ability) to control important outcomes (Williams and Deci 1996; Williams et al. 1998). As older adults experience chronic conditions and their consequences and other challenges, effectiveness in self-management of health, health care and daily living requires both the experience of autonomy and feelings of competence (Williams et al. 2004; McCallion and Ferretti 2017). Further, reductions in the ability and possibilities to exercise self-determination whether initiated by self or others (professionals, caregivers and society at large) have consequences for:

1. Sense of and actual experience of health and well-being
2. Stressfulness of situations
3. Increasing dependence
4. Deterioration in the ability to perform tasks (Breitholtz et al. 2013)

Success in supporting self-determination in older age requires commitment of professionals and caregivers, balancing of safety, purposeful efforts for involvement in decision-making and ensuring the views of the ageing person matter (Breitholtz et al. 2013; Ekelund et al. 2014; McCallion and Ferretti 2017).

For nursing and social care staff, much effort is focused on managing the consequences of chronic diseases by ensuring adherence to recommended protocols and the pursuit of health behaviour change (McCallion and Ferretti 2015). Models for care such as the Chronic Care Model (Wagner et al. 2001) build upon proactive individuals actively managing their conditions in collaboration with thoughtful care practice teams of healthcare professionals and community supports encouraging and underpinning the individual's actions (Wagner et al. 2001). Hibbard et al. (2010) have raised that while healthcare professionals are supportive of individuals taking and following through on instructions and advice, they do not treat individuals as partners in care. As people age with an intellectual disability a readiness to acknowledge the centrality of self-determination seems critical.

A key issue is that a majority of older adults (including people with intellectual disabilities) wish to remain in their own homes and communities throughout their ageing years (Pynoos et al. 2009; McCallion and Ferretti 2017). The right balance in staffing, environmental modification and support of families caring rather than transfer to increasingly formal services increases the informal supports likely to be critical to remaining there (Sabia 2008). Considerations of ageing in place emphasise the importance of the fit between one's home and the individual. The person environment fit is both subjective (housing-related identity) and objective (housing-related autonomy) and mediated by the individual's changing independence, needs and challenges to connectedness to others (McCallion 2014). There are three considerations: (1) environmental press (changing circumstances and declining functional abilities make independence and remaining in place more difficult); (2) environmental richness (personal and technological supports to increase their ability to remain within the home); and (3) person-environment fit (congruence between needs and capacity of home to support those needs) (Wahl et al. 2012). Often, attention is paid to practical services and physical aspects of homes. However, there is also a need for consideration of social relationships and community connections (Cannuscio et al. 2003). Staying connected with one's supports contributes to the individual's better health and contributes to independent, fulfilling and self-determined ageing in place (Tang and Lee 2011; McCallion and Ferretti 2017).

Palliative Care and End of Life

Palliative care is most often delivered to people with diseases such as cancer (Fahey-McCarthy et al. 2008) as curative care becomes more futile and increasingly as death approaches but also where typical trajectories of dying are understood well enough to prepare for death (Clark 2007). The model has not always been well-translated for dementia where ambiguity is reported in understanding differences between palliative care and high-quality, person-centred care in a more general sense (McCarron et al. 2011). Equitable access to palliative care services for people with intellectual disabilities requires steps that include changes to service delivery, recognition of differing communication needs, greater professional vigilance for signs of serious illness and end of life, and support for the people who matter to the person with an intellectual disability, including training in symptom management in collaboration with service providers (European Association for Palliative Care 2015; Tuffrey-Wijne et al. 2017). This has not always been well achieved. End-of-life care should also take account of others who may be grieving after the death of an individual, including other service users or paid carers as well as family members (Fahey-McCarthy et al. 2008). New models are needed and are being increasingly developed that facilitate social care and nursing staff being both supported and becoming leaders in care, building collaborative relationships with hospital and palliative care specialty staff; care teams that include the person, their peers and their family; and support networks for all who journey with the person including aftercare and ensuring that desired last days are realised (Ferretti et al. 2022; McCarron et al. 2022; Stancliffe et al. 2022).

By way of concluding the chapter the following vignette helps to illustrate many of the points raised.

Vignette

Joseph represents many people with intellectual disabilities now aged in their 60s and 70s. They have had the opportunity to make decisions, to have a variety of life experiences and to have built relationships with friends, family and staff. End of life may perhaps be coming at an earlier age than is usually true for the general population and chronic illness may be more frequent and earlier onset. However, living the desired life, last days and even death for people with intellectual disabilities is both possible and something to be supported.

As Joseph approached his last days he sat with his brother, his key worker and his friends from both his day program, his old neighbourhood and his current group home. Breathing was now difficult and laboured but he had been helped to understand how to manage for himself the oxygen mask he now needed. An armchair from his family home that he always liked sitting in was in his room and each day he was helped to sit there. A consultation with an occupational therapist had helped train both staff and family to position him in the chair most comfortably and so as not to impair his breathing. Joseph also appreciated some other objects from home that his brother Ian had brought. Joseph, Ian and his friends Niamh and Sally liked to sit each day and talk about old days, old places and people gone but not forgotten. June, the key worker, had developed a memory book for Joseph with pictures that then became the starting off point for conversations. As part of Joseph's individualised plan he had taken several trips in the previous years using his saved money to visit places on his "bucket list", often places remembered, and a beach known from a postcard that Ian had sent many years ago and which had pride of place in Joseph's room. Although travel was now more difficult his key worker was working to arrange a trip to Joseph's day program from 15 years earlier that he and Sally had both attended. Sally was also included in the trip plans. "This must be what they mean by retirement", Joseph said, "Doing things you like, being with friends, surrounded by people you care about. It's a good life".

Conclusion

This chapter has given an insight into the importance of considering ageing for people with intellectual disabilities. As the ageing population grows, there are notable concerns about health, changes in function and the potential for loneliness and isolation and often unwelcome transitions to other settings. Growing older successfully and ageing in place are considered and the right to self-determination and how this might be supported are also considered. Approaches to care are emphasised with prevention, health promotion and supports rather than "treatment" of ageing highlighted. It is evident services are changing and the challenges are recognised. The need to shift to recognising a greater likelihood of ageing independently and with family rather than in out-of-home and provider-based care is discussed. Furthermore, this chapter offers some thoughtful reflective questions and highlights key concepts for the reader.

Reflective Questions

- Considering the material you have just reviewed, has this made you consider ageing differently for people with intellectual disability?
- How might this influence you in your work supporting those individuals who age with an intellectual disability?
- How can the various approaches to care be applied in your practice?

Key Concepts Discussed

- Ageing with disadvantages
- Premature ageing
- Ageing—the impact on physical and mental health
- Approaches to care in ageing
- Social networks and supports
- Family caregiving
- Ageing in the community as opposed to ageing in community-based services
- Self-determination
- Palliative care and end of life

References

Adams N, Grieder DM (2005) Treatment planning for person-centred care. Elsevier, Burlington, MA

Bigby C (1997) When parents relinquish care. The informal support networks of older people with intellectual disability. J Appl Intellect Disabil Res 10, 4:333–344

Bigby C, McCallion P, McCarron M (2014) Serving an elderly population. In: Agran M, Brown F, Hughes C, Quirk C, Ryndak D (eds) Equality and full participation for individuals with severe disabilities: a vision for the future. Paul H. Brookes, Baltimore, MD, pp 319–348

Breitholtz A, Snellman I, Fagerberg I (2013) Older people's dependence on caregivers' help in their own homes and their lived experiences of their opportunity to make independent decisions. Int J Older People Nursing 8:139–148

Cannuscio C, Block J, Kawachi I (2003) Social capital and successful aging: the role of senior housing. Ann Intern Med 139(Supplement 2):395–399

Clark D (2007) From margins to centre: a review of the history of palliative care in cancer. Lancet Oncol 8(5):430–438. https://doi.org/10.1016/S1470-2045(07)70138-9

Coppus AM, Evenhuis HM, Verberne GJ, Visser FE, Oostra BA, Eikelenboom P, Van Gool WA, Van Duijn CM (2008) Survival in elderly persons with Down syndrome. J Am Geriatr 56(12):2311–2316

Ekelund C, Dahlin-Ivanoff S, Eklund K (2014) Self-determination among older people—a concept analysis. Scand J Occup Ther 21:116–124

European Association for Palliative Care (2015) Consensus norms for palliative care of people with intellectual disabilities in Europe: EAPC White Paper. Retrieved from: www.learningdisabilityanddementia.org/uploads/1/1/5/8/11581920/eapc-white-paper-id_full-version_april2015.pdf

Evenhuis HM, Hermans H, Hilgenkamp TI, Bastiaanse LP, Echteld MA (2012) Frailty and disability in older adults with intellectual disabilities: results from the healthy ageing and intellectual disability study. J Am Geriatr Soc 60:934–938

Fahey-McCarthy E, McCallion P, Connaire K, McCarron M (2008) Supporting persons with intellectual disability and advanced dementia: fusing the horizons of intellectual disability, palliative and person-centred dementia care. Trinity College Dublin, Dublin. Accessed from: https://nursing-midwifery.tcd.ie/assets/publications/pdf/fusing-horizons-ofcare.pdf

Ferretti LA, McCarron M, McCallion P (2022) Building shared end-of-life supports and cross-training for hospice/palliative and intellectual disability services providers. In: Stancliffe R, Weise M, McCallion P, McCarron M (eds) End of life and people with intellectual and developmental disability—contemporary issues, challenges, experiences and practice. Palgrave Macmillan, London, pp 211–233. https://doi.org/10.1007/978-3-030-98697-1_8

Fujiura GT (2012) Structure of I/DD households in the U.S.: the family in 2010. Paper presented at the American Association on Intellectual and Developmental Disabilities, Charlotte, North Carolina

Haveman M, Heller T, Maaskant M, Lee L, Shooshtari S, Strydom A (2009) Health risks in older adults with intellectual disabilities: a review of studies (IASSID report). Retrieved from: http://www.IASSID.org. Sept 2022

Heslop P, Blair PS, Fleming PJ, Hoghton MA, Marriott AM, Russ LS (2014) The Confidential Inquiry into premature deaths of people with intellectual disabilities in the UK: a population-based study. Lancet 383(9920):889–895

Hewitt A, Lightfoot E, Bogenschutz M, McCormack K, Sedlezky L, Doljanic R (2010) Parental caregivers' desires for Lifetime Assistance Planning for future supports for their children with Intellectual and Developmental Disabilities. J Fam Soc Work 13(5):420–434. https://doi.org/10.1080/10522158.2010.514678

Hibbard JH, Collins PA, Mahoney E, Baker LH (2010) The development and testing of a measure assessing clinician beliefs about patient self-management. Health Expect 13:65–72

Hilgenkamp M, Reis D, Wijck D, Evenhuis H (2012) Physical activity levels in older adults with intellectual disabilities are extremely low. Res Dev Disabil 33:477–483

Jackson R, Howe N, Nakashima K (2011) Global aging preparedness index. Center for Strategic and International Studies, Washington, DC

Kaneda T (2006) Health care challenges for developing countries with aging populations. Population Reference Bureau, Washington, DC

Kirkendall AM, Waldrop D, Moone RP (2012) Caring for people with intellectual disabilities and life-limiting illness: merging person-centred planning and patient-centered, family-focused care. J Social Work End Life Palliat Care 8(2):135–150. https://doi.org/10.1080/15524256.2012.685440

Kitwood TM (1997) Dementia reconsidered: the person comes first. Open University Press

Lightfoot E, McCallion P (2015) Older adults and developmental disabilities. In: Berkman B, Kaplan D (eds) Handbook of social work in health & aging, 2nd edn. Oxford University Press, New York, pp 489–499

Lightfoot E, McCallion P (2016) Older adults and developmental disabilities. In B. Berkman & D. Kaplan (Eds.). Handbook of Social Work in Health & Aging. 2nd edn. Oxford University Press, New York, pp 489–499

McCallion P (2014) Aging in place. In: Whitfield K, Baker T (eds) Handbook of minority aging. Springer, New York, pp 277–290

McCallion P, Ferretti LA (2015) Building capacity for self-management interventions: the challenges. J Nurs Care 4(6):1–2. https://doi.org/10.4172/2167-1168.1000308

McCallion P, Ferretti LA (2017) Understanding, supporting and safeguarding self-determination as we age. In: Wehmeyer ML, Shogen KA, Little TD, Lopez SJ (eds) Development of self-determination through the life-course. Springer, Dordrecht

McCallion P, Kolomer SR (2003) Aging persons with developmental disabilities and their aging caregivers. In: Berkman B, Harootyan L (eds) Social work and health care in an aging world. Springer, New York, pp 201–225

McCallion P, McCarron M (2015) People with disabilities entering the third age. In: McConkey R, Gilligan R, Iriarte EG (eds) Disability in a global age: a human rights based approach. Palgrave Macmillan, London

McCallion P, Toseland RW (1993) Empowering families of adolescents and adults with developmental disabilities. Fam Soc 74(10):579–589. https://doi.org/10.2307/585095

McCallion P, Ferretti L, Park J (2013) Financial issues and an aging population: responding to an increased potential for financial abuse and exploitation. In: Birkenmaier J, Curley J, Sherraden M (eds) Financial education & capability: research, education, policy and practice. Oxford University Press, New York, pp 129–155

McCallion P, Jokinen N, Janicki MP (2017a) Aging. In: Wehmeyer ML, Brown I, Percey M, Shogren KA, Fung M (eds) A comprehensive guide to intellectual and developmental disabilities. Paul Brookes Press, Baltimore, MD

McCallion P, Hogan M, Santos FH, McCarron M, Service K, Stemp S, Keller S, Fortea J, Bishop K, Watchman K, Janicki MP, Working Group of the International Summit on Intellectual Disability and Dementia (2017b) Consensus statement of the International Summit on Intellectual Disability and Dementia related to end-of-life care in advanced dementia. J Appl Res Intellect Disabil 30(6):1160–1164. https://doi.org/10.1111/jar.12349

McCallion P, Ferretti L, Beange H, McCarron M (2019) Epidemiological issues. In: Prasher VP, Janicki MP (eds) Physical health of adults with intellectual disabilities. Wiley, London, pp 9–26

McCallion P, Ferretti LA, McCarron M (2021) The emergence of aging with long-term disability populations. In: Putnam M, Bigby C (eds) Handbook on ageing with disability. Taylor & Francis, London

McCarron M, McCallion P, Fahey-McCarthy E, Connaire K (2011) The role and timing of palliative care in supporting persons with intellectual disability and advanced dementia. J Appl Res Intellect Disabil 24(3):189–198. https://doi.org/10.1111/j.1468-3148.2010.00592.x

McCarron M, Swinburne J, Burke E, McGlinchey E, Carroll R, McCallion P (2013) Patterns of multimorbidity in an older population of persons with an intellectual disability: results from the Intellectual Disability Supplement to the Irish Longitudinal Study on Ageing (IDS-TILDA). Res Dev Disabil 34:521–527

McCarron M, McCallion P, Reilly E, Mulryan N (2014) A prospective 14-year longitudinal follow-up of dementia in persons with Down syndrome. J Intellect Disabil Res 258:61–70

McCarron M, McCallion P, Reilly E, Dunne P, Carroll R, Mulryan N (2017) A prospective 20 Year longitudinal follow-up of dementia in persons with Down syndrome. J Intellect Disabil Res 61(9):843–852. https://doi.org/10.1111/jir.12390

McCarron M, Sheerin F, Roche L, Ryan AM, Griffiths C, Keenan P, Doody O, D'Eath M, Burke E, McCallion P (2018) Shaping the future of intellectual disability nursing in Ireland. Health Services Executive, Dublin. https://www.inmo.ie/attachment.aspx?doc=4970

McCarron M, Allen A, Mulryan N, Leigh M, O'Reilly L, McCarthy C, Dunne P, Reilly E, McCallion P (2022) Living and dying well with dementia. In: Stancliffe R, Weise M, McCallion P, McCarron M (eds) End of life and people with intellectual and developmental disability—contemporary issues, challenges, experiences and practice. Palgrave Macmillan, London, pp 179–209. https://doi.org/10.1007/978-3-030-98697-1_7

McCausland D, McCallion P, Carroll R, McCarron M (2020) The nature and quality of friendship for older adults with an intellectual disability in Ireland. J Appl Res Intellect Disabil. https://doi.org/10.1111/jar.12851

McKenzie N, Mirfin-Veitch B, Conder J, Brandford S (2017) "I'm still here": exploring what matters to people with intellectual disability during advance care planning. J Appl Res Intellect Disabil 30(6):1089–1098. https://doi.org/10.1111/jar.12355

Niemiec RM, Shogren KA, Wehmeyer ML (2017) Character strengths and intellectual and developmental disability: a strengths-based approach from positive psychology. Educ Training Autism Dev Disabil 52(1):13–25

Nirje B (1969) The normalisation principle and human management implications. In: Kugel R, Wolfensberger W (eds) Changing patterns in residential services for the mentally retarded. Presidents Committee on Mental Retardation, Washington, DC, pp 179–195

O'Brien J, O'Brien CL (1998) A little book about person centered planning. Inclusion Press, Toronto

Pynoos J, Caraviello R, Cicero C (2009) Lifelong housing: the anchor in aging-friendly communities. Generations 33(2):26–32

Rowe J, Kahn R (1998) Successful aging. Random House, New York

Sabia JJ (2008) There's no place like home. A hazard model analysis of aging in place among older homeowners. Res Aging 30:3–35

Schoufour J, Echteld M, Evenhuis H (2012) Frailty in eldery with intellectual disabilities. J Intellect Disabil Res 56:661

Sheerin F, McCallion P, McCarron M (2021) Responding to changing workforce realities: one profession's experience. In: Putnam M, Bigby C (eds) Handbook on ageing with disability. Taylor & Francis, London

Stancliffe RJ, Wiese MY, Read S, Jeltes G, Clayton JM (2017) Assessing knowledge and attitudes about end of life: evaluation of three instruments designed for adults with intellectual disability. J Appl Res Intellect

Disabil 30(6):1076–1088. https://doi.org/10.1111/jar.12358

Stancliffe R, Weise M, McCallion P, McCarron M (2022) Experience of end-of-life issues by people with intellectual disability. In: Stancliffe R, Weise M, McCallion P, McCarron M (eds) End of life and people with intellectual and developmental disability—contemporary issues, challenges, experiences and practice. Palgrave Macmillan, London, pp 29–57. https://doi.org/10.1007/978-3-030-98697-1_2

Tang F, Lee Y (2011) Social support networks and expectations for aging in place and moving. Res Aging 33:444–464

Tuffrey-Wijne I, Rose T, Grant R, Wijne A (2017) Communicating about death and dying: developing training for staff working in services for people with intellectual disabilities. J Appl Res Intellect Disabil 30(6):1099–1110. https://doi.org/10.1111/jar.12382

van Schrojenstein Lantman-De Valk HM, Metsemakers JF, Haveman MJ, Crebolder HF (2000) Health problems in people with intellectual disability in general practice: a comparative study. Fam Pract 17(5):405–407

Verdonschot MML, de Witte LP, Reichrath E, Buntinx WH, Curfs LM (2009) Community participation of people with an intellectual disability: a review of empirical findings. J Intellect Disabil Res 53(4):303–318

Wagner EH, Austin BT, Davis C, Hindmarsh M, Schaefer J, Bonami A (2001) Improving chronic illness care: translating evidence into action. Health Aff (Millwood) 20:64–78

Wahl H-W, Iwarsson S, Oswald F (2012) Aging well and the environment: toward an integrative model and research agenda for the future. The Gerontologist 52(3):306–316

Weise M (2022) End-of-life resources. In: Stancliffe R, Weise M, McCallion P, McCarron M (eds) End of life and people with intellectual and developmental disability—contemporary issues, challenges, experiences and practice. Palgrave Macmillan, London, pp 29–57

Williams GC, Deci EL (1996) Internalization of biopsychosocial values by medical students: a test of self-determination theory. J Pers Soc Psychol 70:767–779

Williams GC, Freedman ZR, Deci EL (1998) Supporting autonomy to motivate glucose control in patients with diabetes. Diabetes Care 21:1644–1651

Williams GC, McGregor HA, Zeldman A, Freedman ZR, Deci EL (2004) Testing a self-determination theory process model for promoting glycemic control through diabetes self-management. Health Psychol 23:58–66

Wolfensberger W (1985) An overview of social role valorisation and some reflections on elderly mentally retarded persons. In: Janicki M, Wisniewski H (eds) Aging and developmental disabilities: issues and approaches. Paul Brookes Publishing, Baltimore

Zendell A (2011) Decision-making processes among siblings caring for adults with intellectual or developmental disabilities. Unpublished Dissertation, University at Albany

Intellectual Disability, Mental Health and Mental Disorders

11

Sandra Fleming and Carlos Peña-Salazar

Chapter Topics

- The concept of mental health, quality of life for people with intellectual disability and its relationship with mental health disorders and problem behaviours
- The prevalence of mental health disorders in people with intellectual disabilities
- The classification and assessment of mental disorders in the person with intellectual disability
- Access to services
- The recovery model in supporting the person with intellectual disability and a mental health condition
- Recognition and management of common mental disorders

S. Fleming (✉)
School of Nursing & Midwifery, Trinity College Dublin, The University of Dublin, Dublin, Ireland
e-mail: flemins@tcd.ie

C. Peña-Salazar
Mental Health and Intellectual disability services, Parc Sanitari Sant Joan de Deu, Barcelona, Spain

Neurology Department, Parc Sanitari Sant Joan de Deu, Barcelona, Spain

Teaching, Research & Innovation Unit, Parc Sanitari Sant Joan de Deu, Barcelona, Spain

Center for Biomedical Research in Epidemiology and Public Health Network (CIBERESP), Madrid, Spain
e-mail: carlosmanuel.pena@sjd.es

Introduction

People with intellectual disability experience the same range of mental health issues and mental disorders as their non-intellectually disabled peers. The risk factors for developing a mental disorder for both populations are the same; however, the person with intellectual disability can be more vulnerable to developing mental disorders due to: (a) biological factors, for example, behavioural phenotype, neurological disorders such epilepsy and endocrinological disorders; (b) psychological factors, for example, limited problem-solving capacity and poor self-esteem; and (c) social factors, such as lack of meaningful experiences and under- or over-stimulating environment (Deb et al. 2001a). If not identified, diagnosed and treated in a timely fashion, mental health issues and mental disorders can negatively impact the quality of life (QoL) of the person with intellectual disabilities.

The Concept of Mental Health and Quality of Life for People with Intellectual Disability and Its Relationship with Mental Disorders and Problem Behaviours

A mental disorder is defined as "syndromes characterised by clinically significant disturbance in an individual's cognition, emotional

© The Author(s), under exclusive license to Springer Nature Switzerland AG 2023
F. Sheerin, C. Doyle (eds.), *Intellectual Disabilities: Health and Social Care Across the Lifespan*,
https://doi.org/10.1007/978-3-031-27496-1_11

regulation, or behaviour that reflects a dysfunction in the psychological, biological, or developmental processes that underlie mental and behavioural functioning. These disturbances are usually associated with distress or impairment in personal, family, social, educational, occupational, or other importance areas of functioning" (World Health Organization 2019). Historically it was claimed that people with an intellectual disability did not experience mental health disorders with the changes seen in the person's behaviour attributed to the person's intellectual disability (Smiley and Cooper 2003). It is only in the last 40 years that there is an awareness that not only do people with intellectual disability experience the same range of mental health disorders as seen in their non-intellectually disabled peers, but they are more vulnerable to and have a higher prevalence rate of these disorders (Cooper et al. 2007; Mazza et al. 2020).

The World Health Organization (WHO) conceptualises mental health as a "state of mental well-being that enables people to cope with the stresses of life, realize their abilities, learn well and work well, and contribute to their community" (World Health Organization 2022, p. 8). The focus of mental health is not about the absence of illness, it is individualised to each person and influences how the person feels, thinks about and values themselves and others. Factors such as societal structures, cultural values, the everyday experience of the person and their ability to communicate, develop and sustain relationships, cope with change and the stresses of life, e.g. transitions, disappointments and enjoy life, all impact on a person's mental health. Mental health is a basic human right (WHO 2022), fundamental to our overall health and wellbeing, and helps one to connect, function, cope and thrive (Fig. 11.1).

Whilst having good mental health helps us to make good decisions and cope with everyday stressors of life, poor mental health can impact on a person's ability to recognise the need for and be able to access the support(s) they require to improve their wellbeing (WHO 2022). When compared to their peers in the general population, people with intellectual disability may be at increased risk of having poorer mental health (Deb et al. 2001a) due to health inequalities which can impact on a person's resilience and ability to cope with everyday life events.

A person's mental health and wellbeing is not static, it can change over time due to factors that impact on one's mental health and wellbeing and

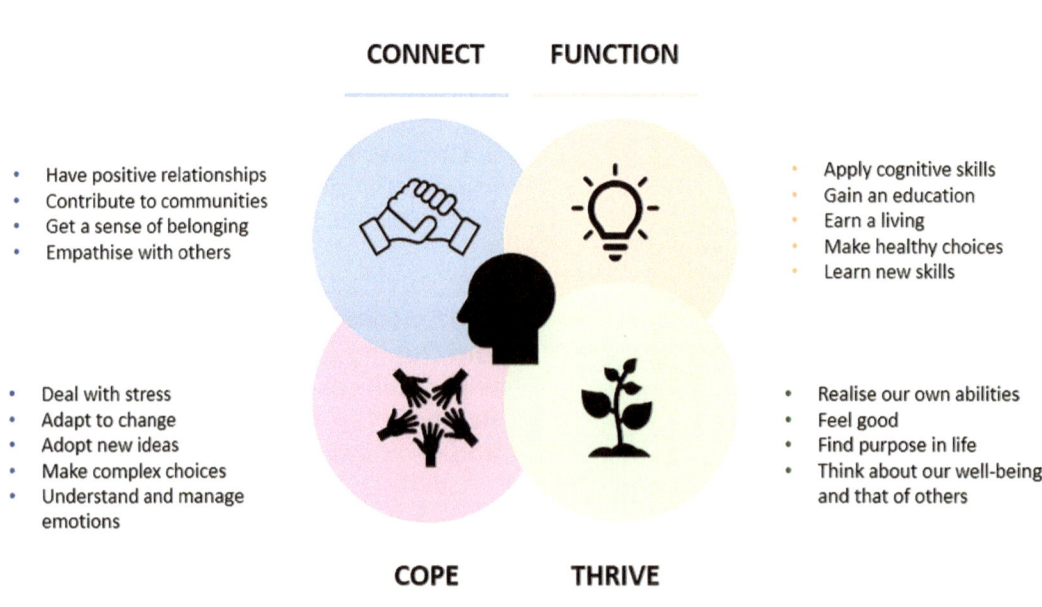

CONNECT   **FUNCTION**

- Have positive relationships
- Contribute to communities
- Get a sense of belonging
- Empathise with others

- Apply cognitive skills
- Gain an education
- Earn a living
- Make healthy choices
- Learn new skills

- Deal with stress
- Adapt to change
- Adopt new ideas
- Make complex choices
- Understand and manage emotions

- Realise our own abilities
- Feel good
- Find purpose in life
- Think about our well-being and that of others

COPE   **THRIVE**

Fig. 11.1 Mental health: helping us to connect, function, cope and thrive. (Based on WHO 2022, p. 11)

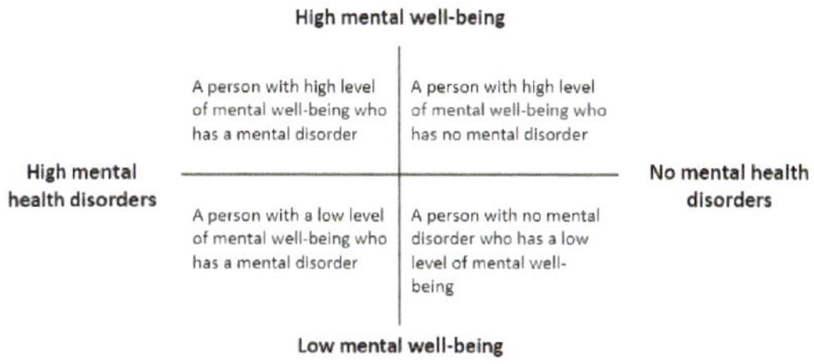

Fig. 11.2 The relationship between mental wellbeing and mental health disorders. (Based on Tudor 1996)

Table 11.1 Instruments to assess quality of life for people with intellectual disability

Name of instrument	Used for
Gencat Scale (Verdugo et al. 2010)	All people with intellectual disabilities but mainly people with mild and moderate intellectual disability
San Martin Scale (Verdugo et al. 2014)	People with severe and profound intellectual disability
Quality of life in Late Stage Dementia (QUALID) (Weiner et al. 2000)	People with severe and profound intellectual disability

so the person may experience a change in their mental health. Therefore, it is more apt to view mental health on a continuum from a high to a low level of wellbeing (Tudor 1996). Mental health does not imply or indicate absence of mental disorders nor is having a mental disorder synonymous with having poor mental wellbeing. Whilst a person with a mental disorder may be more prone to experiencing mental health and wellbeing on the lower aspect of the continuum, they can also experience good mental health whilst presenting with a mental disorder as indicated in Fig. 11.2.

The QoL of people with intellectual disabilities has been the subject of attention in numerous studies in the last two decades (Schalock and Verdugo 2002), as these individuals are considered to have potentially lower QoL than the general population (Golubović and Skrbić 2013; Simes and Santos 2016). The World Health Organization (2012, p. 2) defines QoL as "individuals' perceptions of their position in life in the context of the culture and value systems in which they live and in relation to their goals, expectations, standards and concerns". Due to its inherent complexity QoL is difficult to measure rigorously, since it is influenced by many factors (Schalock and Verdugo 2002). It may be disguised by factors such as age, sensory and motor limitations, medical comorbidity, mental illness, nutritional problems (Petry et al. 2009) and from being institutionalised (Sines et al. 2012).

There are a number of different QoL models, but two of the most widely used are My Life: Personal Outcomes Index (The Seniors 2011) and Schalock and Verdugo's multidimensional model (2002). Although there are no specific instruments to measure the QoL of people with

intellectual disability and challenging behaviour, self-reported and proxy assessment tools have been developed to measure QoL based on the foregoing and other models (Townsend-White et al. 2012). To further assess QoL in people with intellectual disability, it is crucial to consider some factors such as the high prevalence of medical and psychiatric comorbidity (10–60% of the cases) (Cooper et al. 2007; Koskentausta et al. 2007), behavioural disorders (Cohen et al. 2010), psychopharmacological treatments and housing, which often play a role in QoL. Table 11.1 identifies some instruments used to assess QoL in people with intellectual disabilities.

A review of the existing literature on the influence of challenging behaviour and/or psychiatric disorders on the QoL of people with intellectual disability revealed a scarcity of studies on this subject. In a sample of 138 subjects with varying degrees of intellectual disability (from borderline to moderate), Horovitz et al. (2014) found significantly reduced QoL in those affected by an associated mental illness. Similarly Koch et al. (2015) and Scheifes et al. (2016) found impaired QoL in subjects with associated mental illness and challenging behaviour and those treated with high doses of psychotropic drugs, mainly due to their frequent secondary effects. In an adult sample population of 142 people with different degrees of intellectual disability, Peña-Salazar et al. (2018) found QoL was worse in people living in residential care homes and in people who presented higher rates of problem behaviour, but no association was found with mental disorders.

In summary, wellbeing and quality of life are complex concepts in people with intellectual disabilities. Place of residence plays a key role in the QoL, while medical and psychiatric comorbidity, including problem behaviour, has a clear negative influence in QoL. Therefore, to improve QoL for the person with intellectual disability who has mental disorders and or problem behaviours, it is necessary to promote an active integration into society to get involved in activities that are interesting and meaningful to them and to live where and with whom they want (National Institute for Health and Care Excellence (NICE) 2016). A correct identification of medical and psychiatric problems, and therefore a correct treatment of them, will collaborate to achieve a better QoL.

Prevalence of and Vulnerability to Mental Disorders in People with Intellectual Disabilities

The reported prevalence of mental disorders in adults with intellectual disability is about 33% (Mazza et al. 2020) and the rate of underdiagnosed psychiatric disorders in this population is nearly 30% (Peña-Salazar et al. 2017). Mazza et al. (2020) systematic review found that mood disorders are the most prevalent psychiatric disorders, followed by anxiety disorders and schizophrenia. Cooper et al. (2007) found autism spectrum disorders as the most prevalent disorder in adults with intellectual disability, followed by affective and anxiety disorders. The estimated prevalence is similar in children and adolescents (38%) with attention-deficit/hyperactivity disorders, conduct disorders and anxiety disorders being the most prevalent (Buckley et al. 2020).

Depressive disorders (Peña-Salazar et al. 2018; Cooper et al. 2007), psychosis, personality disorder and autism (Deb et al. 2001a; Turygin et al. 2013) were found as the most frequent mental disorders in adults with mild/moderate intellectual disability. In people with severe/profound intellectual disability, anxiety disorders (Peña-Salazar et al. 2017) and psychosis (Rojahn et al. 2004) were the most prevalent disorders. Kozlowski et al. (2011) found that 61.8% of the

individuals with severe intellectual disability scored positively in two or more dimensions of the DASH-II scale, representing a psychiatric multimorbidity.

Genetic mutations or behavioural phenotypes are key factors in the high prevalence of psychiatric disorders in this population (Blackwood et al. 2008; Thygesen et al. 2018). Social exclusion, socioeconomic factors (Emerson et al. 2004) and childhood trauma also play an important role. Numerous well-known biological and environmental factors, which work as triggers of psychiatric disorders, are frequently present in people with intellectual disabilities.

A possible explanation for this high rate of psychiatric disorders in people with severe/profound intellectual disability could be the frequent brain damage seen in this population, such as agenesis of the corpus callosum (Mohapatra et al. 2015), schizencephaly (Melo et al. 2013) and lissencephaly (Chang et al. 2007), as well as cerebral atrophy, leucomalacia and hypoxic and traumatic damage. Such neurological damage could facilitate, via the breakdown of integrative cerebral functioning, the onset of mental disorders in general. The high proportion of epilepsy among people with a psychiatric comorbidity could be viewed as a common pathway that makes people with intellectual disability more vulnerable to both mental and neurological disorders (Matsuura et al. 2005; Sperli et al. 2009; Peña-Salazar et al. 2022). Moreover, the high prevalence of mental disorders in people with severe/profound intellectual disability could reflect the difficulties in diagnosing mental disorders in this group (Borthwick-Duffy 1994; Rush and Frances 2000). The limitations in communicating thoughts and feelings among people with severe/profound intellectual disability (Matson et al. 1999) and the quite different clinical features of mental disorders in this population (Walton and Kerr 2016) could lead to diagnostic overshadowing as a propensity to overlook real psychopathological phenomena among people with intellectual disability, causing a biased assessment of mental comorbidity (Jopp and Keys 2001) and diagnostic inaccuracy (Smiley and Cooper 2003).

Differentiating Between Mental Health Disorders and Challenging Behaviours

Challenging behaviour has been defined as culturally abnormal behaviour(s) of such an intensity, frequency or duration that the physical safety of the individual or others is placed in serious jeopardy or seriously limits the use or leads to denial of access to ordinary community facilities (Emerson and Einfeld 2011). The prevalence of behavioural disorders in the population with intellectual disability ranges from 30% to 60% (Cohen et al. 2010). In people with mild/moderate intellectual disability prevalence is about 45.3% (Schützwohl et al. 2016), and in individuals with severe/profound intellectual disability, the rate could be even higher (Sheehan et al. 2015).

Studies on the co-occurrence of mental disorder and intellectual disability have found very divergent figures (Munir 2016; Nettelbladt et al. 2009). This lack of consistency between challenging behaviour and psychiatric disorders has been explained as being due to diagnostic difficulties (Salvador-Carulla and Novell-Alsina 2002), the use of different diagnostic criteria (Cooper et al. 2007) and the existence of functional "precursors" of challenging behaviour. Furthermore, it is of interest to highlight the heterogeneity of the population assessed due to the variety of syndromes, different localisations and causes of brain damage, most of which have an unclear aetiology (Chiurazzi and Pirozzi 2016; Mehregan et al. 2016) and multiple behavioural phenotypes (Nyhan 1972).

While psychiatric disorders and challenging behaviour have typically been investigated separately, some studies have focused on the relationship between both conditions in individuals with intellectual disability. Peña-Salazar et al. (2018) in 91 adults with different degrees of intellectual disability found that challenging behaviour was more frequent among people with mild/moderate intellectual disability and comorbid mental disorders, with depressive disorders the most frequent disorder related with challenging behaviour. Newman et al. (2015) found a positive association between severe challenging behaviour and psychiatric comorbidity in a study assessing children with fragile X syndrome and different degrees of intellectual disability. Tsiouris et al. (2011) and Newman et al. (2015) reported more challenging behaviour among individuals with intellectual disability and psychiatric comorbidity in comparison with people with intellectual disability not suffering from a mental disorder. This association was stronger among people suffering from affective disorders (Moss et al. 2000; Reiss and Rojahn 1993).

Classification and Diagnosis of Mental Health Disorders in the Person with Intellectual Disability

It is possible to assess a psychiatric disorder in people with mild intellectual disability using ICD 11 or DSM 5 criteria, but for people with more severe intellectual disabilities, specialised criteria such as the DM-ID 2 (Diagnostic Manual of Intellectual Disability) or DC-LD criteria (Royal College of Psychiatrists 2001) are recommended.

DM-ID 2 was created by the National Association for the Dually Diagnosed (2017) in association with the American Psychiatric Association (APA). The DM-ID 2 criteria were designed as a companion of the DSM 5 with the aim to achieve a more accurate diagnosis in this population.

DC-LD criteria is a classification system providing operationalised diagnostic criteria for psychiatric disorders, intended for use with adults with moderate to profound learning disabilities. It may also be used in conjunction with the ICD 11 and DSM 5 manuals in a complementary way, when working with adults with mild learning disabilities.

Use of Assessment and Screening Instruments

There are a number of screening and assessment instruments that have been adapted (Table 11.2) for use in the diagnosis of mental health disorders in the person with an intellectual disability. A screening tool can be used by a health professional to identify the possibility of a particular disorder before referring on for assessment. An

Table 11.2 Screening and assessment instruments

Screening instruments	Assessment instruments
Moss-PAS (Check) (Moss 2019) is a 25-item screening checklist that aims to help staff and carers to identify and monitor the person considered to be at risk for mental health problems. The checklist includes threshold scores that indicate if the person requires referral for assessment using the Moss-Pass (ID) or Moss-PAD (Diag ID)	**Diagnostic Assessment for the Severely Handicapped II (DASH-II) scale** (Matson et al. 1991) was created to assess mental disorders in the population with severe/profound intellectual disability. It consists of 96 items following the criteria of the DSM-IV-TR (American Psychiatric Association 2000)
Glasgow Depression Scale for people with intellectual Disability (GDS-LD) (Cuthill et al. 2003) is a series of 20 self-rating questions asking a participant about their experiences in the previous week with possible scores from 0 to 40 **The Carer Supplement (GDS-CS)** (Cuthill et al. 2003) is a 16-item questionnaire with possible scores from 0 to 32. If a score of 13 or more is calculated in the GDS-LD or GDS-LD, the person is referred for mental health consultation	**Moss-Pass (ID)** (Moss 2019) a clinical interview (formerly Mini PAS-ADD) fully compliant with DSM 5 and ICD 11 is an assessment instrument that assesses across seven diagnostic areas to detect and measure change in the mental health of the person with intellectual disabilities and limited language
Glasgow Anxiety Scale for people with intellectual Disability (GAS-ID) (Mindham and Espie 2003) is a series of 27 questions asking a participant about their experiences in the previous week resulting in a range of possible scores from 0 to 54. If a score of 15 or more is calculated in the GAS-LD, the person is referred for mental health consultation	**The Moss-PAS (Diag ID)** (Moss and Friedlander 2020) is a semi-structured clinical interview developed from the PAS-ADD Clinical Interview. It is primarily designed for people who have limited language skills to contribution to an interview. It has separate sets of questions for the person with intellectual disability and informants. The interview produces criterion-by-criterion diagnoses under both ICD 11 and DSM 5
HoNOS-LD is designed for use with people with an intellectual disability and with mental health needs, irrespective of their degree of disability, to monitor their response to treatment; it consists of 18 items that are each graded from 0, no problem, to 4, severe problem. Its primary aim is to measure change in an individual over two or more points in time as a measurement of outcome for therapeutic interventions. The HoNOS-LD measures global outcomes and not inputs	**Diagnostic Assessment for the Severely Handicapped II (DASH-II) scale** (Matson et al. 1991) was created to assess mental disorders in the population with severe/profound intellectual disability. It consists of 96 items following the criteria of the DSM-IV-TR (American Psychiatric Association 2000)

assessment instrument is used by a professional, for example, a clinical psychiatrist or psychologist, experienced in diagnosing mental health disorders in people with intellectual disability, to establish the nature of the disorder and develop an appropriate treatment plan for the person.

Challenges in Identifying and Diagnosing Mental Health Issues in the Person with Intellectual Disability

Diagnostic Overshadowing

Diagnostic overshadowing is a tendency for professionals to assign psychopathological symptoms to a mental/cognitive condition rather than to a psychiatric comorbidity (Reiss et al. 1982). The limitations in communicating thoughts and feelings among people with intellectual disability (Matson et al. 1999) and the quite different clinical features of mental disorders in the population with intellectual disability (Walton and Kerr 2016) could lead to diagnostic overshadowing as a propensity to overlook real psychopathological phenomena among people with intellectual disability, causing a biased assessment of mental comorbidity (Jopp and Keys 2001) and diagnostic inaccuracy (Smiley and Cooper 2003). To minimise and overcome diagnostic overshadowing in people with intellectual disability, it is necessary to have a detailed knowledge of mental health concerns in people with intellectual disability and to understand the differences in symptomatology between people with and without intellectual disability.

The PAS-ADD scale covers the whole range of intellectual disability and has higher specificity for people with mild and moderate intellectual disability, whereas the DASH-II was designed to assess mental disorders in people with severe and profound intellectual disability. The correlation between the PAS-ADD and the DASH-II is stronger for the sum scores than for each individual scale (Myrbakk and von Tetzchner 2008).

Mental Health Service Provision

Historically in Ireland, the UK and other international countries, services for people with intellectual disability were mainly delivered in large institutional type settings. The advent of the normalisation movement in the 1970s prompted a fundamental rethinking and reshaping of the way services were delivered for people with intellectual disabilities. This resulted in a move from institutional congregated-based settings to the development of community integrated-based services and an assumption that the health needs of the person would be provided in the community by mainstream health services. However, due to issues such as an already considerable workload, lack of specialist training for professionals and absence of specific mental health diagnostic tools for this population, it soon became apparent that all the mental health needs of this populace could not be catered for by mainstream mental health services (HSE Mental Health Services 2021; Holt et al. 2000). This called for a rethink of how timely equitable access to mental health support and services could be achieved for the person with intellectual disability.

Countries responded in different ways to the move to non-congregated service provision; consequently various configurations of service delivery models for people with intellectual disability and mental health issues exist. These range from care delivered solely in mainstream health-care services and specialised care delivered by intellectual disability services to integrated care with mental health services (HSE Mental Health Services 2021; Royal College of Psychiatrists 2020; Department of Developmental Disability

Neuropsychiatry 2014; Chaplin 2009). Despite the dearth of empirical evidence and lack of consensus on what model of provision is the best to address the mental health needs of this population, international models of service recommend that people with intellectual disability should be able to access mental health services in the same way as the general population and have access to integrated specialist services within mainstream services when required (HSE Mental Health Services 2021; Courtenay 2018; NICE 2016; Sheehan and Paschos 2013; Chaplin 2011), requiring intellectual disability and mental health services to work in partnership in meeting the needs of this populace.

Accessing Mental Health Services: Barriers and Enablers

When compared to the general population people with intellectual disability experience poorer mental health service provision, incongruent with the high prevalence rate of mental disorders observed in this population (McCarthy and Boyd 2002; Whittle et al. 2018; Department of Developmental Disability Neuropsychiatry 2014). While it is recognised that people with intellectual disabilities should have timely access to mental health care and services (HSE Mental Health Services 2021; Hsieh et al. 2020), health disparity in accessing appropriate and equitable mental health services for the person with intellectual disability still exists (Holt et al. 2000; Ramsay and Dodd 2018; Whittle et al. 2018; Department of Developmental Disability Neuropsychiatry 2014). People with and without intellectual disability can experience barriers when trying to access appropriate mental health services (Royal College of Psychiatrists 2020) but people with intellectual disability face additional barriers trying to access mental health services (Walton et al. 2022; HSE Mental Health Services 2021; Hsieh et al. 2020; Ahlström et al. 2020; Whittle et al. 2018; Ramsay and Dodd 2018; Department of Developmental Disability Neuropsychiatry 2014). Whittle et al. (2018) identified barriers related to the availability of services and

Table 11.3 Barriers and enablers (based on Whittle et al. 2018, p. 84)

Domain of access	Barriers	Enablers
Service availability	Limited and scarce services	Innovative models of service delivery
	Logistical and geographical issues	
Utilisation of services and barriers to access	Organisational barriers	Clear referral pathways
	Siloing of service sectors	Established protocols
	Competing service models	Single point of access Interagency collaboration
	Failure of interagency communication	Education
	Inconsistent eligibility criteria	
	Conflict and competition between services	
	Transition	
	Unclear referral pathways	
	Identification of need	
	Lack of help seeking	
Relevance, effectiveness and access	Diagnostic overshadowing	Capacity building
	Misidentification of mental disorder	Up-skilling and training service providers
	Clinical knowledge deficits	
Equity and access	Severity of intellectual disability	None identified
	Social determinants	

the utilisation of service and barriers to effectiveness, equity and access. In addition to the barriers identified in Table 11.3 people with intellectual disability do not tend to self-refer to mental health services (Hsieh et al. 2020), may not be able to navigate their way unaided through these services or have the expressive language to enable them to articulate their emotions and feelings. As this can hinder the establishment of a reliable diagnosis, they are reliant on their caregivers and families to be able to identify signs and symptoms indicative of mental health issues, so that referral to appropriate services can be expedited. A skilled workforce, who understands the needs of the person with intellectual disability and how mental health issues present in this population, is vital to the delivery high-quality care (Courtenay 2018). If caregivers and clinicians do not have the knowledge and skills to recognise the signs and symptoms of the mental health issue, it may go unrecognised (Costello and Bouras 2006) leading to the propensity for diagnostic overshadowing whereby the persons presenting signs and symptoms are attributed to their intellectual disability (Reiss et al. 1982) as opposed to a mental health disorder. Having an association with an intellectual disability service provider can also result in the person experiencing difficulty accessing mainstream mental health services (Ramsay and Dodd 2018), particularly in relation to confusion pertaining the roles and responsibilities of each service in relation to who provides the assessments, draws up the care plan and provides the day-to-day support for the person (Donner et al. 2010).

Enabling access and appropriate care can be facilitated by addressing the shortage of skilled clinicians in this area of practice (Ramsay and Dodd 2018; Donner et al. 2010), improving existing staff education and training opportunities and utilising innovative models of service delivery, such as tele-psychiatry models and stepped care to maximise resources according to the needs of the individual (Whittle et al. 2018), in conjunction with a multidisciplinary interagency collaborate approach with clear referral pathways (HSE Mental Health Services 2021; Walton et al. 2022).

Models of Service

Internationally the key guiding principles of mental health service provision for people with intellectual disabilities are underpinned by human rights, inclusion, person-centred approach, recovery-orientated practice and promoting independence and evidence-based treatment (Department of Health (UK) 2001; Department of Developmental Disability Neuropsychiatry 2014; HSE Mental Health Services 2021) (Table 11.4).

Table 11.4 Guiding principles of mental health services for people with intellectual disabilities

Human rights	Without discrimination, people have a right to the highest achievable standard of health and health care
Inclusion	People have a right to timely, full participation in all facets of community life, including access to mainstream and specialist mental health services as required
Person-centred approach	The person should be seen as an active participant in their care and involved in all aspects of their care and decision-making processes, working in partnership with service
Recovery-orientated practice	Promotion of a culture of hope and empowers and supports the person to build on their strengths so that they can stay well and take control of their lives
Promoting independence	Taking cognisance of the person's age and capacity, acknowledge the person autonomy and provide the supports require to maximise their independence
Evidence-based treatment	The best available evidence should be used by mental health professionals when proving interventions so that the best possible outcome for the person can be achieved

It is beyond the scope of this chapter to address international service models in detail; thus, an outline of the English and Irish models will be provided. In England the development of mental health specialist services for people with intellectual disabilities has been informed by policies such as No Health without Mental Health (Department of Health (UK) 2011), Guidance for commissioners of mental health services for people with learning disabilities (Joint Commissioning Panel for Mental Health 2013) and Achieving Better Access to Mental Health Services by 2020 (Department of Health (UK) 2014) in conjunction with NICE guidelines (NICE 2016). These services are generally well developed and are provided through multidisciplinary teams comprising of health and social work professionals who work in partnership with mainstream health services to deliver high-quality mental health care for the individual (Fig. 11.3). Variations in models of service delivery exist which reflect local needs and the current services in situ.

In Ireland, similar to other European countries, the provision of mental health services for people with intellectual disability has been limited, with a geographical bias towards the provision of services in larger urban areas (Holt et al. 2000). As in the UK the development of mental health intellectual disability (MHID) services has been informed by international best practice and key

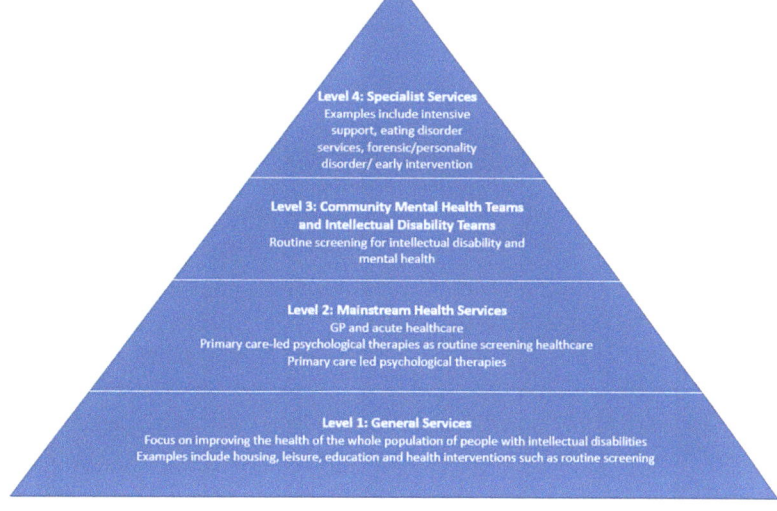

Fig. 11.3 Service organisation model to meet the mental health needs of people with intellectual disabilities in England. (Based on Royal College of Psychiatrists 2020, p. 11)

Fig. 11.4 Integrated person-centred care for people with intellectual disability and mental health problems. (Based on HSE Mental Health Services 2021, p. 40)

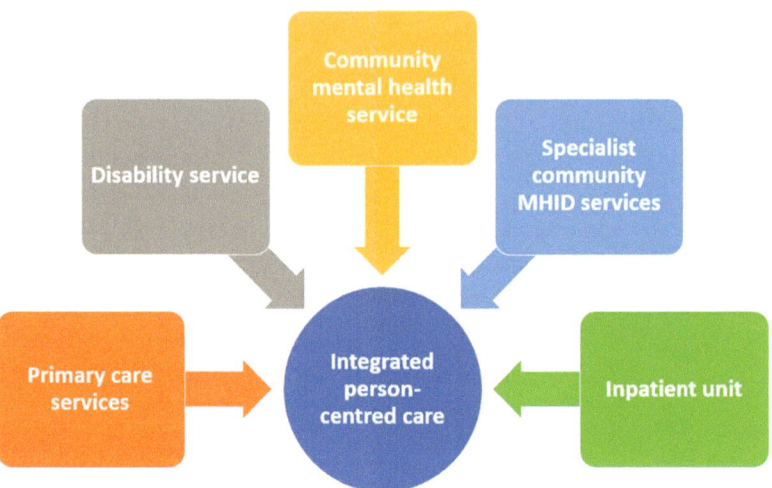

national and international policies and conventions. The National Disability Authority (2003) and the Irish College of Psychiatrists (2004) identified the shortcomings in service delivery and made recommendations for the development of mental health multidisciplinary services to address the deficits. A Vision for Change (Department of Health and Children 2006) recommended that people with intellectual disability should have access to services similar to the general population and endorsed the development of specialist, catchment-specific community-based teams. Despite the above recommendations progress in developing services has been slow; thus, a service improvement plan has been implemented to address the shortcomings and to develop these community-based MHID teams (HSE Mental Health Services 2021) and implement the National Model of Service (Fig. 11.4).

Both models of care recognise that people have varying levels of needs and they may move up or down or between these tiers depending on the care they require to manage their mental health difficulties.

Recovery-Orientated Approach to Practice

The concept of recovery in mental health services emerged in the 1980s in response to studies that showed the course of severe mental illness was not one of predestined deterioration for the individual, but that people could recover and have a meaningful life. It differs from rehabilitation, which focuses on services to enable the person to adapt to their mental disorder, in that the emphasis is on the lived experience of the person and how they come to accept and overcome the challenges presented by their mental disorder (Jacobson 2003). Implementing the recovery approach requires a rethinking of how services are structured and delivered to meet the needs of their client group. Recovery is personal to the person; it cannot be practised by mental health services and staff, but staff and services can create the conditions to support and empower the person in their recovery and conversely prevent conditions that are not amenable for recovery (Shepherd et al. 2008).

While universally there is no consensus on the definition of recovery, one of the founders of the recovery movement describes it "as a deeply personal, unique process of changing one's attitudes, values, feelings, gaols, skills, and/or roles. It is a way of living satisfying, hopeful, and contributing life even with limitations caused by illness. Recovery involves the development of new meaning and purpose in one's life as one grows beyond the catastrophic effects of mental illness" (Anthony 1993, p. 527). The premise of recovery is that the person who has a mental health disorder can develop skills to enable them to manage their mental health disorder, empower them to stay well and take more control of their lives so that they can live meaningfully (Jay et al. 2017; Trustam et al. 2022). It is specific to the person's own individual journey and necessitates a change in the person's attitudes, values, self-belief and skills to promote their level of wellness and improve their quality of life (Anthony 1993; Higgins 2008). The person is supported to identify triggers that might cause a change in their mental health and, in their individualised plan, identify the internal and external resources they can utilise to minimise or eliminate these triggers and stay well, within the limitations they may have from their disorder. Recovery-orientated practice is not just about the need for clinical recovery or symptom relief; it includes psychological recovery, the creation of a meaningful and fulfilling life and a positive self-identity underpinned by hopefulness and self-belief (Andresen et al. 2003). The Department of Developmental Disability Neuropsychiatry (2014) and HSE Mental Health Services (2021) identify that due to the complexity of supports that the person with intellectual disability may have, additional resources

and effort may be required when adopting a recovery-orientated approach to care.

Key Concepts Underpinning the Recovery Approach

Recovery is about supporting the person to have their own personal goals and create a satisfying and meaningful life, irrespective of any continuing or returning mental health issues they may experience. It recognises the person's right to have a good life, have a home and meaningful education and/or work and establish good relationships with their family, friends and their community (Finnerty 2019). The Copeland Center for Wellness and Recovery (2022) identifies five key concepts of recovery (Fig. 11.5).

Recovery-orientated practice is not just about the need for clinical recovery or symptom relief; it includes psychological recovery, the creation of a meaningful and fulfilling life and a positive self-identity underpinned by hopefulness and self-belief (Andresen et al. 2003). While there is

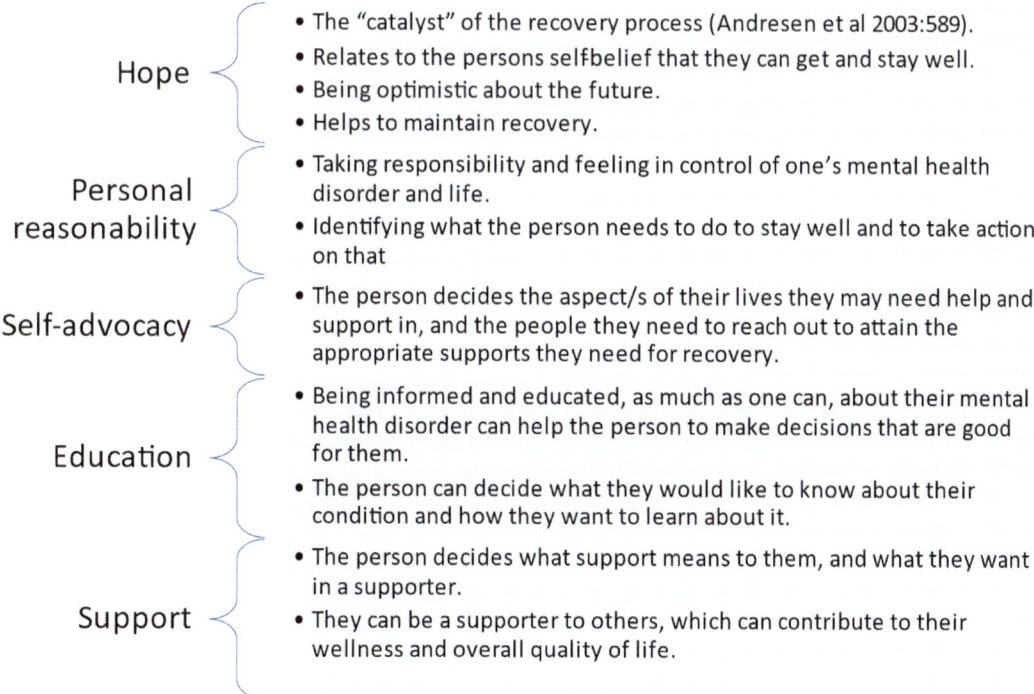

Fig. 11.5 Five key concepts of recovery

a dearth of literature on recovery and the person with intellectual disability presenting with mental health disorders, the guiding vision of national and international mental health policy stresses the importance of all aspects of mental health services to be underpinned by a recovery-orientated approach to practice (Department of Health and Children 2006; Department of Health (UK) 2009; Department of Developmental Disability Neuropsychiatry 2014). Handley et al. (2012) contend that the principles of recovery are similar to the values underpinning person centredness which has informed policy and practice within intellectual disability services for many years particularly in relation to community participation and social inclusion. Indeed, when adopting a recovery-orientated approach to care Trustam et al. (2022) found that the recovery experience of people with intellectual disabilities was similar to that of the general population.

Composition of Mental Health Intellectual Disability Teams

Staff working in mainstream mental health services with people with intellectual disabilities identified that they did not have the specialist skills to meet the needs of this service user group (Slevin et al. 2008). Providing a service where staff are not adequately prepared to address the persons needs impacts on the person being able to receive equitable care and can be seen as a violation of their human rights. Likewise, Chaplin (2009) reported that providing mainstream mental health services for people with intellectual disabilities, without incorporating intellectual disability-specific input, was seen as creating a negative environment and was inadequate in meeting the needs of the person with intellectual disability. Sheehan and Paschos (2013) found that providing specialist services within mainstream mental health services was more appropriate than providing solely mainstream services. Specialist mental health services for people with intellectual disability should be provided by Mental Health Intellectual Disability (MHID) teams (HSE Mental Health Services 2021) who have appropriate skills and experience to provide

specialist mental health services to this service user group. The team should be composed of key professionals from psychiatry, nursing, psychology, speech and language therapy, social work and occupational therapy, as required, as well as administration support. They typically have a smaller caseload and a higher staff to service user ratio to enable them to adapt the specific services required to the suit the person's communication and cognitive capacity and complex needs.

These teams should complement the services provided by disability services, primary care and community mental health teams and support the person with intellectual disability in their specialist mental health assessment. This may involve developing and utilising accessible information formats and reasonable adjustments, as required by the person, so that they are prepared for their assessment and, with the involvement of the person, their family and carers, develop the person's personal mental health care plan. They agree that realistic and meaningful (to the person) recovery-focused goals and intervention(s) and prescribed medication, if required, provide specific carer and staff education and training, monitor and evaluate progress and liaise with intellectual and mental health services. As the person improves, they support the person by working with them in developing a recovery discharge plan to enable the person to stay well.

Mental Health Disorders Common in the People with Intellectual Disability

As mentioned previously mood and anxiety disorders are the most prevalent mental health disorders seen in adults with intellectual disability, and attention-deficit hyperactive disorders are the most prevalent mental health disorders in children. The person with mild intellectual disability usually presents with the same range of symptoms of mental disorders as seen in the general population and diagnosis can be made using the ICD 11 and DSM 5 standardised measures (Lunsky and Palucka 2004). As the diagnostic symptoms identified in the ICD 11 and DSM 5 manuals may not be identifiable in people with moderate to profound intellectual disabilities, clinically diagnosing these disorders for this group can be challenging. It is therefore more appropriate for skilled practitioners with diagnostic expertise in this area to use the DM-ID 2 or DC-LD diagnostic criteria to establish the diagnosis. The person with moderate to severe intellectual disability generally does not have the skills to seek help when they experience mental health problems or they may not be able to recognise, articulate or understand their inner emotions and so are reliant on carers and families to pick up on the observable signs of the disorder and refer onwards (Jahoda 2020). Screening tools such as the GAD-LD (Cuthill et al. 2003) and the GAS-LD (Mindham and Espie 2003) can be used by carers to identify possible signs of the mental disorder that the person may be presenting with and can indicate if diagnostic assessment is required (Hermans and Evenhuis 2010).

Depression

Depression is a mood disorder referring to "a wide range of mental health problems characterised by the absence of a positive affect (a loss of interest and enjoyment in ordinary things and experiences), low mood and a range of associated emotional, cognitive, physical and behavioural symptoms" (National Collaborating Centre for Mental Health 2011, p. 14). It differs from the person's normal emotions that they may experience in response to stressful or challenging everyday events, such as feeling down or depressed, in that the person's low mood is persistent in duration (for at least 2 weeks) and intensity, low across all aspects of the person's life and unresponsive to situations that are known to normally lift the person's mood (Unwin et al. 2019).

Factors Associated with Depression in the Person with Intellectual Disability

The onset of depression has been shown to be predicted by a number of biopsychosocial factors. Underlying chronic health conditions, such

as diabetes mellitus and heart failure, are among the conditions, especially in the older person, associated with an increase in depressive symptoms (Hermans and Evenhuis 2013; Bond et al. 2020; Hsieh et al. 2020). Higher rates of depression are seen in people with genetic conditions such as Down syndrome and Prader-Willi syndrome, as well as those who have associated epilepsy and autism (Tromans et al. 2020). Exposure to one or more negative life events in the previous year, such as change of staff, loss or decline in mobility, problems with fellow residents and having a mild physical illness, is associated with depression, particularly in the person of advancing age (Hermans and Evenhuis 2012). In individuals with mild and or moderate intellectual disabilities, adverse psychosocial factors such as poor self-esteem, self-criticism, negative automatic thoughts, social comparison and deficits in social and interpersonal skills have been shown to be possible risk factors for depression (McGillivray and McCabe 2007).

Presentation of Depression

Smiley and Cooper (2003) identified that some of the signs and symptoms associated with depression are observed in both the general and intellectual disability populations whilst others are specific to their group (Table 11.5).

Diagnosis

In accordance with the NICE guidelines (NICE 2016), a clinical diagnosis of depression is made following a full physical assessment and a review of the person's medication to rule out any underlying conditions. A screening tool such as the GDS-LD can be utilised before a formal diagnostic assessment such as the DC-LD category IIIB4.1 depressive episode is completed.

The presentation of depression in the person with intellectual disability can vary according to their level of intellectual disability (Marston et al. 1997). The person with severe intellectual disability may not be able to self-report, recognise or express their feelings in relation to some

Table 11.5 Signs and symptoms of depression observed in the general and intellectual disability populations

Signs and symptoms of depression	Observed in the general and intellectual disability population	Observed in the general population but uncommon, particularly in the person with severe intellectual disability	Observed in people with intellectual disability but not included in ICD 11 or DSM 5
	Depressed, irritable and labile mood Loss of energy, anhedonia Onset or increase in the following: Sleep disturbances and appetite or weight disturbances Psychomotor agitation and retardation	Guilt Suicidal ideations, worthlessness and low self-esteem	Onset or increase in problem behaviour, self-injurious behaviours and aggression Tearfulness, increased social withdrawal or isolation Reduced speech and communication, loss of skills Increase in somatic complaints

of the features of depression such as guilt, anhedonia and suicidal ideations or feelings of worthlessness (Smiley and Cooper 2003; Walton and Kerr 2016); consequently a formal diagnosis of depression may not be possible, and the disorder may go unrecognised and undiagnosed (Lunsky and Palucka 2004). In the absence of the person being able to provide an account of their emotional symptoms, depression in the person with severe or profound intellectual disability may be made on the presence of behaviour equivalents such as disturbed sleep pattern, irritability, aggression, social withdrawal and deterioration in skills (Janowsky and Davis 2005).

Therapeutic Interventions

The management of depression and anxiety for the person with intellectual disability necessitates a biopsychosocial multidisciplinary collaborate approach, in partnership with the person, their carers and family, based on best available evidence (NICE 2016; Tromans et al. 2020). The person's mental health plan should be developed in accordance with the NICE guidelines on depression (NICE 2009), generalised anxiety disorder and panic disorder in adults (NICE 2020) and mental health problems in people with learning disabilities (NICE 2016). The therapeutic interventions offered to the person can be pharmacological, psychological or a combination of both, with the least intrusive, most effective treatment option being provided first. It is beyond the scope of this

chapter to provide a detailed account of all the pharmacological and psychological interventions that can be used in the treatment of depression and anxiety and so a brief overview will be provided.

Psychological Interventions

Despite the high prevalence rate of depression in people with intellectual disability, the evidence base for the psychological interventions in the treatment of depression in this population is scarce, particularly in relation to people with severe or profound intellectual disability. The psychological intervention should be informed by the outcome of the person's mental health assessment and tailored to the individual to take account of their cognitive level, communication needs and any sensory, neurological or physical impairments they may have as well as the amount of support they may require practising and applying the skills (NICE 2016). However, while a number of psychological interventions are available to the general population, not all of the interventions can be modified or adapted for all people with an intellectual disability due to the person's cognitive or communication limitations, e.g. adapted cognitive behavioural therapy (CBT) requires the person to discuss their feelings, thoughts and attitudes and thus is more suited to the person with mild to moderate intellectual disabilities (Knight et al. 2019; Hamers et al. 2018). NICE (2016) recommends the use of adapted CBT to treat depression in the person with mild intellectual disability. Bakken's (2021) systematic review of psychosocial treatments of depression in the people with intellectual disabilities found that modified CBT showed the best outcome for the treatment of severe depression. In their systematic review of non-pharmacological interventions for adults with intellectual disabilities and depression, Hamers et al. (2018) reviewed studies pertaining to five different modalities: CBT, exercise interventions, behavioural therapy, bright light therapy and social problem-solving skills programme. CBT was the most studied modality in the treatment of depression. Of the eight studies reviewed, seven studies identified that depressive symptoms decreased as a result of CBT and in six of these studies the improvements were still seen on follow-up. Two studies explored exercise intervention, both of which found exercise to have positive results. However, exercise may not be an option for some people who have complex mobility impairments. In the three studies reviewed using behaviour therapy, depressive symptoms were seen to decrease and this decrease maintained at follow-up in two of the studies. Sample sizes were small, though, and the majority of the study participants had a mild intellectual disability with only one study also including people with a moderate intellectual disability. Three case studies were reviewed that investigated bright light therapy with people who had a profound intellectual disability. They received this therapy over a 12-week period, and whilst improvements on the person's mood were observed and maintained at 3-week review, they were not maintained at the 8-week review. One study in the review investigated the use of social problem-solving skills programme for three people with mild intellectual disabilities, and two of the three participants showed a reduction in their depressive symptoms, which were maintained at their 4-week review. Most of the studies reviewed had a small number of participants who have a mild or moderate intellectual disability so it is difficult to know how effective these modalities, even when modified, may be for people with severe or profound intellectual disabilities. Bakken (2021) suggests that therapies such as sensory therapy, systematic gardening and animal-assisted therapy shown to be beneficial in the general population may be beneficial in the treatment of depression in people with severe and profound intellectual disabilities and could be investigated.

Pharmacological Interventions

When prescribing pharmacological interventions for mental health disorders, NICE (2016) recommends adhering to the specific NICE guideline specific to that disorder and the principles therein. Pharmacological interventions may not be the first-line treatment option for less severe forms of depression, and if required medication should only be prescribed by professionals with expertise in treating mental health disorders in people with intellectual disability. People with intellectual disabilities have a high incidence of comorbidities which can include epilepsy, mental health disorders and chronic physical health conditions among others, all of which may necessitate the use of medication in the treatment of these conditions, thus increasing the likelihood of polypharmacy particularly those in the older age group (Eady et al. 2015; O'Dwyer et al. 2016). Psychoactive medications are regularly prescribed for the treatment of depression, and while they have been shown to decrease some of the symptoms associated with the mental disorder, they can have negative side effects and can interact with other medications the person may be prescribed (Eady et al. 2015). To negative these adverse effects, when prescribing medications NICE (2016) recommends that the lowest effective dose of antidepressant to treat the symptoms is prescribed and potential drug to drug interactions need to be ascertained, particularly those medications that may lower the seizure threshold in the person with epilepsy. The person's risk for noncompliance, carer monitoring responsibilities relating to identifying benefits and side effects, the person's consent and their education needs pertaining to the medication and medication review all need to be planned and adjusted to suit the person's needs. Some of the antidepressant groups of drugs are outlined in Table 11.6.

Table 11.6 Pharmacological interventions for the treatment of depression (National Collaborating Centre for Mental Health 2019; HSE 2021)

Antidepressant group	Mode of action	Therapeutic effect	Side effects	Contraindicated in
Selective serotonin reuptake inhibitors (SSRIs) First-line pharmacological intervention	Inhibit the reuptake of serotonin into the presynaptic neurone, thereby increasing serotonin activity and neurotransmission	Consistent across the SSRIs and develops 2–4 weeks after commencement of treatment (HSE 2021)	The most common side effects are nausea, diarrhoea, headache and sexual dysfunction	The person with poorly controlled epilepsy (HSE 2021)
Serotonin noradrenaline reuptake inhibitors (SNRIs)	Inhibit serotonin reuptake and also inhibit the reuptake of noradrenaline and increase the availability of neurotransmitters	Develops from 2 to 6 weeks after commencement of treatment	Similar to SSRIs and also constipation, dry mouth and sweating	The person with uncontrolled blood pressure
Tricyclic antidepressants (TCAs)	Improve noradrenergic and serotonergic neurotransmission by inhibiting the reuptake of monoamine neurotransmitters into the presynaptic neuron	Develops 2–4 weeks after commencement of treatment	Cause anticholinergic side effects, for example, dry mouth, constipation and urinary retention	Prescribed with caution in the person with cardiovascular disease as they can cause sedation, sinus tachycardia and postural hypotension

Anxiety Disorder

Anxiety is a common feeling that everyone experiences from time to time and is a normal response to stressful or threating situations. It can be protective and motivational in nature, by helping the person cope in adverse situations, and prepare for forthcoming events, for example, examinations. Apprehension and worrying about situations can trigger anxiety; however, if anxiety occurs in the absence of a trigger, or if the intensity or duration of the anxiety is not commensurate with the reality of the perceived threat or harm, the symptoms of anxiety can be severely distressing for the person, can impact on all aspects of their life and manifest as an anxiety disorder (Reid et al. 2011). Anxiety disorder is a generic term to describe a range of disorders characterised by feelings of fear, apprehension and anxiety and include generalised anxiety disorders, obsessive-compulsive disorder, social phobias, specific phobias, panic disorder, post-traumatic stress disorder and acute stress disorder (NICE 2020).

Factors Associated with Anxiety Disorder in the Person with Intellectual Disability

The person with an intellectual disability may be more predisposed to developing anxiety disorders due to a combination of biopsychosocial factors. Anxiety symptoms are associated with Fragile X syndrome, Williams syndrome and Prader-Willi and Rubinstein-Taybi syndromes (Cooray and Hiremath 2020), and people with autism spectrum disorder have an increased risk for developing anxiety (Hsieh et al. 2020). Increasing age can also be associated with anxiety symptoms, especially where the person has an underlying chronic physical health condition (Hermans and Evenhuis 2012; Bond et al. 2020), has sleep difficulties and reports feelings of loneliness (Bond et al. 2020). Increase in symptoms of anxiety in both older and younger adults is also shown to be associated with experiencing recent or changing life events in the past year (Reid et al. 2011; Hermans and Evenhuis 2012; Bond et al. 2019;

Hsieh et al. 2020). The person's ability to cope with stressful life situations, such as death or illness of a friend, family member or self, and changes in staff are among some of the life events that have been associated with an increase in the person's anxiety levels (Hermans and Evenhuis 2012; Bond et al. 2019). Other factors, including lack of daytime occupation and employment, low education level and having communication impairment which may affect the person's ability to report or describe their complex emotions, have been shown to contribute to the anxiety levels of the person with intellectual disability (Reid et al. 2011; Bond et al. 2019).

Presentation of Anxiety Disorder

Anxiety can manifest as psychological, cognitive, physiological and behavioural symptoms. Cognitive and psychological symptoms can include fearful apprehension, excessive and repetitive worrying, lack of concentration and irritability. Physiological symptoms can include an increase in somatic complaints, dry mouth, epigastric discomfort, sweating, headache, dizziness, chest pain, palpitations, muscular tension, insomnia, diarrhoea and increased micturition (Deb et al. 2001b; Cooray and Bakala 2005). Most of these above symptoms require the person to be able to verbalise and report these complex feelings and emotions. Symptoms of anxiety, in people with severe or profound intellectual disability who do not have the cognitive or linguistic ability to report their feelings of anxiety, will most likely be manifested in changes in the person's behaviour (Matson et al. 1997) and are reliant on primary caregivers to observe and report the behaviour changes. These anxiety-related observable behaviours can include the person taking short breaths, trembling or shaking, becoming upset, hides or shields face with unfamiliar people or situations, crying, withdrawal, easily fatigues, exaggerated startle response and sleep problems (Matson et al. 1997; Cooray and Bakala 2005).

Diagnosis

Diagnosis of anxiety is made in accordance with the NICE guideline specific to people with intellectual disabilities and mental health disorder (NICE 2016), in conjunction with the clinical guideline on generalised anxiety disorder and panic disorder in adults (NICE 2020). A full review of the person's medication and physical assessment is conducted to exclude any underlying conditions that may be causing the symptoms. A screening tool such as the GAS-LD can be utilised before a formal diagnostic assessment using the DM-ID or DC-LD is completed by a clinician with diagnostic expertise in this area. Before a diagnosis of anxiety can be made, all other explanations for these behavioural changes must be ruled out (Matson et al. 1997).

Therapeutic Interventions

The therapeutic intervention(s) selected should be based on the outcome of the person's multidisciplinary assessment, taking cognisance of the duration and intensity of the symptoms of anxiety and the impact they have on the person's day-to-day life, and tailored to suit the person's needs. Evidence-based psychotherapeutic interventions are effective in the treatment of anxiety disorders (NICE 2014) and are recommended as the first line of treatment for people with mild intellectual disability (NICE 2020). NICE (2020) recommends consulting with a relevant specialist when assessing or offering an intervention to the person with a moderate or severe intellectual disability. In line with the NICE (2014) stepped care approach, the person should be offered the most effective, least intrusive intervention.

Psychological Interventions

Most of the studies on the use of modified psychological interventions in the treatment of anxiety for the person with intellectual disability have been based on case studies, with small sample sizes. Modified interventions such as CBT, relaxation training, reassurance, counselling and self-help have been found to be effective in reducing anxiety (Cooray and Hiremath 2020; Davis et al. 2008).

Pharmacological Interventions

If medication is being prescribed in the treatment of anxiety, it should be prescribed at the lowest possible dose that will achieve the greatest improvements, with minimum side effects (Cooray and Hiremath 2020). If mediation is required an SSRI should be offered after the person has consented to treatment and being informed about the reasons for prescribing, the likely side effects and benefits of treatment (NICE 2020). Davis et al. (2008) in their review of the literature on anxiety found that SSRIs demonstrated efficacy, with mild side effects, in reducing anxiety in people with intellectual disability. Due to their adverse effects benzodiazepines should not be offered for the treatment of anxiety in primary or secondary care, and if prescribed it should only be as a temporary measure during a crisis (NICE 2020) while longer-term interventions are being established (Cooray and Hiremath 2020).

Attention-Deficit/Hyperactivity Disorder

Attention-deficit/hyperactivity disorder (ADHD) is a neurodevelopmental disorder "characterized by a persistent pattern of inattention and/ or hyperactivity-impulsivity that interferes with functioning or development" (Perera 2018: 213). While ADHD is associated with children, it can persist into adolescence and adulthood (Al-Khudaira et al. 2019).

Aetiology of ADHD

There is no identified single cause of ADHD; it is influenced by non-inherited factors, multiple genes and their interplay (Thapar et al. 2012). It is associated with genetic syndromes that have

concomitant intellectual disability and ADHD symptoms such as Rubinstein-Taybi syndrome, Tuberous Sclerosis Complex and Fragile X (Royal College of Psychiatrists 2021; Reilly and Holland 2011; Thapar et al. 2012). There is a higher rate of ADHD in siblings of affected parents and a higher concordance rate in monozygotic twins when compared to dizygotic twins, signifying inherited factors (Thapar et al. 2012). It is also associated with mental health and neurodevelopmental disorders such as depressive disorder, bipolar affective disorder, anxiety disorder and autism spectrum disorder (ASD) (Royal College of Psychiatrists 2021; Al-Khudaira et al. 2019; Thapar et al. 2012; Reilly and Holland 2011). There are a number of environmental factors associated with ADHD; these include prenatal exposure to maternal alcohol; tobacco and drug use; low birth weight and prematurity; infection; exposure to toxin, for example, lead; and psychosocial adversity (Thapar et al. 2012).

Presentation

If the person is mostly assisted by family or carers when carrying out their day-to-day activities, it might be difficult to ascertain if the person had difficulty remembering their daily activities, or if they lose items necessary to perform certain tasks and so the manifestation of inattention may not be apparent (Perera et al. 2022). The hyperactive and impulsive symptoms are apparent in the person's behaviour and in keeping with the diagnostic criteria must occur across two or more settings to prevent misdiagnosis (Perera et al. 2022). These can include impatience and difficulty in waiting their turn or for things to happen, seeking immediate gratification, difficulty in remaining seated, difficulties in getting to sleep, pacing the room during the day and sometimes night, high energy, distracted in busy environments and restlessness.

Diagnosis

Diagnosis can only be made after a detailed assessment by a skilled clinician with expertise in ADHD (NICE 2018; Perera 2018, p. 215).

Diagnosing ADHD in the person with intellectual disability can present challenges for the clinician as the primary signs of ADHD can be manifestations of the intellectual disability (Raji and Javaid 2022). Other challenges include differentiating between the symptoms of ADHD and comorbid mental health and neurodevelopmental disorders such as depressive disorder, bipolar affective disorder, anxiety disorder and ASD (Raji and Javaid 2022; Royal College of Psychiatrists 2021; Al-Khudaira et al. 2019; Reilly and Holland 2011) and the availability of only one intellectual disability-specific ADHD screening and assessment tool (Royal College of Psychiatrists 2021). Also challenging for the clinician is how to measure the level of inattention in the person with intellectual disability. This is one of the core symptoms associated with ADHD (Perera et al. 2022) and not generally something the person may complain about.

Managing ADHD

The severity of the person's ADHD symptoms and the impact they have on the person's life need to be taken into consideration by the multidisciplinary team when developing the person's management plan and should address the behavioural, psychological, educational and occupational needs specific to the individual (NICE 2018). Perera et al. (2022) recommend a three-pronged holistic approach to care for the person with intellectual disability who has ADHD which addresses psychoeducation, pharmacological treatment and behavioural and psychological interventions.

Psychoeducation

Psychoeducation is a psychosocial intervention that can help the person and their family/carers to be involved in the person's care by developing an understanding of ADHD, the diagnosis, how the symptoms of ADHD manifest in the person's behaviours and functional impairments and the impact ADHD has on different aspects of the person's life (Perera et al. 2022; Royal College of Psychiatrists 2021). Psychoeducation can help carers to think constructively about ADHD

and provides them with the opportunity to be involved in the person's care and in the development of positive behaviour support plans to manage ADHD (Royal College of Psychiatrists 2021).

Pharmacological Treatments

The use of pharmacological treatments for ADHD in the general population is well established but the evidence base on the effectiveness of pharmacological treatments for the person with intellectual disability and ADHD is scarce (Miller et al. 2020). As per NICE (2018) guidelines, medication for ADHD should only be prescribed by a health-care professional with expertise in diagnosing and managing ADHD. Stimulant and non-stimulant medications are the NICE (2018) recommended pharmacological treatment options for ADHD. The two main stimulant medications are methylphenidate and dexamphetamine; they block the reuptake of dopamine and noradrenaline and are the NICE (2018) recommended first-line treatments for ADHD. Non-stimulant medications include atomoxetine, clonidine and guanfacine, of which atomoxetine is the NICE (2018) recommended second-line pharmacological option. Atomoxetine is a noradrenaline reuptake inhibitor and clonidine and guanfacine are alpha 2 agonists that modulate the release of dopamine and noradrenaline (Royal College of Psychiatrists 2021). Miller et al. (2020) review of the pharmacotherapy treatment of ADHD in the person with intellectual disability found supporting evidence for the use of both methylphenidate and atomoxetine but recommends that further research evaluating the efficacy of these medications for ADHD for people with intellectual disability is required.

While ADHD medications reduce the core symptoms of ADHD, hyperactivity, inattention and impulsiveness and have a positive effect on the person's daily functioning and quality of life (Perera 2018), they can also have side effects. The most common side effects associated with methylphenidate include sleep disturbances, anorexia, weight loss, anxiety and irritability. Dexamphetamine side effects include mood liability and irritability. The common adverse effects of atomoxetine include drowsiness, gastrointestinal upset and irritability, and clonidine and guanfacine are associated with drowsiness and transient sedation (Miller et al. 2020).

Behavioural and Psychological Interventions

Modified CBT can reduce the core symptoms of ADHD (Royal College of Psychiatrists 2021). Other strategies that can be used to minimise the core symptoms in settings where ADH symptoms are most likely to occur can include reducing auditory distraction by moving to a quieter environment or through the use of noise cancelling headphones and decreasing the amount of visual distractions by modifying the environment, for example, repositioning of furniture in the classroom and breaking tasks into smaller achievable goals (Perera et al. 2022; Royal College of Psychiatrists 2021). Although not supported by strong evidence physical activity incorporated into the person's day-to-day activities can help in managing symptoms of hyperactivity and can be incorporated into the person's care plan.

Conclusion

This chapter explored the concept of mental health, quality of life for people with intellectual disability and its relationship with mental health disorders and problem behaviours. The classification of and prevalence of mental health disorders in people with intellectual disabilities were identified and the some of the complexities associated with accessing mental health services were addressed. The presentation of and management of some of the common mental health disorders most prevalent in people with intellectual disability was outlined.

Key Concepts Discussed

The person with intellectual disability:

- The person experiences the same range of mental health issues and disorders as seen in the general population.
- They are more vulnerable to developing mental health disorders due to biopsychosocial factors.

- It is possible to use ICD 11 and DSM 5 diagnostic criteria to diagnose mental health disorders in the person with mild intellectual disability but not for the person with moderate to profound intellectual disability.
- The person should be in receipt of services underpinned by the guiding principles of mental health service provision for people with intellectual disabilities.

References

Ahlström G, Axmon A, Sandberg M, Hultgvist J (2020) Specialist psychiatric health care utilization among older people with intellectual disability—predictors and comparisons with the general population: a national register study. BMC Psychiatry 20:70. https://doi.org/10.1186/s12888-020-02491-6

Al-Khudaira R, Perera B, Solomou S, Courtenay K (2019) Adults with intellectual disability and attention deficit hyperactivity disorder: clinical characteristics and medication profiles. Br J Learn Disabil 47(2):145–152. https://doi.org/10.1111/bld.12265

American Psychiatric Association (2000) diagnostic and statistical manual of mental disorders. DSM-IV. Washington, American Psychiatric Association

Andresen R, Oades L, Caputi P (2003) The experience of recovery from schizophrenia: towards an empirically validated stage model. Aust N Z J Psychiatr 37(5):586–594. https://doi.org/10.1046/j.1440-1614.2003.01234.x

Anthony WA (1993) Recovery from mental illness: the guiding vision of the mental health service system in the 1990s. Psychosoc Rehabil J 16(4):11–23. https://doi.org/10.1037/h0095655

Bakken TL (2021) Psychosocial treatment of major depression in people with intellectual disabilities. Improvements within the last four decades: points of view. Int J Dev Disabil 67(5):366–370. https://doi.org/10.1080/20473869.2021.1969498

Blackwood DHR, Thiagarajah T, Malloy P, Pickard BS, y Muir, W. J. (2008) Chromosome abnormalities, mental retardation and the search for genes in bipolar disorder and schizophrenia. Neurotox Res 14:113. https://doi.org/10.1007/BF03033803

Bond L, Carroll R, Mulryan N, O'Dwyer M, O'Connell J, Monaghan R, Sheerin F, McCallion P, McCarron M (2019) The association of life events and mental ill health in older adults with intellectual disability: results of the wave 3 Intellectual Disability Supplement to The Irish Longitudinal Study on Ageing. J Intellect Disabil Res 63(5):454–465. https://doi.org/10.1111/jir.12595

Bond L, Carroll R, Mulryan N, O'Dwyer M, O'Connell J, Monaghan R, Sheerin F, McCallion P, McCarron

M (2020) Biopsychosocial factors associated with depression and anxiety in older adults with intellectual disability: results of the wave 3 Intellectual Disability Supplement to The Irish Longitudinal Study on Ageing. J Intellect Disabil Res 64(5):368–380. https://doi.org/10.1111/jir.12724

Borthwick-Duffy SA (1994) Epidemiology and prevalence of psychopathology in people with mental retardation. J Consult Clin Psychol 62(1):17–27

Buckley N, Glasson EJ, Chen W, Epstein A, Leonard H, Skoss R, Jacoby P, Blackmore AM, Srinivasjois R, Bourke J, Sanders RJ, Downs J (2020) Prevalence estimates of mental health problems in children and adolescents with intellectual disability: a systematic review and meta-analysis. Aust N Z J Psychiatr 54(10):970–984. https://doi.org/10.1177/0004867420924101

Chang B, Duzcan F, Kim S et al (2007) The role of RELN in lissencephaly and neuropsychiatric disease. Am J Med Genet 144B:58–63

Chaplin R (2009) Annotation: new research into general psychiatric services for adults with intellectual disability and mental illness. J Intellect Disabil Res 53(3):189–199. https://doi.org/10.1111/j.1365-2788.2008.01143.x

Chaplin R (2011) Mental health services for people with intellectual disabilities. Curr Opin Psychiatry 24(5):372–376. https://doi.org/10.1097/YCO.0b013e3283472524

Chiurazzi P, Pirozzi F (2016) Advances in understanding—genetic basis of intellectual disability. F1000Res 5:Faculty Rev-599

Cohen IL, Tsiouris JA, Flory MJ, Kim S-Y, Freedland R, Heaney G, Pettinger J, Ted Brown W (2010) A large scale study of the psychometric characteristics of the IBR modified overt aggression scale: findings and evidence for increased self-destructive behaviors in adult females with autism spectrum disorder. J Autism Dev Disord 40(5):599–609. https://doi.org/10.1007/s10803-009-0908-z

Cooper S, Smiley E, Morrison J, Williamson A, Allan L (2007) Mental ill-health in adults with intellectual disabilities: prevalence and associated factors. Br J Psychiatry 190(1):27–35. https://doi.org/10.1192/bjp.bp.106.022483

Cooray S, Bakala A (2005) Anxiety disorders in people with learning disabilities. Adv Psychiatr Treat 11(5):355–361. https://doi.org/10.1192/apt.11.5.355

Cooray S, Hiremath A (2020) Anxiety and related disorders in people with intellectual disability. In: Bhaumik S, Alexander R (eds) Oxford textbook of the psychiatry of intellectual disability. Oxford University Press, Oxford, pp 129–139

Copeland Center for Wellness & Recovery (2022) What is WRAP. 21 Feb 2022. Retrieved from: https://www.wellnessrecoveryactionplan.com/what-is-wrap/

Costello H, Bouras N (2006) Assessment of mental health problems in people with intellectual disabilities. Isr J Psychiatry Relat Sci 43(4):241–251. Available at: https://pubmed.ncbi.nlm.nih.gov/17338443/

Courtenay K (2018) Special edition: mental health and intellectual disabilities in Europe. Adv Ment Health Intellect Disabil 12(3/4):89–90. https://doi.org/10.1108/AMHID-07-2018-069

Cuthill FM, Espie CA, Cooper SA (2003) Development and psychometric properties of the Glasgow depression scale for people with a learning disability: individual and carer supplement versions. Br J Psychiatry 182(4):347–353. https://doi.org/10.1192/bjp.182.4.347

Davis E, Atezaz Saeed S, Antonacci DJ (2008) Anxiety disorders in persons with developmental disabilities: empirically informed diagnosis and treatment. Psychiatry Q 79(3):249–263. https://doi.org/10.1007/s11126-008-9081-3

Deb S, Thomas M, Bright C (2001a) Mental disorder in adults with intellectual disability. 1: prevalence of functional psychiatric illness among a community-based population aged between 16 and 64 years. J Intellect Disabil Res 45(6):495–505

Deb S, Matthews T, Holt G, Bouras N (2001b) Practice guidelines for the assessment and diagnosis of mental health problems in adults with intellectual disability. Pavilion, Brighton

Department of Developmental Disability Neuropsychiatry (2014) Accessible mental health services for people with an intellectual disability: a guide for providers. Department of Developmental Disability Neuropsychiatry. ISBN: 978-0-7334-3431-0

Department of Health (UK) (2001) Valuing people, a new strategy for learning disability for the 21st century [Cm 5086]. The Stationery Office, London. Retrieved from: https://assets.publishing.service.gov.uk/government/uploads/system/uploads/attachment_data/file/250877/5086.pdf. Accessed 21 Feb 2022

Department of Health (UK) (2009) New Horizons: Towards a shared vision for mental health: consultation. Retrieved from: https://www.nhs.uk/NHSEngland/NSF/Documents/NewHorizonsConsultation_ACC.pdf. Accessed 12 Nov 2021

Department of Health (UK) (2011) No health without mental health: a cross-government mental health outcomes strategy for people of all ages. Department of Health, London. Retrieved from: https://assets.publishing.service.gov.uk/government/uploads/system/uploads/attachment_data/file/138253/dh_124058.pdf. Accessed 13 Nov 2021

Department of Health (UK) (2014) Achieving better access to mental health services by 2020. Department of Health, London. Retrieved from: https://assets.publishing.service.gov.uk/government/uploads/system/uploads/attachment_data/file/361648/mental-health-access.pdf. Accessed 13 Nov 2021

Department of Health and Children (2006) A vision for change: report of the expert group on mental health policy. Stationary Office, Dublin

Donner B, Mutter R, Scior K (2010) Mainstream inpatient mental health care for people with intellectual disabilities: service user, carer and provider experiences. J Appl Res Intellect Disabil 23:214–225. https://doi.org/10.1111/j.1468-3148.2009.00527.x

Eady N, Courtenay K, Strydom A (2015) Pharmacological management of behavioral and psychiatric symptoms in older adults with intellectual disability. Drugs Aging 32(2):95–102. https://doi.org/10.1007/s40266-014-0236-7

Emerson E, Einfeld SL (2011) Challenging behaviour. Cambridge University Press, New York

Emerson E, Hatton C, Thompson T, Parmenter T (2004) International handbook of applied research in intellectual disabilities. Wiley & Sons, Chichester. 656 pp. ISBN: 0471497096

Finnerty S (2019) Rehabilitation and recovery Mental Health Services in Ireland 2018/2019. Mental Health Commission, Dublin. Retrieved from: https://www.mhcirl.ie/publications/rehabilitation-and-recovery-mental-health-services-ireland-2018/2019. Accessed 22 Feb 2022

Golubović S, Skrbić R (2013) Agreement in quality of life assessment between adolescents with intellectual disability and their parents. Res Dev Disabil 34(6):1863–1869. https://doi.org/10.1016/j.ridd.2013.03.006

Hamers PCM, Festen DAM, Hermans H (2018) Non-pharmacological interventions for adults with intellectual disabilities and depression: a systematic review. J Intellect Disabil Res 62(8):684–700. https://doi.org/10.1111/jir.12502

Handley E, Southwell O, Steel J (2012) Recovery and intellectual disabilities: a review. Adv Ment Health Intellect Disabil 6(4):192–198. https://doi-org.elib.tcd.ie/10.1108/20441281211236625

Health Service Executive (2021) Medicines Management Programme. Preferred drugs selective serotonin reuptake inhibitors (SSRIs) & serotonin noradrenaline reuptake inhibitors (SNRIs) for the treatment of depression. Health Service Executive, Dublin. Retrieved from: https://www.hse.ie/eng/services/publications/clinical-strategy-and-programmes/ssris-snris-for-the-treatment-of-depression.pdf. Accessed 18 Jan 2022

Hermans H, Evenhuis HM (2010) characteristics of instruments screening for depression in adults with intellectual disabilities: systematic review. Res Dev Disabil 31:1109–1120. https://doi.org/10.1016/j.ridd.2010.04.023

Hermans H, Evenhuis HM (2012) Life events and their associations with depression and anxiety in older people with intellectual disabilities: results of the HA-ID study. J Affect Disord 138(1–2):79–85. https://doi.org/10.1016/j.jad.2011.12.025

Hermans H, Evenhuis HM (2013) Factors associated with depression and anxiety in older adults with intellectual disabilities: results of the healthy ageing and intellectual disabilities study. Int J Geriatr Psychiatry 28(7):691–699. https://doi.org/10.1002/gps.3872

Higgins A (2008) A recovery approach within the Irish mental health service: a framework for development. Mental Health Commission, Dublin

Holt G, Costello H, Bouras N, Diareme S, Hillery J, Moss S, Rodriguez-Blazquez C, Salvador L, Tsiantis J,

Weber G, Dimitrakaki C (2000) BIOMED-MEROPE project: service provision for adults with intellectual disability: a European comparison. J Intellect Disabil Res 44(Part 6):685–696

Horovitz M, Shear S, Mancini LM, Pellerito VM (2014) The relationship between Axis I psychopathology and quality of life in adults with mild to moderate intellectual disability. Res Dev Disabil 35(1):137–143. https://doi.org/10.1016/j.ridd.2013.10.014

HSE Mental Health Services (2021) Mental health services for adults with intellectual disabilities. National Model of Service. Health Service Executive, Dublin. Retrieved from: http://hdl.handle.net/10147/628948. Accessed 22 Feb 2021

Hsieh K, Scott HM, Murthy S (2020) Associated risk factors for depression and anxiety in adults with intellectual and developmental disabilities: five-year follow up. Am J Intellect Dev Disabil 125(1):49–63. https://doi.org/10.1352/1944-7558-125.1.49

Irish College of Psychiatrists (2004) Proposed model for the delivery of a mental health service to people with intellectual disability. Irish College of Psychiatrists, Dublin

Jacobson N (2003) Defining recovery: an interactionist analysis of mental health policy development, Wisconsin 1996-1999. Qual Health Res 13(3):378–393. https://doi.org/10.1177/1049732302250334

Jahoda A (2020) Depression and people with a learning disability: a way forward. Tizard Learn Disabil Rev 25(1):13–21. https://doi.org/10.1108/TLDR-03-2019-0010

Janowsky DS, Davis JM (2005) Diagnosis and treatment of depression in patients with mental retardation. Curr Psychiatry Rep 7:421–428. https://doi.org/10.1007/s11920-005-0062-z

Jay L, Macadam B, Gardner P, Mahboub L (2017) Hope headquarters: recovery college. Health Promot J Aust 28:170–173. https://doi.org/10.1071/HE17034

Joint Commissioning Panel for Mental Health (JCPMH) (2013) Guidance for commissioners of mental health services for people with learning disabilities. Joint Commissioning Panel for Mental Health, London. Retrieved from: https://www.basw.co.uk/resources/guidance-commissioners-mental-health-services-people-learning-disabilities. Accessed 13 Nov 2021

Jopp DA, Keys CB (2001) Diagnostic overshadowing reviewed and reconsidered. Am J Ment Retard 106(5):416–433

Knight R, Jahoda A, Scott K, Sanger K, Knowles D, Dagnan D, Hastings RP, Appleton K, Cooper S, Melville C, Jones R, Williams C, Hatton C (2019) "Getting into it": people with intellectual disabilities' experiences and views of behavioural activation and guided self-help for depression. J Appl Res Intellect Disabil 32(4):819–830. https://doi-org.elib.tcd.ie/10.1111/jar.12571

Koch AD, Vogel A, Becker T, Salize HJ, Voss E, Werner A, Arnold K, Schützwohl M (2015) Proxy and self-reported Quality of Life in adults with intellectual disabilities: impact of psychiatric symptoms, problem behaviour, psychotropic medication and unmet needs. Res Dev Disabil 45–46:136–146. https://doi.org/10.1016/j.ridd.2015.07.022

Koskentausta T, Iivanainen M, Almqvist F (2007) Risk factors for psychiatric disturbance in children with intellectual disability. J Intellect Disabil Res 51(Pt 1):43–53. https://doi.org/10.1111/j.1365-2788.2006.00871.x

Kozlowski AM, Matson JL, Sipes M et al (2011) The relationship between psychopathology symptom clusters and the presence of comorbid psychopathology in individuals with severe to profound intellectual disability. Res Dev Disabil 32(5):1610–1614

Lunsky Y, Palucka AM (2004) Depression in intellectual disability. Curr Opin Psychiatry 17(5):359–363. https://doi.org/10.1097/01.yco.0000139970.52813.f2

Marston GM, Perry DW, Roy A (1997) Manifestations of depression in people with intellectual disability. J Intellect Disabil Res 41(Pt 6):476–480. https://doi.org/10.1111/j.1365-2788.1997.tb00739.x

Matson JL, Gardner WI, Coe DA, Sovner R (1991) A scale for evaluating emotional disorders in severely and profoundly mentally retarded persons. Development of the Diagnostic Assessment for the Severely Handicapped (DASH) scale. Br J Psychiatry 159:404–409. https://doi.org/10.1192/bjp.159.3.404

Matson JL, Smiroldo BB, Hamilton M, Baglio CS (1997) Do anxiety disorders exist in persons with severe and profound mental retardation? Res Dev Disabil 18(1):39–44. https://doi.org/10.1016/s0891-4222(96)00036-4

Matson JL, Rush KS, Hamilton M et al (1999) Characteristics of depression as assessed by the Diagnostic Assessment for the Severely Handicapped-II (DASH-II). Res Dev Disabil 20(4):305–313

Matsuura M, Adachi N, Muramatsu R et al (2005) Intellectual disability and psychotic disorders of adult epilepsy. Epilepsia 46(1):11–14

Mazza MG, Rossetti A, Crespi G, Clerici M (2020) Prevalence of co-occurring psychiatric disorders in adults and adolescents with intellectual disability: a systematic review and meta-analysis. J Appl Res Intellect Disabil 33(2):126–138. https://doi.org/10.1111/jar.12654

McCarthy J, Boyd J (2002) Mental health services and young people with intellectual disability: is it time to do better? J Intellect Disabil Res 46(3):250–256. https://doi.org/10.1046/j.1365-2788.2002.00401.x

McGillivray J, McCabe MP (2007) Early detection of depression and associated risk factors in adults with mild/moderate intellectual disability. Res Dev Disabil 28(1):59–70. https://doi.org/10.1016/j.ridd.2005.11.001

Mehregan H, Najmabadi H, Kahrizi K (2016) Genetic studies in intellectual disability and behavioral impairment. Arch Iran Med 19(5):363–375

Melo M, Albuquerque S, Luz J et al (2013) Schizencephaly and psychosis: a rare association. Case Rep Med 2013:210868

Miller J, Perera B, Shankar R (2020) Clinical guidance on pharmacotherapy for the treatment of attention-deficit hyperactivity disorder (ADHD) for people with intellectual disability. Expert Opin Pharmacother 21(15):1897–1913. https://doi.org/10.1080/14656566.2020.1790524

Mindham J, Espie CA (2003) Glasgow anxiety scale for people with an intellectual disability (GAS-ID): development and psychometric properties of a new measure for use with people with mild intellectual disability. J Intellect Disabil Res 47(1):22–30. https://doi.org/10.1046/j.1365-2788.2003.00457.x

Mohapatra S, Panda U, Sahoo A et al (2015) Neuropsychiatric manifestations in a child with agenesis of the corpus callosum. J Neurosci Rural Pract 6(3):456

Moss S (2019) Moss-PAS ID. Pavilion Publishing, Middlesex

Moss S, Friedlander R (2020) Moss-PAS (Diag-ID). Pavilion Publishing, Middlesex

Moss S, Emerson E, Kiernan C et al (2000) Psychiatric symptoms in adults with learning disability and challenging behaviour. Br J Psychiatry 177:452–456

Munir KM (2016) The co-occurrence of mental disorders in children and adolescents with intellectual disability/intellectual developmental disorder. Curr Opin Psychiatry 29(2):95–102

Myrbakk E, von Tetzchner S (2008) Screening individuals with intellectual disability for psychiatric disorders: comparison of four measures. Am J Ment Retard 113(1):54–70

National Association for the Dually Diagnosed (2017) In: Fletcher RJ, Barnhill J, Cooper SA (eds) DM-ID-2: diagnostic manual, intellectual disability: a textbook of diagnosis of mental disorders in persons with intellectual disability. National Association for the Dually Diagnosed. https://thenadd.org/products/dm-id-2/

National Collaborating Centre for Mental Health (2011) Common mental health disorders identification and pathways to care. National clinical guideline number 123. The British Psychological Society and The Royal College of Psychiatrists, Leicester and London

National Collaborating Centre for Mental Health (2019) Depression the treatment and management of depression in adults. National clinical practice guidance 90. The British Psychological Society and The Royal College of Psychiatrists, Leicester and London

National Disability Authority (2003) Review of access to mental health services for people with an intellectual disability. National Disability Authority, Dublin. Retrieved from: http://hdl.handle.net/10147/251418. Accessed 22 Nov 2021

National Institute for Health and Care Excellence (NICE) (2009) Depression in adults: recognition and management. Clinical guideline. National Institute for Health and Clinical Excellence, London. Retrieved from: www.nice.org.uk/guidance/cg90. Accessed 22 Nov 2021

National Institute for Health and Care Excellence (NICE) (2014) Anxiety disorders quality standard. National Institute for Health and Clinical Excellence,

London. Retrieved from: https://www.nice.org.uk/guidance/qs53/resources/anxiety-disorders-pdf-2098725496261. Accessed 22 Nov 2021

National Institute for Health and Care Excellence (NICE) (2016) Mental health problems in people with learning disabilities: prevention, assessment and management. NICE Guideline (NG54). National Institute for Health and Clinical Excellence, London. Retrieved from: https://www.nice.org.uk/guidance/ng54. Accessed 22 Nov 2021

National Institute for Health and Care Excellence (NICE) (2018) Attention deficit hyperactivity disorder: diagnosis and management. National Institute for Health and Clinical Excellence, London. Retrieved from: https://www.nice.org.uk/guidance/ng87/resources/attention-deficit-hyperactivity-disorder-diagnosis-and-management-pdf-1837699732933. Accessed 22 Nov 2021

National Institute for Health and Care Excellence (NICE) (2020) Generalised anxiety disorder and panic disorder in adults: management. National Institute for Health and Clinical Excellence, London. Clinical guideline. Retrieved from: https://www.nice.org.uk/guidance/cg113/resources/generalised-anxiety-disorder-and-panic-disorder-in-adults-management-pdf-35109387756997. Accessed 22 Nov 2021

Nettelbladt P, Goth M, Bogren M et al (2009) Risk of mental disorders in subjects with intellectual disability in the Lundby cohort 1947-97. Nord J Psychiatry 63(4):316–321

Newman I, Leader G, Chen J et al (2015) An analysis of challenging behavior, comorbid psychopathology, and attention-deficit/hyperactivity disorder in fragile X syndrome. Res Dev Disabil 38:7–17

Nyhan WL (1972) Behavioral phenotypes in organic genetic disease: presidential address to the Society for Pediatric Research, May 1, 1971. Pediatr Res 6(1):1–9

O'Dwyer M, Peklar J, McCallion P, McCarron M, Henman M (2016) Factors associated with polypharmacy and excessive polypharmacy in older people with intellectual disability differ from the general population: a cross-sectional observational nationwide study. BMJ Open 6:e010505. https://doi.org/10.1136/bmjopen-2015-010505

Peña-Salazar C, Arrufat Nebot F, Fontanet A, García-León N, Más S, Roura Poch P, Santos López J (2017) Underdiagnosis of mental disorder in the population with intellectual disability: prevalence study in population with different degrees of intellectual disabilities. Siglo Cero Spanish Mag Intellect Disabil 48(3):27–39. https://doi.org/10.14201/scero20174832739

Peña-Salazar C, Arrufat F, Fontanet A, Font J, Mas S, Roura-Poch P, Santos JM (2018) The role of mental health and challenging behaviour in the quality of life in people with intellectual disabilities in Spain. Adv Ment Health Intellect Disabil 12(1):34–43. https://doi.org/10.1108/AMHID-06-2017-0022

Peña-Salazar C, Alfonso-Ramos M, Arroyo-Uriarte P, Serrano-Blanco A, Aznar-Lou I (2022) Is epilepsy related to psychiatric disorders in people with intellectual disability? A systematic review. J Intellect Disabil. https://doi.org/10.1177/17446295221116506. Advance online publication

Perera B (2018) Attention deficit hyperactivity disorder in people with intellectual disability. Ir J Psychol Med 35(3):213–219. https://doi.org/10.1017/ipm.2018.7

Perera B, McCarthy J, Courtenay K (2022) Assessing and managing attention-deficit hyperactivity disorder in people with intellectual disability. BJPsych Adv 28:363. https://doi.org/10.1192/bja.2022.23

Petry K, Maes B, Vlaskamp C (2009) Measuring the quality of life of people with profound multiple disabilities using the QOL-PMD: first results. Res Dev Disabil 30(6):1394–1405. https://doi.org/10.1016/j.ridd.2009.06.007

Raji O, Javaid S (2022) Successful diagnosis of attention deficit hyperactivity disorder in later life of an adult with intellectual disability: a case report. Br J Learn Disabil 50:1–8. https://doi-org.elib.tcd.ie/10.1111/bld.12446

Ramsay H, Dodd P (2018) Mental health services for people with intellectual disability in Ireland: evidence, barriers and opportunities. Adv Ment Health Intellect Disabil 12(3/4):105–113. https://doi-org.elib.tcd.ie/10.1108/AMHID-03-2018-0016

Reid KA, Smiley E, Cooper SA (2011) Prevalence and associations of anxiety disorders in adults with intellectual disabilities. J Intellect Disabil Res 55(2):172–181. https://doi.org/10.1111/j.1365-2788.2010.01360.x

Reilly C, Holland N (2011) Symptoms of attention deficit hyperactivity disorder in children and adults with intellectual disability: a review. J Appl Res Intellect Disabil 24(4):291–309. https://doi.org/10.1111/j.1468-3148.2010.00607.x

Reiss S, Rojahn J (1993) Joint occurrence of depression and aggression in children and adults with mental retardation. J Intellect Disabil Res 37(3):287–294

Reiss S, Levitan G, Szyszko J (1982) Emotional disturbance and mental retardation: diagnostic overshadowing. Am J Ment Defic 86(6):567–574

Rojahn J, Matson JL, Naglieri JA et al (2004) Relationships between psychiatric conditions and behavior problems among adults with mental retardation. Am J Ment Retard 109(1):21–33

Royal College of Psychiatrists (2001) DC-LD: diagnostic criteria for psychiatric disorders for use with adults with learning disabilities/mental retardation. Occasional paper OP 48. Royal College of Psychiatrists, London

Royal College of Psychiatrists (2020) Mental health services for adults with mild intellectual disability. College Report. Royal College of Psychiatrists, London. Retrieved from: https://www.rcpsych.ac.uk/docs/default-source/improving-care/better-mh-policy/college-reports/college-report-cr226.pdf?sfvrsn=8220109f_2. Accessed 18 Jan 2022

Royal College of Psychiatrists (2021) Attention deficit hyperactivity disorder (ADHD) in adults with intellectual disability. College Report. Royal College of Psychiatrists, London. Retrieved from:

https://www.rcpsych.ac.uk/improving-care/campaigning-for-better-mental-health-policy/college-reports/2021-college-reports/ADHD-in-adults-with-intellectual-disability-CR230. Accessed 18 Jan 2022

Rush AJ, Frances A (2000) Expert consensus guideline series: treatment of psychiatric and behavioral problems in mental retardation. Am J Ment Retard 105(3):159–226

Salvador-Carulla L, Novell-Alsina R (2002) Guía Práctica de la Evaluación Psiquiátrica en el Retraso Mental [in Spanish]. Aula Medica Ediciones, Madrid

Schalock RL, Verdugo MA (2002) Handbook on quality of life for human service practitioners, 1st edn. American Association on Mental Retardation, Washington, DC

Scheifes A, Walraven S, Stolker JJ, Nijman HLI, Egberts TCG, Heerdink ER (2016) Adverse events and the relation with quality of life in adults with intellectual disability and challenging behaviour using psychotropic drugs. Res Dev Disabil 49–50:13–21. https://doi.org/10.1016/j.ridd.2015.11.017

Schützwohl M, Koch A, Koslowski N et al (2016) Mental illness, problem behaviour, needs and service use in adults with intellectual disability. Soc Psychiatr Psychiatr Epidemiol 51(5):767–776

Sheehan R, Paschos D (2013) A comparison of different models to meet the mental health needs of adults with intellectual disabilities. Adv Ment Health Intellect Disabil 7(3):161–168. https://doi-org.elib.tcd.ie/10.1108/20441281311320747

Sheehan R, Hassiotis A, Walters K et al (2015) Mental illness, challenging behaviour, and psychotropic drug prescribing in people with intellectual disability: UK population based cohort study. Br Med J 351:1–9

Shepherd G, Boardman J, Slade M (2008) Making recovery a reality. Sainsbury Centre for Mental Health, London. Retrieved from: Making recovery a reality policy paper.pdf (centreformentalhealth.org.uk). Accessed 13 Nov 2021

Simes C, Santos S (2016) Comparing the quality of life of adults with and without intellectual disability. J Intellect Disabil Res 60(4):378–388. https://doi.org/10.1111/jir.12256

Sines D, Hogard E, Ellis R (2012) Evaluating quality of life in adults with profound learning difficulties resettled from hospital to supported living in the community. J Intellect Disabil 16(4):247–263. https://doi.org/10.1177/1744629512463840

Slevin E, Truesdale-Kennedy M, McConkey R, Barr O, Taggart L (2008) Community learning: disability teams: developments, composition and good practice: a review of the literature. J Intellect Disabil 12(1):59–79. https://doi.org/10.1177/1744629507083583

Smiley E, Cooper SA (2003) Intellectual disabilities, depressive episode, diagnostic criteria and Diagnostic Criteria for Psychiatric Disorders for Use with Adults with Learning Disabilities/Mental Retardation (DC-LD). J Intellect Disabil Res 47(Suppl 1):62–71. https://doi.org/10.1046/j.1365-2788.47.s1.26.x

Sperli F, Rentsch D, Despland PA et al (2009) Psychiatric comorbidity in patients evaluated for chronic epilepsy: a differential role of the right hemisphere? Eur Neurol 61(6):350–357

Thapar A, Cooper M, Jefferies R, Stergiakouli E (2012) What causes attention deficit hyperactivity disorder? Arch Dis Childhood 97(3):260–265. https://doi.org/10.1136/archdischild-2011-300482

The Seniors (2011) My life: personal outcomes index. The Seniors, Edmonton

Thygesen JH, Wolfe K, McQuillin A, Viñas-Jornet M, Baena N, Brison N, D'Haenens G, Esteba-Castillo S, Gabau E, Ribas-Vidal N, Ruiz A, Vermeesch J, Weyts E, Novell R, Buggenhout GV, Strydom A, Bass N, Guitart M, Vogels A (2018) Neurodevelopmental risk copy number variants in adults with intellectual disabilities and comorbid psychiatric disorders. Br J Psychiatr 212(5):287–294. https://doi.org/10.1192/bjp.2017.65

Townsend-White C, Pham ANT, Vassos MV (2012) Review: a systematic review of quality of life measures for people with intellectual disabilities and challenging behaviours. J Intellect Disabil Res 56(3):270–284. https://doi.org/10.1111/j.1365-2788.2011.01427.x

Tromans S, Umar A, Torr J, Alexander R, Bhaumik S (2020) Depressive disorders in people with intellectual disability. In: Bhaumik S, Alexander R (eds) Oxford textbook of the psychiatry of intellectual disability. Oxford University Press, Oxford, pp 105–116

Trustam E, Chapman P, Shanahan P (2022) Making recovery meaningful for people with intellectual disabilities. J Appl Res Intellect Disabil 35(1):252–260. https://doi.org/10.1111/jar.12944

Tsiouris JA, Kim SY, Brown WT et al (2011) Association of aggressive behaviours with psychiatric disorders, age, sex and degree of intellectual disability: a large-scale survey. J Intellect Disabil Res 55(7):636–649

Tudor K (1996) Mental health promotion paradigms and practice. Routledge, London

Turygin N, Matson JL, Konst M, Williams L (2013) The relationship of early communication concerns to developmental delay and symptoms of autism spectrum disorders. Dev Neurorehabil 16(4):230–236. https://doi.org/10.3109/17518423.2012.756950

Unwin GL, Deb S, John R (2019) Depression. In: Matson J (ed) Handbook of intellectual disabilities: integrating theory, research and practice. Springer, Cham

Verdugo M, Arias B, Gomez LE, Schalock RL (2010) Development of an objective instrument to assess quality of life in social services: reliability and validity in Spain. Int J Clin Health Psychol 10(1):105–123

Verdugo MA, Gomez LE, Arias B, Navas P, Schalock RL (2014) Measuring quality of life in people with intellectual and multiple disabilities: validation of the San Martin scale. Res Dev Disabil 35(1):75–86. https://doi.org/10.1016/j.ridd.2013.10.025

Walton C, Kerr M (2016) Severe intellectual disability: systematic review of the prevalence and nature of presentation of unipolar depression. J Appl Res Intellect Disabil 29(5):395–408. https://doi.org/10.1111/jar.12203

Walton C, Medhurst D, Madhavan G, Shankar R (2022) The current provision of mental health services for individuals with mild intellectual disability: a scoping review. J Ment Health Res Intellect Disabil 15(1):49–75. https://doi.org/10.1080/19315864.2021.1992549

Weiner MF, Martin-Cook K, Svetlik DA, Saine K, Foster B, Fontaine CS (2000) The quality of life in late-stage dementia (QUALID) scale. J Am Med Direct Assoc 1(3):114–116

Whittle EL, Fisher KR, Reppermund S, Lenroot R, Trollor J (2018) Barriers and enablers to accessing mental health services for people with intellectual disability: a scoping review. J Ment Health Res Intellect Disabil 11(1):69–102. https://doi.org/10.1080/19315864.2017.1408724

World Health Organization (2012) Programme on mental health: WHOQOL user manual, 2012 revision. WHO, Geneva. https://www.who.int/publications/i/item/WHO-HIS-HSI-Rev.2012-3. Accessed 16 Sep 2022

World Health Organization (2019) International classification of diseases 11th revision. World Health Organisation, Geneva. https://icd.who.int/browse11/l-m/en#/http%3A%2F%2Fid.who.int%2Ficd%2Fentity%2F334423054. Accessed 23 May 2022

World Health Organization (2022) World mental health report: transforming mental health for all. WHO, Geneva. Licence: CC BY-NC-SA 3.0IGO. https://www.who.int/publications/i/item/9789240049338. Accessed 17 Jun 2022

Part IV

Integrating Health and Social Perspectives

The Social Contract of Care for People with an Intellectual Disability

12

Damien Brennan and Maureen D'Eath

Chapter Topics

- This chapter considers the responsibility of care provision for people with intellectual disabilities.
- Furthermore, the impacts of social policies of deinstitutionalisation and de-congregation on caregiving are reflected.
- The impact of changing family structure on caregiving in family homes is also discussed.

Introduction

This chapter explores the social contract for care provision within the contemporary post-institutional context, with specific reference to intellectual disability. The extensive use of congregated settings of confinement as a means of managing the care needs of people with intellectual disability was dehumanising, abusive and wrong, and the cessation of this approach to caregiving is most welcome. Over the past 50 years a social policy reorientation towards de-congregation and deinstitutionalisation has shifted caregiving away from large built environments to community settings.

The social policy prioritisation of care within the community has occurred during a time when family units have also undergone significant changes. Wide-scale sociological dynamics, such as greater gender equality, increased control of fertility, increased participation of women within the formal labour market, emigration, migration and labour mobility and macro-economic factors such as decreased affordability of living spaces have all impacted on the role, function and makeup of family units. This in turn has impacted on the capacity to provide care within the family unit at a time when social policy is emphasising the increased role of the family as an entity that can provide long-term care. The social contract for care encapsulates the relationship between the nation state, the family and the individual who requires care. Within the post-institutional policy era there remains uncertainty regarding this social contract for care, specifically what the expectations, roles and responsibility of the family are.

The wide-scale utilisation of large residential institutions as a societal response to the needs of people with an intellectual disability was common across Europe and most of the Western world during the nineteenth and twentieth centuries. The proliferation of institutions for people with intellectual disability was one aspect of an era of great confinement, with similar congregated settings being utilised as a controlling response for a spectrum of human

D. Brennan (✉) · M. D'Eath
School of Nursing and Midwifery,
Trinity College Dublin, Dublin, Ireland
e-mail: dbrennan@tcd.ie

© The Author(s), under exclusive license to Springer Nature Switzerland AG 2023
F. Sheerin, C. Doyle (eds.), *Intellectual Disabilities: Health and Social Care Across the Lifespan*,
https://doi.org/10.1007/978-3-031-27496-1_12

experiences such as mental health problems, disability, childhood destitution, poverty, control of sexuality and disapproved pregnancy and birth. During that era of extensive incarceration there was a shared social view that this was a rational "care" response, enacted for the better good of the confined individual. This approach to social intervention was administered by multiple structures and systems including governments, church organisations, philanthropic and voluntary organisations and the private market. The process of admission and long-term confinement within these institutions was made possible by the cooperation of families and local communities in collaboration with the staff and professionals employed within these settings.

The contemporary revisionist historical account of institutions of confinement is damning. The impulse within society to construct human experiences as "deviant" or "abnormal" is now heavily condemned, while the act of institutional confinement is now understood as a direct violation of the most basic of human rights. Since the late twentieth century, social policies across the Western world have embraced a process of deinstitutionalisation (Bredewold et al. 2020), have advocated for a much broader acceptance of diverse human realities and have advanced community-based interventions to respond to specific care needs.

The specific field of intellectual disability has been part of this drive to de-institutionalise. Alongside the scaling down and closure of institutional buildings, there has been a widespread progressive movement to reframe the social construction of people with intellectual disability, emphasising their equal rights as citizens within societies that embrace diversity. The provision of care for people with intellectual disability within this new policy context has shifted away from institutional settings to the domestic setting, primarily care within the family home provided by the family. This chapter explores this shift of care provision, with specific focus on how the family is situated within this new social contract for care provision.

The Social Contract for Care

The social contract for care encapsulates how care provision is understood and mediated, specifically the expected and routinised roles and responsibilities between the individual who requires care, the family and the nation state. Such care provision operates within dynamic political and cultural contexts resulting in a wide diversity of systems and expectations regarding care provision across different jurisdictions. Care "is central to the boundaries drawn between state and family, as seen in the formal definitions of family obligations" (Leira and Saraceno 2002, p. 10); it embodies a society's vision of care and presents unique issues for public policy (Daly 2002). While all welfare states accept some public responsibility for care, they differ in how this responsibility is assigned and in the underlying assumptions and conditions of this responsibility which they undertake this responsibility (Knijn and Kremer 1997).

In his seminal work, Esping-Andersen (1990, 1999) proposed a classification of welfare regimes according to the extent to which they support or replace family care. Although Esping-Andersen's typology has been extensively debated, critiqued and modified (Powell et al. 2019), it still stands as a useful framework through which to overview welfare regimes. Coining the terms familialist and de-familialist, Esping-Andersen defined the first as a state that "assigns a maximum of welfare obligations to the household", whereas de-familialist policies are those that "lessen individuals' reliance on the family; that maximise individuals' command of economic resources independently of familial or conjugal reciprocities" (Esping-Andersen 1999, p. 45).

Esping-Andersen (1999) identified three ideal welfare regimes: liberal, conservative and social-democrat, underpinned by the principles of:

- Decommodification: the extent to which welfare is dependent on the market
- Social stratification: the state's role in maintaining or breaking down social stratification
- The public private mix (Bambra 2007)

Liberal welfare regimes have minimal, residual social welfare expenditure and rely on the market economy and private provision; the ideological underpinning of such regimes is that of freedom. Conservative welfare regimes offer certain benefits arising from social insurance which is usually employment based. Individuals excluded from the labour force are ineligible for the benefits and such regimes thereby reinforce the male breadwinner model. Social-democrat regimes are characterised by universal social programmes based on citizenship which serve to minimise dependence on the market and collectivise familial responsibilities. Other theorists have since added the Latin or Southern welfare regime to Esping-Andersen's typology as a fourth ideal regime (Saint-Arnaud and Bernard 2003). This welfare regime is the most familialist, with few redistributive social policies and with family support dependent on the primary breadwinner (Saint-Arnaud and Bernard 2003).

While there is a wide diversity of specific social welfare and policy orientations in individual countries, a broad application of Esping-Andersen's typology suggests that Anglo-Saxon countries are largely market-based, Southern European and Japanese regimes are predominantly familialist and Nordic countries are highly de-familialist with much of the welfare delivered by the state. Saraceno (2016) distinguished between supported familialism, prescribed familialism and familialism by default with the latter occurring in countries wherein no services or allowances are available to replace or support family care. In 2019, Le Bihan et al. took up the proposals of Saraceno (2016) and those of Leitner (2003) to distinguish between supported and unsupported familialism in the context of weak service policies. They explain:

> In both cases, families are considered responsible for care and expected to provide it. Under unsupported familialism, policies do not recognise families' need for support. Under supported familialism, families are helped in taking up care. The fact that these support measures also represent an enforcement of familialism is due to lack of services and not necessarily to the existence of explicit informal care supporting schemes (Le Bihan et al. 2019, p. 581).

Interestingly, a high level of formal state provision of care does not reduce the extent of informal care provided by family and friends; rather it reduces the intensity of care and changes the type of care given. Verbakel (2017) examined how the prevalence rates of informal caregiving and intensive caregiving (defined as providing at least 11 hours of care weekly) vary between European countries and the relationship of informal and intense caregiving to the countries' formal long-term care provision and family care norms. Informal caregiving was most prevalent in countries with the most generous long-term care provisions, but these countries had a low prevalence of intensive caregiving. Family care norms were found to be positively related to intensive caregiving but not to the likelihood of informal caregiving. The author concluded that:

> … less generosity of formal long-term care provisions was also related to fewer informal caregivers in total. Since especially intensive caregiving is burdensome, … low levels of formal long-term care provisions might bring risks. Overtaxed informal caregivers may provide lower-quality care, may dropout as caregivers, and may even become in need of care themselves. Therefore, a situation in which 'many caregivers do a little each' may be a more sustainable situation for the healthcare system. This study's results suggested that such a situation is most common in countries with generous formal long-term care provisions. (Verbakel 2017, p. 10)

Defamilialisation and degenderisation may be seen as "two sides of the same coin" (Chybalski and Marcinkiewicz 2021, p. 400). The Nordic countries' highly defamilialistic public service models are characterised by comprehensive public social services provided universally as a right of citizenship and by high levels of gender equality in the paid workforce. By contrast, the traditionally highly familialistic regimes of Southern European countries exhibit a more gendered division of family roles with a lower rate of female participation in the paid workforce. Familialism locates the responsibility for the family within the family, and in general, familialisatic regimes reflect and reinforce traditional gendered roles and a male breadwinner/female homemaker (carer) model of economic and family life.

Ironically, according to Jensen (2008), women can only experience defamilialisation through being commodified:

> Therefore, the great paradox becomes that the only way for women to gain independence from the family realm is by being commodified by the market (Jensen 2008, p. 157).

The social policy orientation of any specific nation state is directly impacted by, but also frames, the public perception and normalisation of expected roles within the family with regard to care provision. However, family units are not static entities and changing family structures directly impacts on the capacity for care provision at any point in time.

Demographic Shifts and Care Capacity Within the Family

The right of individuals to access care has advanced over the past decades; however, during this time the capacity for caregiving within family units has altered in response to the changing demographic profiles. Within the European context a right to long-term care was jointly proclaimed in 2017 by the European Parliament, the Council of the EU and the EC. Principle 18 of the European Pillar of Social Rights asserts that everyone has the right to affordable long-term care of good quality, in particular homecare and community-based services. A right to care for those who need such presupposes that there will be people to provide the care; currently 80% of long-term care in Europe is provided by family or other informal carers. However, the demographic structure of Western society is changing rapidly (Eurostat 2020). The European population is ageing, and historically low fertility rates and increased life expectancy are resulting in a declining proportion of people of working age. These developments are likely to have profound implications across all sectors of society including health and social care systems (Eurostat 2020). The family unit itself has also undergone significant changes in recent decades. There are now more single-parent families and double-income households than ever before, and family members are more mobile and may not live close to their family home. The world of work has also undergone a transformation from that upon which welfare states were built wherein "a Fordist economy guarantees decent pay and secure employment" (Lister 2001, p. 93). The previously prevailing, breadwinner model wherein mothers took care of the home and family while fathers worked in paid employment, paying taxes and receiving the social insurance benefits of pensions and social assistance when required, has increasingly given way to an adult worker model. Lewis (2007) argues that the assumption that all adults will be financially independent and active in the labour market is paralleled in the restructuring of welfare states to an extent that it constitutes a "new social settlement" (p. 272). Hoffmann and Rodrigues (2010) describe as a "key policy challenge" the European drive to expand the workforce by increased female and older person participation and the importance of also "trying to avoid a 'drying out' of the family care pool" (p. 4). Thus, the provision of informal care is characterised as a barrier to female participation in the paid labour force and a hinderance to a nation's economic expansion (International Confederation of Trade Unions 2018), and those providing family care are characterised as economically "inactive":

> Caring responsibilities are reasons for inactivity for almost 31% of inactive women, while this is only the case for 4.5% of men. Taking action is not only a question of fairness, but it is also an economic imperative: we estimate the economic loss due to the gender employment gap amounts to around €370 billion per year (European EU 2019, npn).

While the reorientation of care away from large institutional settings to the community is most welcome, the capacity for care provision within communities is heavily reliant on the assumed existence of a large pool of carers, who are predominately female carers within family units. Within the field of intellectual disability this raises tensions between social policy expectations, the rights of the person with an intellectual disability to access care and the assumption that family members will be in a position to provide care and indeed the assumption that family members will want to take on this role.

Social Policies of Deinstitutionalisation and Its Impact on Family-Based Care for People with Intellectual Disability

As set out above, the social contract for care operates within a complex and dynamic social process influenced by the social welfare orientation of the state, national social policy, the demographic profile and the cultural expectations of families. During the past 30 years this has raised profound questions regarding the long-term care of people with intellectual disability. Intellectual disability is one of the most prevalent and enduring disabilities across all countries and the question of where the responsibility for care lies is highly pertinent to the lives of people with intellectual disability. The dynamics for care provision for people with an intellectual disability have radically altered and are now framed within concepts of human rights. Milestones marking the establishing of the civil and human rights of people with disabilities include the United Nations Declaration on the Rights of Mentally Retarded People in 1971, the Declaration on the Rights of Disabled Persons in 1975 and the Americans with Disabilities Act in 1990. In 2006 the United Nations Convention on the Rights of Persons with Disabilities (UNCRPD) became the first legally enforceable international instrument to address the rights of people with disabilities and signatories committed:

> …to promote, protect and ensure the full and equal enjoyment of all human rights and fundamental freedoms by all persons with disabilities, and to promote respect for their inherent dignity (Article 1).

Although largely incomplete, the process of deinstitutionalisation has taken place in most Western countries. Bredewold et al. (2020) describe Novella's (2010) account that:

> The move towards deinstitutionalisation started in the 1950s in the UK, the USA and Italy and then rapidly spread to the remainder of continental

Europe, Scandinavia and the Antipodes. (Bredewold et al. 2020, p. 84)

At its simplest, deinstitutionalisation constituted the closure of large, congregated settings and the relocation of the residents of those settings into the community, a policy described by Mansell and Beadle-Brown as "the most significant policy development in intellectual disability in the post-war period" (Mansell and Beadle-Brown 2010, p. 104).

However, deinstitutionalisation also entailed the ideals of normalisation, social inclusion and participation of people with disabilities (Chung et al. 2018). A contrast between welfare regimes can be illustrated by the way in which deinstitutionalisation and normalisation were operationalised in Sweden and in the UK. The "normalisation principle" underpins the Swedish disability policy and the deinstitutionalisation of people with intellectual disability was completed in the 1990s. As in other Nordic countries, Swedish young people move out of the family home early in their adult lives and few adults continue to live with their parents, and since deinstitutionalisation, this is also the case for adults with an intellectual disability. An adult with intellectual disability living at home with their parents is non-normative, and Engwall (2019) asserts that such a living arrangement "violates social norms and disability policy ambitions" (p. 119).

Parker (1990) argues that in the UK the concept of "community care" originally covered a range of provisions including community hospitals, hostels, day hospitals, residential homes, day centres and domiciliary support (Parker 1990). However, by the 1980s community care had been re-defined as care by the community—family and neighbours with state support—rather than care provided by the state in the community (Allen 2000). Feminist scholars characterised community care policies as "regressive and patriarchal, effectively transferring responsibility from the state to the family and, within the family, to women" (Fine 2006, p. 603), and it is argued that community care is often a synonym for family care (Power 2016). Within contemporary post-institutionalised society, the predominant reality for most people with intellectual disability is to live with their families. Within this context, family carers of people with intellectual disability may be strongly reliant on formal supports, particularly day and respite services, to sustain their ability to care (Brennan et al. 2016). Indeed, family carers have been reported to have concerns about the impact of deinstitutionalisation on family life (Tabatabainia 2003) and may fear an increased burden of care when their family member is moved into the community (O'Doherty et al. 2016).

These policy changes are converging to place greater emphasis than ever before on the need for future care planning for adults with an intellectual disability and their family carers. Within contemporary society, people with and intellectual disabilities are now living longer, including those with profound intellectual and multiple disabilities (McCarron et al. 2011; García-Domínguez et al. 2020); hence, there is a growing population of people with intellectual disabilities. This tension between deinstitutionalisation and family capacity to provide care can be illustrated by an exploration of Ireland as a case study.

The Changing Nature of the Social Contract for Care: Ireland as a Case Study

Ireland is an interesting country to serve as a case study for considering the social contract for care, particularly because of the speed at which Ireland has undergone social, cultural and financial transformations over recent decades which have directly impacted on the makeup and dynamic of family structures. During this period of time Irish social policy for people with intellectual disability moved from a system of institutional-based care to care within the community. This case study of Ireland as a nation state highlights the importance of the social contract for care evolving with societal and policy changes, so as to avoid a fundamental mismatch between policy and lived reality, which can result in a devaluing of both care givers and care recipients.

When Ireland achieved its independence in 1922, the fledgling State left much of the nation's health and social services to religious and voluntary bodies who were largely funded by the State which then distanced itself from the administration of the services. This included large-scale institutional provision for people with intellectual disability. Ireland's constitution reflects the patriarchal society of 1937 in which women were firmly subordinated to men (Brady 2012). Article 41.2 of the Constitution recognised "that by her life within the home, woman gives to the State a support without which the common good cannot be achieved" and asserted that mothers should not be forced by economic necessity to engage in labour to the neglect of their duties in the home. Whereas this clause did allude to the vital role of care within a society, its highly gendered nature frames care in the private sphere and exempts men from care responsibilities.

With regard to care within the community, the social thinking of the Catholic Church was underpinned by the "fundamental", "unshaken" and "unchangeable" principle of subsidiarity which demands that care should be given by those closest to the individual who needed that care (Timonen and Doyle 2008), and this principle of subsidiarity dovetailed neatly with the Irish State's reluctance to involve itself in personal and family issues. Indeed, the 1970 Health Act explicitly restricted state provision of home care service to those who were not being supported by voluntary organisations, families or neighbours (Murphy and Turner 2017). Today, Ireland's care system is distinct from that of any other European or Nordic country with the legacy of a fragmented health and social care system. This unique health system is a mix of limited public provision and state-funded provision delivered through third-party organisations and, increasingly, through private market provision, alongside familialistic welfare regime that locates care primarily as a family issue.

Care within the family setting has thus been historically situated as a private matter and as one that was not the concern of the State (Smith 2012). Nevertheless, Ireland also experienced large-scale institutional confinement of those whose needs fell outside the perceived norms, including those with intellectual disability or mental illnesses (Brennan 2014).

Unlike in some EU countries, family members in Ireland have no formal legal obligation to provide care. However, where a person is deemed to have assumed a responsibility for care, criminal sanction may be taken against them if they fail to provide such care and are considered to have been criminally neglectful. In an Appeal Court decision in 2016, Mr Justice Birmingham stated that the general position in Ireland is "that there is no obligation to care for another"; however, a duty to care "might be derived from the assumption of a responsibility to act" (vLex n.d.). Thus, informal carers have a responsibility to care to a legally acceptable standard of proficiency, and, although an "unassuming feature of everyday life" (Bryant and Garnham 2016, p. 2), caring is also an unbounded responsibility which can restrict and dominate all other roles in life. Informal carers, in general, sustain Ireland's long-term care system (Russell et al. 2019). The limited availability of appropriate supports hindered public provision of care services and strict eligibility criteria for services amount to familiarisation by default, with family members as the default caregivers. Although the experiences of families caring for people with intellectual disabilities will mirror the experiences of carers in other contexts, a number of features also distinguish these carers including the longevity of the caring relationship (Taggart et al. 2012; Mahon et al. 2019), the impact of ageing on both the caregiver and the care recipient and concerns about the future of the care recipient when the caregiver dies or is no longer in a position to continue caring.

Whereas in the past the availability of a pool of (mainly) females to provide care in family homes in the community was facilitated by Ireland's strong male breadwinner/female homemaker model, Ireland's contemporary long-term care paradigm is increasingly based on a model of family structure that no longer exists. Driven by a perceived economic imperative of the Irish state, women were increasingly encouraged to enter the paid workforce since the 1990s. Arising from this, Ireland's traditional strong male breadwinner model has given way to a dual-breadwinner model or adult-worker model. However, the absence of an available, reliable and accessible care infrastructure may exclude many family carers from the choice to participate in the paid workforce. A Eurofound (2015) report on reconciling care and employment highlighted this contradiction:

> In sharp contrast to the progress made in raising awareness of the rights of workers with care responsibilities for children, public awareness and policies relative to workers with care responsibilities for adults and elderly relatives have been extremely limited. A double approach is needed to improve the situation of working carers: more publicly funded support infrastructures and improving the rights of workers with care responsibilities, including receiving compensation for the foregone earnings (Eurofound 2015, p. 85).

The increased participation of women in the paid workforce, an increase in the age of retirement, shrinking family sizes, greater geographical distances between family members and an ageing and predominantly rural population all challenge the sustainability of a care system reliant on unpaid family-based carers (Broese Van Groenou and De Boer 2016; Marking 2017; Murphy and Turner 2017). In recent decades Ireland's policy paradigm for the care of people with intellectual disability has followed international trends in espousing deinstitutionalisation and community care. Ireland is one of very few European countries with a database of persons with an intellectual disability which contains up-to-date data on demographic details, current service provision and future service needs (Dodd et al. 2010). From this data, the Irish Department of Health anticipates that the number of young adults with an intellectual disability will grow by one third by 2032 and the number of those aged over 55 years will grow by a quarter by that date (Department of Health 2021). It further projects that the number of adults with intellectual disability who are living with family members will be 20% higher by 2032 than it was in 2017 (Department of Health 2021).

The mismatch between the prevailing social contract for care in Ireland and the needs of both caregivers and care recipients is evident. However, there are indications that the sentiment of the citizens of Ireland may be driving a new era of greater valuing of caregivers necessitating a new contract of care. A recent study by Teahan et al. (2021) in the context of dementia reported that the Irish public were not only in favour of greater support for carers but were also willing to pay more tax to fund this. Similarly, a Citizens' Assembly on Gender Equality unanimously voted in 2021 to replace Article 4.2 of the constitution with a provision that is not gender specific and which "obliges the State to take reasonable measures to support care within the home and wider community". The Irish process of Citizens' Assembly brings together a representative body of citizens to discuss and consider important legal and policy issues and to make recommendations to the legislature (Citizens' Information 2022). The vote of the Citizens' Assembly should herald a fundamentally important national debate on the social contract for care in Ireland leading to a shared and explicit understanding about where, and with whom, the responsibility for care resides.

Ireland as a nation state provides an interesting case study that illustrates the intersecting tensions between social policy orientation towards community-based care, a changing national demographic profile, shifting family structure, improved gender equality and an increasingly rights-based approach for care of people with intellectual disability.

Discussion

Sharing risks across society is the basis of the welfare state, indicating a collective responsibility for the risk of hardships during a lifetime. An emerging rights-based and more respectful paradigm of care for people with intellectual disability, a welcome increase in the life span of people with intellectual disability and transformations in social, economic and cultural norms have converged to foreground the importance of examining the adequacy of the current social contract for care.

Fineman (2001) asserts that the work of care preserves and perpetuates society, creating a social debt "that binds each and every member of society" (p. 1411). Many carers derive great benefits from providing care and family care is embedded in relationships and mutuality, and reciprocity of care may be a particularly important feature of the lives of parents of people with intellectual disability as they age (Knox and Bigby 2007; Ryan et al. 2014; McKenzie and McConkey 2016; Gant and Bates 2019). However, caring can have significant negative physical, psychological, social and financial impacts on family carers including those who care for family members with intellectual disability (Pinquart and Sörensen 2007; O'Reilly et al. 2008; Dawson et al. 2016; Grey et al. 2018). Because so much family care is intrinsically motivated, carers have little bargaining or negotiating power, and where care is central to the personal identities of family carers, they are vulnerable to lack of respect and material supports (Lynch et al. 2009). Gordon-Bouvier argues:

> the state does not value those who perform caregiving labour. Instead, its institutions, including law, are structured to marginalise care, depicting it as a labour of love with little value outside the private family unit. (Gordon-Bouvier 2019, p. 165)

Family care for people with intellectual disability may span decades. The neoliberal social policy shift towards an adult worker model focusses on individual autonomy and independence through employment, and many social policy responses such as Carers Leave are underpinned by a conceptualisation of care as "a temporary stage in an otherwise employment centred life course" (Pfau-Effinger 2005, p. 322) and therefore does not accommodate those for whom caregiving spans a lifetime.

Care is the most basic of human needs, without which humans will not only fail to flourish but will fail to survive (Lynch and Walsh 2009). Accepting that care is a "universal activity that binds us all" (Williams 2002, p. 487) is to recognise that that dependency is a fundamental feature of being human. In contrast to the neoliberal approach, the ethic of care approach envisions individuals as existing within interdependencies and with multiple responsibilities to each other and also to themselves (Hill 2015). Where the right to receive and give care has an ethical value, it also has an intrinsic value. If the responsibility for care is equally distributed within societies rather than being located within individuals and families, then high-quality and accessible formal care services will be a sine qua non of social policy (Hill 2015). Where the state does not explicitly accept the responsibility to share care, it defaults to the family. A residualist approach to care ignores the obligation of society not to exploit individuals who provide care, to attend to caregivers' wellbeing and to support caregivers to survive and thrive (Kittay 1999).

Conclusion

Across much of Western Europe, North America and Australia, the inhumanity of the institutionalisation of people with intellectual disability is largely a feature of the past. As a consequence of better health care, people with intellectual disabilities are living longer, and to varying degrees people with intellectual disability are taking their place as citizens within their communities. The post-institutional era has also witnessed significant change in demographics and in the nature of family structure. The assumption that a continued and unconditional supply of family-based caring labour will be provided within the homeplace may no longer be tenable in the social and economic environment of the twenty-first century. A distinguishing feature of the care of people with intellectual disability is the duration of this care which, on the death of a parent, can span generations. Family members may provide care as an act of love and from a sense of family solidarity, but where that care is unbounded or exceeds that capacity of family members to provide, it may also be burdensome and detrimental to the caregiver. As this century progresses, a new social contract for care is required to address the fundamental question as to where the responsibility for the long-term care of people with intellectual disability resides.

Reflective Questions

- Consider the people with intellectual disability you work with. How is their care provision influenced by the social policy of deinstitutionalisation and de-congregation?
- Examine the approach to family caregiving you are familiar with. How does this support the person with intellectual disability to live in the family home and/or a move to independent living?

Key Concepts Discussed

- The social contract for care in society
- The capacity for caregiving within family structures
- Social policies of deinstitutionalisation and de-congregation

References

Allen A (2000) Negotiating the role of expert carers on an adult hospital ward. Sociol Health Illn 22:149–171

Bambra C (2007) Going beyond the three worlds of welfare capitalism: regime theory and public health research. J Epidemiol Community Health 61(12):1098–1102. https://doi.org/10.1136/jech.2007.064295

Brady A (2012) The constitution, gender and reform: improving the position of women in the Irish constitution. National Women's Council of Ireland, Dublin

Bredewold F, Hermus M, Trappenburg M (2020) 'Living in the community' the pros and cons: a systematic literature review of the impact of deinstitutionalisation on people with intellectual and psychiatric disabilities. J Soc Work 20(1):83. https://doi.org/10.1177/1468017318793620

Brennan D (2014) Irish insanity 1800–2000. Routledge, New York

Brennan D, Murphy R, McCallion P, Griffiths M, McCarron M (2016) Understanding family strategies that enable long-term and sustainable home environments for older people with an intellectual disability. Trinity College Dublin, Dublin

Broese Van Groenou MI, De Boer A (2016) Providing informal care in a changing society. Eur J Ageing 13:271–279

Bryant L, Garnham B (2016) Bounded choices: the problematisation of longterm care for people ageing with an intellectual disability in rural communities. J Rural Stud 51:259–266

Chung H, Filipovič Harst M, Rakar T (2018) Provision of care, whose responsibility and why? In: Taylor-Gooby P, Leruth B (eds) Attitudes, aspirations and welfare. Palgrave Macmillan

Chybalski F, Marcinkiewicz E (2021) Incorporating pro-family and profemale components into empirical welfare state classification: some new evidence for European countries. Innov Eur J Soc Sci Res 34(3):399–421. https://doi.org/10.1080/13511610.2021.1909461

Citizens' Information (2022) Citizens' assembly. https://www.citizensinformation.ie/en/government_in_ireland/irish_constitution_1/citizens_assembly.html. Accessed 22 Aug 2022

Daly M (2002) Care as a good for social policy. J Soc Policy 31(2):251–270. https://doi.org/10.1017/S0047279401006572

Dawson F, Shanahan S, Fitzsimons E, O'Malley G, Mac GN, Bramham J (2016) The impact of caring for an adult with intellectual disability and psychiatric comorbidity on carer stress and psychological distress. J Intellect Disabil Res 60(6):553–563. https://doi.org/10.1111/jir.12269

Department of Health (2021) Disability capacity review to 2032 a review of disability social care demand and capacity requirements up to 2032. Government Publications, Dublin

Dodd P, Craig S, Kelly F et al (2010) An audit of the Irish national intellectual disability database. Res Dev Disabil 31:446–451

Engwall K (2019) Why live together? The stories of co-living parents and adult children with intellectual disabilities. Nordic Soc Work Res 9(2):118–130. https://doi.org/10.1080/2156857X.2018.1463285

Esping-Andersen G (1990) The three worlds of welfare capitalism. Polity Press, Cambridge

Esping-Andersen G (1999) Social foundations of post-industrial economies. Oxford University Press, New York

Eurofound (2015) Working and caring: reconciliation measures in times of demographic change. Publications Office of the European Union, Luxembourg

EU (2019) A new start to support work-life balance for parents and carers. Available from: https://ec.europa.eu/social/BlobServlet?docId=17583&langId=de

Eurostat (2020) Ageing Europe looking at the lives of older people in the EU. Publications Office of the European Union, Luxembourg

Fine MD (2006) A caring society? Care and the dilemmas of human service in the twenty-first century. Palgrave Macmillan, Basingstoke

Fineman M (2001) Contract and care. Chicago-Kent Law Rev 76(3):1403–1440

Gant V, Bates C (2019) 'Cautiously optimistic': older parent-carers of adults with intellectual disabilities—responses to the care act 2014. J Intellect Disabil 23(3):432–445. https://doi.org/10.1177/1744629519870437

García-Domínguez L, Navas P, Verdugo MÁ, Arias VB (2020) Chronic health conditions in aging individuals with intellectual disabilities. Int J Environ Res Public Health 17:3126. https://doi.org/10.3390/ijerph1709312

Gordon-Bouvier E (2019) Relational vulnerability: the legal status of cohabiting carers. Fem Leg Stud 27(2):163–187. https://doi.org/10.1007/s10691-019-09404-3

Grey JM, Totsika V, Hastings RP (2018) Physical and psychological health of family carers co-residing with an adult relative with an intellectual disability. J Appl Res Intellect Disabil 31(S2):191–202. https://doi.org/10.1111/jar.12353

Hill TJ (2015) Family caregiving in aging populations. Palgrave Macmillan, New York

Hoffmann F, Rodrigues R (2010) Informal carers: who takes care of them? Soc Sci Med 61(3):697–708

International Confederation of Trade Unions (2018) Care work and care jobs for the future of decent work. International Confederation of Trade Unions, Geneva

Jensen C (2008) Worlds of welfare services and transfers. J Eur Soc Policy 18(2):151–162. https://doi.org/10.1177/0958928707087591

Kittay EF (1999) Love's labor: essays on women, equality, and dependency. Routledge, New York

Knijn T, Kremer M (1997) Gender and the caring dimension of welfare states: toward inclusive citizenship. Soc Politics Int Stud Gender State Soc 4(3):328–361

Knox M, Bigby C (2007) Moving towards midlife care as negotiated family business: accounts of people with intellectual disabilities and their families "just getting along with their lives together". Int J Disabil Dev Educ 54(3):287–304. https://doi.org/10.1080/10349120701488749

Le Bihan B, Da Roit B, Sopadzhiyan A (2019) The turn to optional familialism through the market: long-term care, cash-for-care, and caregiving policies in Europe. Soc Policy Admin 53(4):579–595. https://doi.org/10.1111/spol.12505

Leira A, Saraceno C (2002) Care: actors, relationships and contexts. In: Hobson B, Lewis J, Siim B (eds) Contested concepts in gender and social politics. Edward Elgar, Cheltenham, pp 55–66

Leitner S (2003) Varieties of familialism: the caring function of the family in comparative perspective. Eur Soc 5(4):353–375. https://doi.org/10.1080/1461669032000127642

Lewis J (2007) Gender, ageing and the 'new social settlement': the importance of developing a holistic approach to care policies. Curr Sociol 55(2):271–286. https://doi.org/10.1177/0011392107073314

Lister R (2001) Towards a citizens' welfare state. Theory Cult Soc 18(2–3):91–111. https://doi.org/10.1177/02632760122051805

Lynch K, Walsh J (2009) Love, care and solidarity: what is and is not commodifiable. In: Affective equality. Love, care and injustice. Palgrave Macmillan, London, pp 35–53

Lynch K, Baker J, Lyons M (2009) Introduction. In: Affective equality : love, care and injustice. Palgrave Macmillan, London, pp 1–14

Mahon A, Pappas I, Randhawa TE, Vseteckova J (2019) Ageing carers and intellectual disability: a scoping review of literature. Qual Ageing Older Adults

(Early   Access)   20:162.   https://doi.org/10.1108/ QAOA-11-2018-0057

Mansell J, Beadle-Brown J (2010) Deinstitutionalisation and community living: position statement of the comparative policy and practice special interest research group of the International Association for the Scientific Study of Intellectual Disabilities. J Intellect Disabil Res 54(2):104–112. https://doi.org/10.1111/j.1365-2788.2009.01239.x

Marking C (2017) 'Enabling carers to care': making the case for a European Union action plan on carers. Int J Care Caring 1(2):289–292. https://doi.org/10.1332/23 9788217X14951899318087

McCarron M, Swinburne J, Burke E, McGlinchey E, Mulryan M, Andrews V, Foran S, McCallion P (2011) Growing older with an intellectual disability in Ireland 2011: first results from the intellectual disability supplement of the Irish longitudinal study on ageing. School of Nursing and Midwifery, Trinity College Dublin, Dublin

McKenzie J, McConkey R (2016) Caring for adults with intellectual disability: the perspectives of family carers in South Africa. J Appl Res Intellect Disabil 29(6):531–541. https://doi.org/10.1111/jar.12209

Murphy C, Turner T (2017) Formal and informal long term care work: policy conflict in a liberal welfare state. Int J Sociol Soc Policy 37(3/4):134–147

Novella EJ (2010) Mental health care in the aftermath of deinstitutionalisation: a retrospective and prospective view. Health Care Anal 18(3):222–238. https://doi.org/10.1007/s10728-009-0138-8

O'Doherty S, Linehan C, Tatlow-Golden M, Craig S, Kerr M, Lynch C, Staines A (2016) Perspectives of family members of people with an intellectual disability to a major reconfiguration of living arrangements for people with intellectual disability in Ireland. J Intellect Disabil, 20(2):137–151. https://doi.org/10.1177/1744629516636538

O'Reilly D, Connolly S, Rosato M, Patterson C (2008) Is caring associated with an increased risk of mortality? A longitudinal study. Soc Sci Med 67:1282–1290

Parker G (1990) With due care and attention. Family Policy Studies Centre, London

Pfau-Effinger B (2005) Welfare state policies and the development of care arrangements. Eur Soc 7(2):321–347. https://doi.org/10.1080/14616690500083592

Pinquart M, Sörensen S (2007) Correlates of physical health of informal caregivers: a meta-analysis. J Gerontol B 62:126–P137

Powell M, Yörük E, Bargu A (2019) Thirty years of the three worlds of welfare capitalism: a review of reviews. Soc Policy Admin 54:60–87. https://doi.org/10.1111/spol.12510

Power A (2016) Landscapes of care. Routledge, London

Russell H, Grotti R, McGinnity F, Privalko I (2019) Caring and unpaid work in Ireland. Irish Human Rights and Equality Commission and the Economic and Social Research Institute, Dublin

Ryan A, Taggart L, Truesdale-Kennedy M, Slevin E (2014) Issues in caregiving for older people with intellectual disabilities and their ageing family carers: a review and commentary. Int J Older People Nursing 9(3):217–226

Saint-Arnaud S, Bernard P (2003) Convergence or resilience? A hierarchical cluster analysis of the welfare regimes in advanced countries. Curr Sociol 51(5):499–527

Saraceno C (2016) Varieties of familialism: comparing four southern European and East Asian welfare regimes. J Eur Soc Policy 26(4):314–326. https://doi.org/10.1177/0958928716657275

Smith O (2012) How far from a "right to care"? Reconciling care work and labour market work in Ireland. Irish Jurist 47:143–167

Tabatabainia M (2003) Listening to families' views regarding institutionalization & deinstitutionalization. J Intellect Dev Disabil 28(3):241–259. https://doi.org/10.1080/1366825031000150973

Taggart L, Truesdale-Kennedy M, Ryan A, McConkey R (2012) Examining the support needs of ageing family carers in developing future plans for a relative with an intellectual disability. J Intellect Disabil 16(3):217–234

Teahan Á, Walsh S, Doherty E, O'Shea E (2021) Supporting family carers of people with dementia: a discrete choice experiment of public preferences. Soc Sci Med 287:114359. https://doi.org/10.1016/j.socscimed.2021.114359

Timonen V, Doyle M (2008) From the workhouse to the home: evolution of care policy for older people in Ireland. Int J Sociol Soc Policy 28(3/4):76–89. https://doi.org/10.1108/01443330810862151

United Nations (2006) Convention on the rights of persons with disabilities. United Nations, Geneva

Verbakel E (2017) How to understand informal caregiving patterns in Europe? The role of formal long-term care provisions and family care norms. Scand J Public Health 46(4):436–447. https://doi.org/10.1177/1403494817726197

vLex (n.d.) The People (Director of Public Prosecutions) v Joel. Available at: https://ie.vlex.com/vid/the-people-director-of-793864993. Accessed 22 Aug 2022

Williams F (2002) In and beyond new labour: towards a new political ethics of care. Crit Soc Policy 21(4):467–493. https://doi.org/10.1177/026101830102100405

Enabling Families to Support Adults with an Intellectual Disability to Live a Life of Their Choosing

13

Darren McCausland and Mary-Ann O'Donovan

Chapter Topics

Upon reading this chapter, the reader shall have greater appreciation for:

- The role of family in the lives of people with intellectual disability.
- The context for family life and support for people with intellectual disability using theoretical frameworks for general population.
- The changing nature of care and support over the life course.
- Key supports that enable people with intellectual disability to remain living with family should they choose to.

Introduction

Family relationships are fundamental to Quality of Life (QOL) (Schalock et al. 2002). Most people with an intellectual disability live in family settings (Hourigan et al. 2018), and most of those cared for by family wish to continue with these arrangements (McConkey et al. 2006; Bibby 2013; McCausland et al. 2019). For individuals with intellectual disability not living with family, proximity to and regular contact with family nonetheless remain critical factors supporting their social inclusion and community participation (Kozma et al. 2009; McCausland et al. 2018b).

The importance of family for people with intellectual disabilities is enshrined in the United Nations Convention on the Rights of Persons with Disabilities (UNCRPD), which states that 'persons with disabilities and their family members should receive the necessary protection and assistance to enable families to contribute towards the full and equal enjoyment of the rights of persons with disabilities' and which provides the right to an adequate standard of living for individuals and their families, including supports and assistance to protect them from poverty (UN 2006).

Given this, the need to support the families of individuals with intellectual disabilities, to enable them to continue caring for and supporting their loved ones, is clear. However, families face many challenges to this critical role, which jeopardises QOL for themselves and the individuals they support. In this chapter, we will explore some of the areas in which family support is critical for individuals with intellectual disabilities, the supports available to families to enable them in this

D. McCausland (✉)
Trinity College Dublin, Dublin, Ireland e-mail:
dmccaus@tcd.ie

M.-A. O'Donovan
Centre for Disability Studies, University of Sydney, Sydney, NSW, Australia
e-mail: mary-ann.odonovan@sydney.edu.au

© The Author(s), under exclusive license to Springer Nature Switzerland AG 2023

F. Sheerin, C. Doyle (eds.), *Intellectual Disabilities: Health and Social Care Across the Lifespan*,
https://doi.org/10.1007/978-3-031-27496-1_13

role and the challenges faced where needs are not matched by available supports.

Theoretical Context

This section aims to establish the context for family life and support of people with an intellectual disability by exploring the theoretical frameworks relevant to supporting and enabling families. This includes a brief exploration of theories of family, caregiving and the life course.

Family

Giddens and Sutton (2017) defined family as 'a group of individuals related to one another by blood ties, marriage or adoption that form a unit, the adult members of which are responsible for the upbringing of children' (2017, p. 998). Traditional theoretical views of family—which viewed the family as a critical social institution fulfilling important functions for individuals, communities and the wider social system, often within the ideological norm of the nuclear family (Parsons and Bales 1956)—have become less important with the growing diversification more recently of what is considered as 'family' (Giddens and Sutton 2017). Two critical factors in explaining the variation in family life are cultural differences and social divisions such as social class, while individual preferences have also become more important in determining who family are (Cheal 2002). Such diversity also reflects aspirations for more 'democratic relationships', including a focus on increased agency and rights for children and the legitimisation of lesbian, gay, bisexual, transgender and queer (LGBTQ+) relationships (Chambers and Gracia 2022). Challenges to functional and structural views of family emerged through feminist theories in the 1970s and 1980s, which challenged the traditional division of labour and unequal power relationships within families (Giddens and Sutton 2017). From the 1990s, a more accurate way of conceptually framing 'family' was to speak of 'families' instead of 'the family' (Chambers 2012).

An alternative theory about family life suggested that there was no such thing as 'the family', focusing instead on family 'practices', and how people 'do family'—how they do the things which they themselves consider to be familial, suggesting a subjective and socially constructed phenomena rather than conforming to a fixed idea such as the nuclear family (Morgan 2011). Key considerations in this focus on family practices are how individuals experience kinship through everyday practices including intimacy, personal life, labour and caring (Chambers and Gracia 2022). A second theoretical development to emerge in relation to family in recent years is the idea of 'display', meaning the ways in which the status of family is conveyed interpersonally and socially and when people do 'family things' which signify family relationships, including rituals such as family meals, weddings and funerals (Finch 2007), which may be empowering for groups previously excluded from traditional models of 'the family' such as LGBTQ+ couples (Almack 2008; Chambers and Gracia 2022). The exclusion of many people with intellectual disabilities from marriage and formation of their own families has a fundamental impact on their familial network and relationships, with close family relationships often limited to their parents, which is further impacted when they age and lose their parents, leaving a reliance on siblings and their offspring (McCausland et al. 2018b).

Caregiving

In developmental psychology, attachment theory proposed that normal social and emotional development in young children required the development of a relationship with at least one primary caregiver (Ainsworth 1978; Bowlby 1982; Ainsworth and Bowlby 1991) and that this attachment behaviour was complemented by reciprocal caregiving behaviours from the parent (Solomon and George 1996). The concepts within attachment theory have been influential in explaining the formation of caring relationships (Rutter 1995; Schaffer 2004). However, given the complexity of care and competing perspectives within the field, a general theory and definition of care may not be possible (Arber and Ginn 1990; Browne 2010). Distinguishing between caring as a normative activity and activity which goes beyond normative is problematic given that caring is integral to many relationships (Milne and Larkin 2015). However, a number of theories have extended the idea of caring as an activity, something that is done to another person (Ray et al. 2009; Bowlby et al. 2010). Caregiving usually involves the provision of care above what is considered normal, includes supports with activities of daily living (ADLs) and instrumental activities of daily living (IADLs), as well as support accessing healthcare and emotional support; it may be transitional or long term, be part of a close reciprocal relationship and may emerge from a sense of obligation or responsibility (Fine and Glendinning 2005; Hirst 2005; Liu and Gallagher-Thompson 2009; Aggar 2016). Yet, caring and the caregiving relationship requires a complex degree of emotional and moral investment which raises it above mere obligation or responsibility (Noddings 1984; Tronto 1993; Tronto and Fisher 1990; Gilligan 2003; Lynch 2007). For people with intellectual disabilities, families play a critical role in supporting individuals physically, emotionally and materially across the lifespan, supplementing any formal support received by the person (Heller et al. 2021).

The Life Course

Conceptually, the life course 'refers to the age-graded, socially-embedded sequence of roles that connect the phases of life' (Mortimer and Shanahan 2003). The life course is comprised of the various transitions throughout the passage of our lives, influenced by a number of biological, social and psychological factors (Giddens and Sutton 2017). Stages of life course are not experienced universally, with variation through time and place, implying socially constructed phenomena wherein experiences vary with cultural norms and the intersectionality of social divisions such as class, gender and ethnicity (Chatterjee et al. 2001; Elder et al. 2003; Giddens and Sutton 2017). As such, while events and roles throughout the life course may align with age, age alone may not be the best marker of stages in the life course (O'Donovan et al. 2020). The social construction

of the life course experience also aligns with social (UPIAS 1975; Oliver 1990) and biopsychosocial (WHO 2001) concepts of disability which consider how people with impairments are disabled by socially constructed barriers. Social variations through time and place are significant in shaping the lives and barriers faced by people with disabilities throughout their life course, making it difficult to resolve a diversity of experiences within oversimplified linear models (Priestly 2001). Young people with disabilities face particular challenges in making the critical transition into adulthood and therefore experience an extended dependence on their parents (Tisdall 2001). The social construction of adulthood, which sits at the apex of life course progression, contains accepted cultural markers of adult status which signify an idealised adulthood—such as having one's own home, financial autonomy, relationships of choice and parenthood; and while achievement of this is largely shaped by the development of social policies, access to generational rights will be a benchmark for the achievement of human rights by people with disabilities (Priestly 2001). However, often people with disabilities become excluded from the normative life course events (Slota and Martin 2003), with transitions between different stages in the life course especially difficult for people with disabilities and their families (Heller and Harris 2012).

The intersection of theories of family, caregiving and the life course—alongside influential theories within the disability discourse including *Normalisation* (Nirje 1973) and *Social Role Valorisation* (Wolfensberger et al. 1996) and disability frameworks such as the WHO ICF (WHO 2001), which all highlighted the central importance of family relationships and roles—provides a critical context for exploring the role of families in supporting adults with intellectual disability to live a life of their choosing.

Living with Family: Policy and Background

In Ireland, the policy shift away from the historical reliance on large segregated institutional living with a move and expectation for people with disabilities (intellectual disability and other disabilities) to living in smaller community-based settings was instigated in 2011 with the publication of the congregated settings report (HSE 2011) in conjunction with the National Housing Strategy for people with disabilities (Department of the Environment Community and Local Government 2011). With these initiatives there was a renewed and increased focus on the housing needs of people with disability, and in line with the UN Convention the language of rights, choice and independence were cemented with the right of people with disability to choose where they live and who they live with outlined. The congregated settings report specifically called for the move to community living for people with disability, the majority of which had intellectual disability. The National Housing Strategy was broader in focus, incorporating the needs of a range of disability types, and focused mainly on accessing housing through the private rental or social housing stream. It refers to the congregated settings report for people currently living in residential settings and there is a recognition that people with disabilities may not want to live at home forever and that housing assessments should be put in place in these circumstances to support transition to more preferred living arrangement.

The Housing Strategy has been updated with a new Housing for All policy launched in 2022–2027 (Department of Housing Local Government and Heritage 2021) and reinforces the call to end residential congregate settings, while at the same time recognising that with the ageing population the demand for residential care, particularly for people with intellectual disability, is set to grow.

In the caring discourse and policy, carers for people with intellectual disability tend to be invisible. That is, their role as carers over the lifetime of their child is overlooked compared with spousal carers or child carers for ageing parents. There is an implicit expectation from society and policy that parents will continue to care for their adult children with intellectual disability, in a way that is not expected in other care groups. The Carers Strategy does acknowledge the need to

support people to live in their own homes and communities for as long as possible, so in essence it alludes to promoting ageing in place (DoH 2012). The policy states that:

> A key objective of Government policy for older people, children and adults with an illness or a disability is to support them to live in dignity and independence in their own homes and communities for as long as possible. Carers are vital to the achievement of this objective and are considered a backbone of care provision in Ireland. (p. 14)

However, there are no specific policy addressing ageing in place for people with intellectual disability, no specific recognition of carers of adults with intellectual disability and their specific needs and no policy guidance on the future residential needs of adults with intellectual disability living with family. The Housing Strategy does not explicitly address or identify what is needed if the person with disability, specifically the person with intellectual disability, chooses to remain living in the family home. In addition, the congregated settings report does not address the huge future need for residential living recorded on the National Ability Supports System (NASS; formerly National Intellectual Disability Database and National Physical and Sensory Disability Database) for people with intellectual disability living with family. Most recent data (2020) show 31% of people with intellectual disability are living in residential settings with unmet need for residential places recorded for 891 people (Casey et al. 2021). In addition, no current strategy plans for, or outlines resourcing for, the range of services and supports that may be required for a person with intellectual disability to live in the community, independently, semi-independently or with family.

Yet, the majority of people with intellectual disability continue to live with family into adulthood (McConkey et al. 2011; Trip et al. 2019). Kelly et al. (2020) reported a 20% increase in the number of people with intellectual disability living with family, over a 10-year period (2007–2017). The latest data show that 62% of people with intellectual disability (and registered on the NASS) are living with families, with over half of carers aged between 18 and 59 years (Casey et al. 2021).

Aside from living with family into adulthood, families are also the main source of support for people with intellectual disability in Ireland (Chadwick et al. 2013). Supporting families to care at home is said to be a cost-effective way to provide residential care, compared with other forms of residential care (Kelly et al. 2020). Maintaining adults with intellectual disability living with family over the life course is also the preferred option for many families (Kelly et al. 2020). In a survey in Taiwan of ageing carers of older adults with intellectual disability, 61.6% stated their preference was to continue living and ageing with their adult child at home (Chou and Kröger 2022). Families overwhelmingly report wanting to continue caring (Taggart et al. 2012).

People with intellectual disability are living longer and ageing in tandem with ageing carers (Kelly et al. 2020). Thus, the capacity to care for an adult child may be challenged through the carer's own health needs. There is a trend towards more single-parent families, as one parent continues to care following the death of the spouse (McConkey et al. 2011). In a study by Taggart et al. (2012) over half of carers were lone parents.

The strain and burden of caring for a child with a life-long disability is well documented. More recently, the reciprocal nature of the caring relationship and the benefits to the carer are being recognised (Irazabal et al. 2016; Trip et al. 2019). When a family surrenders care, this occurs for a number of reasons, with lack of sufficient and appropriate support or services having a large negative impact on the family's capacity to continue to care (Trip et al. 2019). Evidence shows that families report that they do not get the right amount of supports (Chadwick et al. 2013) and feared a lack of responsiveness from services to the changing needs of their adult child with intellectual disability (Chadwick et al. 2013). This was particularly true of respite, with families reporting no change in service to reflect changing needs (Southby 2017).

Services are important for overall good family QOL (Irazabal et al. 2016). Family well-being and QOL are affected by the availability of supports, with many families playing a role in advocating for supports (Chadwick et al. 2013).

Families also played a role in supporting other families and joining together for advocacy (Chadwick et al. 2013).

However, access to services is not equitable. People with borderline/mild intellectual disability are less likely to be known to services or appear in statistics reporting service use, with people with mild intellectual disability less likely to have access to support needed (Trip et al. 2019; O'Donovan et al. 2020). Geographical inequities are also quite common. Families play a large role in advocating for asking for more should current service provision be rescinded (Chadwick et al. 2013) and gratitude for services and supports they were already in receipt of dominates (Trip et al. 2019). Issue of service fatigue was raised by participants in the study by Trip et al. (2019), and such fatigue can be linked to constant advocacy some parents are required to undertake in order to get appropriate services (Chadwick et al. 2013) as well as lack of clarity and information on who is responsible and where to go for services, leading families being referred onwards (Chadwick et al. 2013; Trip et al. 2019). Access to information about services and within services was a challenge for parents (Chadwick et al. 2013; Southby 2017).

Types of Supports

Maintaining people with intellectual disability living in the family home requires consistent, appropriate and reliable supports for the carer and the individual with intellectual disability. This was specifically raised by family participants in the work of Chadwick et al. (2013, p. 119) where it was stated that 'being provided with flexible and timely support for families at critical times; being offered services, support, entitlements and information without having to fight for them' were key to family well-being and maintaining the caring role and person with intellectual disability at home.

Informal supports to enable the person with intellectual disability to remain living at home with family care were reported as family support (74%), carer good health (67.9%) and religion

(18.8%), while formal supports viewed as essential included day-care provision (65.2%), community intellectual disability team (14.3%), respite (13.4%) and support groups (5.4%) (Taggart et al. 2012).

There are a range of supports that may be required and accessed by families, including day, respite, home help, educational, employment and financial to name a few. The authors explore key areas of support to enable care to continue by the family:

- Day activity
- Respite support
- Home help or home care

Day Activity

In the UK many people with intellectual disability access day supports of some kind (Hatton 2017). Similarly in Ireland, 83% of people with intellectual disability access day services (Casey et al. 2021). Traditional day services have been offered in dedicated buildings. However, there has been a policy to move towards day service 'modernisation', which Hatton (2017) describes as a focus on more innovative day activities and a move away from 'building-based' day services. The analysis by Hatton (2017) illustrated a drop in access to these services in most regions of the UK (with the exception of the North of Ireland). Yet there was not a comparable increase in the uptake and access of non-building-based day services (Hatton 2017). In addition, the author cautions as to interpreting service access numbers overall, stating that though the number of people receiving services may not change, the amount of service received by an individual may change and this is not identifiable in the data (Hatton 2017).

Respite

Respite is the most common type of support generally for family carers of people with intellectual disability (McConkey et al. 2011; Kelly et al. 2020) and is a much-valued service by families

and people with intellectual disability. It has the potential to give the carer and the individual a break from the caring arrangement and prevent the carer from feeling overwhelmed and enhance sustainability of the caring arrangement (McConkey et al. 2011; Chadwick et al. 2013; Irazabal et al. 2016; Southby 2017). Yet oftentimes family carers express feelings of guilt associated with accessing respite (Chadwick et al. 2013; Irazabal et al. 2016; Southby 2017). The benefits to the individual include potential increased independence, social participation and community connection (Southby 2017).

However, demand for respite typically outweighs supply (McConkey et al. 2011) and large variations across geographical regions with regard to access to respite in Ireland were noted (McConkey et al. 2011). In looking at the availability of respite in Ireland, Kelly et al. (2020) found a drop in the number of people respite was available to over a 10-year period (2017–2007). The 2020 data shows 7% of people with intellectual disability had accessed overnight respite. The characteristics of the carer or carer living arrangement was not found to be a predictor of receiving respite (McConkey et al. 2011). In fact, more severe levels of intellectual disability, being older than 20 years of age and having contact with social work supports were predictors of receiving respite care (McConkey et al. 2011). In contrast, Southby (2017) reports how carers who 'shout the loudest' may be more prone to access respite services. This is an important consideration in terms of equity, as due to the disparity between supply and demand, respite is a service that tends to be rationed severely (McConkey et al. 2011). In some cases, respite was found to become an alternative living arrangement for the individual, which puts further pressure on supply (McConkey et al. 2011).

Ensuring respite is a valuable resource requires the service being consistent and timely, as well as being available locally (Southby 2017). Social workers and community nurses play a crucial role in linking families to services and in flagging this need for services within the disability services (McConkey et al. 2011). Non-residential respite is an alternative type of respite but tends to be less known to families and also less valued by those who are aware of it (Southby 2017). Examples of non-residential respite include day trips, holidays and leisure activities (Southby 2017). Just 1% of people with intellectual disability in Ireland (registered on NASS) accessed day respite (Casey et al. 2021), with centre-based respite the most common day respite type.

Home Help/Home Care/ Domiciliary Care

Home help can be an important support to enable families to continue caring at home· but there is limited research on the experience of home care for people with intellectual disability and their families (Hatton 2017). Home supports can include support with personal care, domestic tasks or participation activities, by a paid care worker (Kelly et al. 2020). Similarly, to respite services, demand for home care tends to far exceed the supply, with families not receiving the requisite amount (Kelly et al. 2020).

The numbers availing of home support in Ireland were generally consistent over a 10-year period with a slight drop when comparing use in 2007 and 2017, with people with more severe intellectual disability more likely to access it but disparity in access geographically was an issue as with other services above. People tended to access either home support or respite, and there was a one-third increase in the numbers not receiving either over this time period (Kelly et al. 2020). One factor that is not explicitly addressed is the extent of choice people with intellectual disability and their families have with services. Financial rationing and geographic disparity suggest choice is missing.

The Role of Family in Supporting Decision-Making

Self-determination including decision-making is a critical factor in shaping QOL for people with intellectual disabilities (WHOQOL Group 1998; Schalock et al. 2002). Yet, decision-making and autonomy for this population have historically been restricted with questions around capacity (Commissioner for Human Rights 2012). Here we will look at the role family play in supporting decision-making and self-determination for adults with intellectual disabilities.

Family in Models of Self-Determination and Policy

Wehmeyer (2003) stated that 'self-determination, in essence, refers to *acting* based on *one's own mind or free will*, without external compulsion' (2003, p. 6). Within the intellectual disability literature, an ecological theory of self-determination suggests that the family microsystem plays a critical role in shaping self-determination and in mediating between the individual and society and supporting interactions with the outside world (Abery and Stancliffe 2003; Shogren 2013). Intellectual disability research has also identified that two different types of choice exist, everyday choices and key-life choices, and there is a high degree of interconnectedness between these domains, suggesting that where people make or are supported to make one type of choice, they will be more likely to also exercise choice in the other domain (Tichá et al. 2013; O'Donovan et al. 2017). However, other studies also found that people with intellectual disabilities were more likely to be included in smaller everyday decisions while being excluded from the key decisions in their lives, such as where and with whom they live (Fyson et al. 2007; Antaki et al. 2009; McCarron et al. 2011; McCausland et al. 2018a).

A number of practice models for enhancing independence and inclusion for people with intellectual disabilities, based on supporting decision-making and autonomy, have emerged in recent decades, with family playing a key role in these processes. Models of person-centred planning (Ratti et al. 2016; McCausland et al. 2021a), microboards (Stainton 2016), supported decision-making (Douglas and Bigby 2020) and individualised funding (Fleming et al. 2019) all employ a circle of support approach (Snow 1998) to establish a group of natural supports, including close and extended family, to empower decision-making and self-determination among individuals with intellectual disabilities. An important dimension of models such as these is the idea that supporting decision-making is about more than just the formal and legal decisions and is also an organic process that should be part of daily decision-making (Stainton 2016); and families usually lie at their core, among those 'who know a person intimately as an individual and whose relationship is based on trust and mutuality rather than a professional or contractual relationship' (2016, p. 6).

Research Evidence of Family Supporting Self-Determination

The research has identified that families are a critical factor in decision-making and self-determination for adults with an intellectual disability. IDS-TILDA identified two domains of choice for older adults with an intellectual disability in Ireland, everyday choices and key-life decisions (O'Donovan et al. 2017), and found that that family play an important critical role in supporting decision-making at both levels (O'Donovan et al. 2020). Residence in family settings was associated with greater exercise of choice in key-life decisions by participants; closer proximity to, and more frequent contact with, non-resident family was also associated with increased choice in key-life decisions, and more frequent contact with non-resident family was also associated with increased choice for everyday decisions (McCausland et al. 2018a). An individual's circles of support should become the primary supports in planning and implementing person-centred goals, and that family may play a critical role in this—if the individual chooses (HSE 2018). Studies found that family involvement in person-centred planning improved goal planning and achievement for adults with intellectual disabilities, especially for individuals with more complex support needs; however, family involvement was often limited and not easily achieved in practice (McCarron et al. 2013a; McCausland et al. 2021a).

While there are potential benefits to family supporting decision-making and self-determination for people with intellectual disabilities, the extent to which family support may be a positive influence for promoting self-determination of individuals with intellectual disabilities is mediated by family attitudes and attributes, the quality of the relationship and the decision-making environment (Browning et al. 2021). Studies have identified family characteristics as important in the development of skills to support self-determination, and families mediate the extent to which young people with intellectual disabilities develop such skills (Zhang 2005; Carter et al. 2013). A review by Shogren et al. (2017) identified family attitudes about decision-making as a key factor in shaping decision-making by individuals with intellectual disabilities. Family attitudes, expectations and modelling influence decision-making opportunities for individuals with intellectual disabilities, and decision-making may be restricted depending on family perspectives of capacity and positive risk-taking for the individual (Wennberg and Kjellberg 2010; Timmons et al. 2011; Shogren et al. 2017; Brennan et al. 2018). This suggests that when family play a role in supporting decision-making for adults with intellectual disabilities, they must tread a fine line if they are to facilitate self-determination free from the type of external compulsion Wehmeyer (2003) referred to earlier.

The Role of Family in Supporting Positive Ageing

While early theories of ageing viewed growing older negatively, typified by inactivity and decline, different perspectives emerged in the later twentieth century which highlighted a more active and positive view of ageing (O'Donovan et al. 2020). However, theories of positive ageing, such as that proposed by Rowe and Kahn (1997), where successful ageing included low risk of disease, maintenance of physical and cognitive capacities and continued activity with age, may be challenging for people with intellectual disabilities, who face increasing risks of multimor-bidity (McCarron et al. 2013b; Hussain et al. 2020) and mortality (O'Leary et al. 2018; Doyle et al. 2020; Landes et al. 2021), compared with the general older population. In this context, family play a critical role in supporting the health and well-being of individuals with intellectual disability throughout their life course (Heller et al. 2021), and this may become especially important in later life given their increased risks to health and well-being as well as the earlier onset of certain disease morbidities (Burke et al. 2014) including earlier and elevated risk of dementia for people with Down syndrome (McCarron et al. 2017). McGlinchey et al. (2019) set out a framework of positive ageing indicators for people with intellectual disabilities, highlighting the central role family play in supporting positive ageing across domains of participation, health and security as people age. Wark et al. (2015) identified health, relationships, having a home, opportunities for meaningful activities and choice and control as important factors for positive ageing among people with intellectual disabilities. Reppermund and Trollor (2016) suggested that targeted policies and programmes were needed for those ageing with intellectual disabilities in order for them to achieve the markers of successful ageing—good physical and mental health, healthy lifestyles and behaviours, social interaction and productivity, life satisfaction and access to quality healthcare.

There is a body of research highlighting the importance of family in mediating positive ageing for people with intellectual disabilities across the breadth of these indicators of positive ageing. Family play a critical role in determining the health outcomes of people with intellectual disabilities, and families and carers should be empowered to adequately support their needs (Krahn and Fox 2014). Family support is associated with better health-related QOL (Alonso-Sardón et al. 2019). Preventative healthcare is central to positive ageing, and improved healthcare may prevent avoidable deaths (Hirvikoski et al. 2021). Older women with intellectual disabilities living in family settings were more likely than those in other residence types to have a

mammogram; however, among all older adults, only a few received a flu vaccine or blood cholesterol check compared with those in residential care (McGlinchey et al. 2019). Reliance on family support for healthcare utilisation is common but healthcare encounters must also address family needs as well as those of the individual (Crabb et al. 2020; Hirvikoski et al. 2021). Social support from family is associated with improved physical activity by people with intellectual disabilities (Peterson et al. 2008); yet some living in family settings spend more time being sedentary, and there is a reliance on families to support more active and therefore more positive ageing (Lynch et al. 2022).

With regard to mental health, family support acts as a protective factor for the impact of stress and mediates mental health consequences including preventing depression and supporting recovery from mental illness (Scott and Havercamp 2014). People living in family settings reported a higher level of life satisfaction than others (McGlinchey et al. 2019). Adults with intellectual disabilities living with family reported the lowest risk of reported or diagnosed mental illness and lowest risk of behavioural problems (Scott and Havercamp 2014). However, lack of knowledge among families about how mental health disorders manifest may lead to delays in identifying mental illness in people with intellectual disabilities and ultimately impact access to appropriate services (Costello and Bouras 2006).

The importance of social inclusion and community participation in health and positive ageing has been highlighted in the literature (McGlinchey et al. 2019; McCausland et al. 2021b), underpinning QOL through the life course (WHOQOL Group 1998; Schalock et al. 2002). Once again, family play a critical role in supporting improved inclusion and participation and therefore in achieving positive ageing and maintaining QOL (Bigby 2008; Kozma et al. 2009; Verdonschot et al. 2009; McCausland 2016). However, the importance of family as a support to inclusion and participation highlights the limitations for those whose natural supports including family are more limited, including older adults with intellectual disabilities and those living in residential care settings (Tatlow-Golden et al. 2014; McCausland et al. 2018b). Bigby (2008) identified that close family connections with frequent contacts offered additional monitoring or oversight of the supports provided to relatives with intellectual disabilities in supported community accommodation, but family relationships including frequency of visits may decline over time as family age, thus reducing this oversight.

Clearly a wide range of factors influences positive ageing among people with intellectual disabilities, with family playing a central role in supporting this process.

Future Care Planning

As established earlier and throughout this chapter, families play a critical role in many important dimensions of life for people with intellectual disabilities, throughout their life course and into older age. These supportive and caring relationships offer many mutual benefits for both caregivers and recipients, and most people with intellectual disabilities wish to continue family care arrangements (McConkey et al. 2006; McCausland et al. 2019). However, a significant source of stress and anxiety reported by family carers is the question of who will care for and support their loved ones when they are no longer able to do so themselves (Brennan et al. 2018; Farina et al. 2017; Pryce et al. 2017). Despite this, many studies have reported a lack of future care planning among families, particularly concrete or formal planning for care, accommodation and other specific arrangements (Bowey and McGlaughlin 2005; Heller and Caldwell 2006; McConkey et al. 2006; Dillenburger and McKerr 2009; Heller and Kramer 2009; Weeks et al. 2009; Lunsky et al. 2014; Brennan et al. 2018; Walker and Hutchinson 2019). However, other studies reported that many families have future plans, even though these may be more informal, sometimes aspirational and even unspoken yet understood arrangements within families (Bigby 1996; Pruchno and Patrick 1999; Hewitt et al. 2010; Taggart et al. 2012; Walker and Hutchinson 2018), while these and other approaches may

serve to exclude the individual with intellectual disability from the planning process for fear of causing distress (McCausland et al. 2019).

Factors associated with increased future planning include older caregiver age, caregiver education and training, engagement with formal services and higher support needs of care recipients (Burke et al. 2018). Potential barriers for families in planning for future care needs may include an absence or inadequacy of options including formal services or caregiving successor within the family, reluctance associated with the emotional aspects of future planning, mutual dependence, communication within families and financial difficulties.

Failure to address future care needs may exacerbate the stress and anxiety of carers, but may also have serious impacts for care recipients with intellectual disabilities including the additional emotional distress of crisis or emergency rehousing (Prosser 1997; Gilbert et al. 2008), perhaps coming on top of the bereavement of losing a loved one (Gorfin and McGlaughlin 2004). Given that future care planning is a cause of anxiety for carers, and that failure to plan can have negative outcomes for individuals with intellectual disabilities, there is an obvious need to support families to plan for the future care and support of their loved ones. While there has been a shortage of quality studies evaluating approaches to future planning (Lunsky et al. 2014; Ryan et al. 2014; Brennan et al. 2020), a small number have demonstrated the possibilities for future planning with the right supports in place.

Blue-Banning et al. (2000) identified positive outcomes using a group action planning approach which engaged a support network to share responsibility for decision-making and planning. A case-management approach to planning with families by Bigby et al. (2002) targeted three dimensions—engaging existing services to support continued residence within the family home, effective future planning and enhancing skills of the person with an intellectual disabilities receiving care, resulting in improved planning and preparation for the future as well as improved access to existing services. Botsford and Rule (2004) used a professional-led group psychoeducational programme for older mothers over a 6-week period, resulting in increased awareness and knowledge, more confidence about planning and an increase in planning actions. Heller and Caldwell (2006) instead used a peer-support educational intervention for families, producing a range of positive outcomes including increased planning, reduced caregiver burden and increased daily choice making for individuals with intellectual disabilities. A review by Brennan et al. (2020) concluded that it is possible to improve future planning for families caring for persons with intellectual disabilities if the right resources, time and effort are in place. An intervention by McCausland et al. (2019) used a holistic person-centred approach to improve future planning for individuals and families across a range of life domains, including social activities and interests, interpersonal relationships, work and daily occupation, living arrangements, care and support arrangements, legal arrangements and financial arrangements. Significant factors in determining improved planning included caring capacity (of the individual, of the family and of formal services), as well as readiness of the family to engage in future planning (McCausland et al. 2019), which echoed previous findings (Botsford and Rule 2004; Brennan et al. 2018).

As Heller et al. (2021) noted, recognising the interconnectedness of care recipients and caregivers and addressing factors that mutually affect them will positively impact their family QOL, especially as they age together. While the results of future care planning may envisage diverging outcomes, such outcomes are natural and inevitable, yet planning for them stands to benefit both care recipients and their family caregivers. As such, in addition to the supports highlighted earlier, individuals and families need better support to plan for their futures.

Conclusions

The authors contend that families are a core element in the circle of support for people with intellectual disability across the life course. However, the evidence highlights that this caring relationship is not prioritised in policy or in resource allocation, even though family carers facilitate huge cost savings within the health and social care sector and families play a central role in the health and ageing well of individuals with intellectual disability. In addition, it is well-evidenced that people with intellectual disability and their families are at greater risk of poverty and, unsurprisingly, due to the demands of caring many carers either leave employment, reduce to part-time hours or have never had the opportunity to engage in employment outside the home since the caring role began.

Respite and day services are essential services to maintain the support relationship and to enable the person with intellectual disability to stay living with their family. Without these core supports, the care burden and stress are heightened and the living situation is increasingly unsustainable. There is less evidence on the use and impact of home care and other domiciliary supports, but there are indications of their benefit to families and people with intellectual disability. Across service types it was acknowledged that demand exceeded supply and that rationing of services was common as was geographical inequities in access.

There is a call for more choice in supports and services for families (Kelly et al. 2020). This will require greater resourcing and varying market structure. One approach to stimulate greater choice and control is to provide some mechanism of direct payments or individualised funding, rather than bulk funding to providers. This is available to people with disabilities in countries like the UK and Australia. Individual payments were mentioned by participants in the Chadwick et al. (2013) study as a possible mechanism to have more control over services, while Southby (2017) stated how some parents felt direct payments may facilitate 'creativity' in service access.

As adults with intellectual disability are ageing in tandem with parents, there is an increased need to ensure that both the family carer and person with intellectual disability are supported to age in a place of their choosing, be that together or independent of each other. Future care planning, though important and effective in preventing crisis admissions to potentially inappropriate and unwanted living arrangements for the person with intellectual disability, does not receive the focus required within services and is an area which families are hesitant to engage with.

The recent COVID-19 pandemic raises the importance of future care planning of another kind. During the pandemic there was a rapid move to remote supports, which resulted in increased responsibility falling to parents with day and respite unavailable (Wos et al. 2021). Remote support may be sufficient for some people with intellectual disability and for some types of supports, but it is not a replacement for core supports such as respite and day services. Service providers should take this opportunity to future proof the mechanisms of support for families and people with intellectual disability to ensure they are not forgotten in times of greatest need.

Reflective Questions

- Consider the people with intellectual disability you work with. How does their family connection play a role in their care?
- This chapter identifies a number of supports that may be considered in enabling the person with intellectual disability to remain living with family. Reflecting on these, are you familiar with the supports and how might they assist someone you work with?

Key Concepts Discussed

- Enabling people with intellectual disability to live in the family home is dependent on access to consistent, appropriate and timely services.
- Services are required to support the carer and the person with intellectual disability.
- There is a large unmet need for some services, in particular respite services.
- There is a link between access to services and QOL for the individual and the family.
- Families play a key role in supported decision-making and in development of self-determination.

References

Abery BH, Stancliffe RJ (2003) An ecological theory of self-determination: theoretical foundations. In: Wehmeyer ML, Abery BH, Mithaug DE, Stancliffe RJ (eds) Theory in self-determination. Charles C. Thomas Publisher Ltd., Springfield, IL, pp 25–42

Aggar C (2016) Implications of caregiving. J Austral Rehabil Nurs Assoc 19(2):15–24

Ainsworth M (1978) Pattern of attachment: a psychological study of the strange situation. Erlbaum, Hillsdale, NJ

Ainsworth M, Bowlby J (1991) An ethological approach to personality development. Am Psychol 46(4):333. https://doi.org/10.1037/0003-066X.46.4.333

Almack K (2008) Display work: lesbian parent couples and their families of origin negotiating new kin relationships. Sociology 42(6):1183–1199. https://doi.org/10.1177/0038038508096940

Alonso-Sardón M, Iglesias-de-Sena H, Fernández-Martín LC, Mirón-Canelo JA (2019) Do health and social support and personal autonomy have an influence on the health-related quality of life of individuals with intellectual disability? BMC Health Serv Res 19(1):63. https://doi.org/10.1186/s12913-018-3856-5

Antaki C, Finlay WML, Walton C (2009) Choices for people with intellectual disabilities: official discourse and everyday practice. J Policy Pract Intellect Disabil 6(4):260–266. https://doi.org/10.1111/j.1741-1130.2009.00230.x

Arber S, Ginn J (1990) The meaning of informal care: gender and the contribution of elderly people. Ageing Soc 10(4):429–454

Bibby R (2013) 'I hope he goes first': exploring determinants of engagement in future planning for adults with a learning disability living with ageing parents. What are the issues? Br J Learn Disabil 41(2):94–105

Bigby C (1996) Transferring responsibility: the nature and effectiveness of parental planning for the future of adults with intellectual disability who remain at home until mid-life. J Intellect Dev Disabil 21(4):295–312

Bigby C (2008) Known well by no-one: trends in the informal social networks of middle-aged and older people with intellectual disability five years after moving to the community. J Intellect Dev Disabil 33(2):148–157. https://doi.org/10.1080/13668250802094141

Bigby C, Ozanne E, Gordon M (2002) Facilitating transition: elements of successful case management practice for older parents of adults with intellectual disability. J Gerontol Soc Work 37(3–4):25–43

Blue-Banning MJ, Turnbull AP, Pereira L (2000) Group action planning as a support strategy for Hispanic families: parent and professional perspectives. Ment Retard 38(3):262–275. https://doi.org/10.1352/0047-6765(2000)038<0262:GAPAAS>2.0.CO;2

Botsford AL, Rule D (2004) Evaluation of a group inter-vention to assist aging parents with permanency plan-ning for an adult offspring with special needs. Soc Work 49(3):423–431

Bowey L, McGlaughlin A (2005) Adults with a learning disability living with elderly carers talk about planning for the future: aspirations and concerns. Br J Soc Work 35(8):1377–1392

Bowlby J (1982) Attachment and loss, Attachment, vol 1, 2nd edn. Basic Books, New York

Bowlby S, McKie L, Gregory S, MacPherson I (2010) Interdependency and care over the lifecourse. Routledge, London

Brennan D, Murphy R, McCallion P, McCarron M (2018) "What's going to happen when we're gone?" Family caregiving capacity for older people with an intellec-tual disability in Ireland. J Appl Res Intellect Disabil 31(2):226–235

Brennan D, McCausland D, O'Donovan MA, Eustace-Cook J, McCallion P, McCarron M (2020) Approaches to and outcomes of future planning for family carers of adults with an intellectual disability: a system-atic review. J Appl Res Intellect Disabil. https://doi.org/10.1111/jar.12742

Browne PL (2010) The dialectics of health and social care: toward a conceptual framework. Theory Soc 39(5):575–591. https://doi.org/10.1007/s11186-010-9120-6

Browning M, Bigby C, Douglas J (2021) A process of decision-making support: exploring supported decision-making practice in Canada. J Intellect Develop Disabil 46(2):138–149. https://doi.org/10.31 09/13668250.2020.1789269

Burke E, McCallion P, McCarron M (2014) Advancing years, different challenges: wave 2 IDS-TILDA. Retrieved from Dublin: https://www.tcd.ie/tcaid/assets/pdf/Wave_2_Report_October_2014.pdf

Burke M, Arnold C, Owen A (2018) Identifying the cor-relates and barriers of future planning among parents of individuals with intellectual and developmental dis-abilities. Intellect Dev Disabil 56(2):90–100. https://doi.org/10.1352/1934-9556-56.2.90

Carter EW, Lane KL, Cooney M, Weir K, Moss CK, Machalicek W (2013) Parent assessments of self-determination importance and performance for stu-dents with autism or intellectual disability. Am J Intellect Dev Disabil 118(1):16–31

Casey C, O'Sullivan M, Flanagan N, Fanagan S (2021) Annual report of the National Ability Supports System (NASS) 2020. Retrieved from Dublin: https://www.hrb.ie/fileadmin/2._Plugin_related_files/Publications/2021_publications/NASS/NASS_2020_annual_report.pdf

Chadwick DD, Mannan H, Garcia Iriarte E, McConkey R, O'Brien P, Finlay F, Lawlor A, Harrington G (2013) Family voices: life for family carers of people with intellectual disabilities in Ireland. J Appl Res Intellect Disabil 26(2):119–132

Chambers D (2012) A sociology of family life: change and diversity in intimate relations. Polity Press, Cambridge

Chambers D, Gracia P (2022) A sociology of family life: change and diversity in intimate relations, 2nd edn. Polity Press, Cambridge

Chatterjee P, Bailey D, Aronoff N (2001) Adolescence and old age in twelve communities. J Soc Soc Welfare 28:121

Cheal D (2002) Sociology of family life. Palgrave, Basingstoke

Chou YC, Kröger T (2022) Ageing in place together: older parents and ageing offspring with intellectual disability. Ageing Soc 42(2):480–494

Commissioner for Human Rights (2012) Who gets to decide? Right to legal capacity for persons with intel-lectual and psychosocial disabilities. Retrieved from Strasbourg

Costello H, Bouras N (2006) Assessment of mental health problems in people with intellectual disabilities. Isr J Psychiatry Relat Sci 43(4):241

Crabb C, Owen R, Stober K, Heller T (2020) Longitudinal appraisals of family caregiving for people with dis-abilities enrolled in Medicaid managed care. Disabil Rehabil 42(16):2287–2294. https://doi.org/10.1080/09638288.2018.1557266

Department of Health (2012) The national carers' strat-egy: recognised, supported, empowered. Government of Ireland, Dublin

Department of Housing Local Government and Heritage (2021) Housing for all: a new housing plan for Ireland. Government of Ireland, Dublin

Department of the Environment Community and Local Government (2011) National housing strategy for people with a disability 2011–2016. Government of Ireland, Dublin

Dillenburger K, McKerr L (2009) "40 years is an awful long time": parents caring for adult sons and daughters with disabilities. Behav Soc Issues 18:1

Douglas J, Bigby C (2020) Development of an evidence-based practice framework to guide decision making support for people with cognitive impairment due to acquired brain injury or intellectual disability. Disabil Rehabil 42(3):434–441. https://doi.org/10.1080/09638288.2018.1498546

Doyle A, O'Sullivan M, Craig S, McConkey R (2020) People with intellectual disability in Ireland are still dying young. J Appl Res Intellect Disabil. https://doi.org/10.1111/jar.12853

Elder GH, Johnson MK, Crosnoe R (2003) The emergence and development of life course theory. In: Mortimer JT, Shanahan MJ (eds) Handbook of the life course. Springer, New York, pp 3–19

Farina N, Page TE, Daley S, Brown A, Bowling A, Basset T, Livingston G, Knapp M, Murray J, Banerjee S (2017) Factors associated with the quality of life of family carers of people with dementia: a systematic review. Alzheimers Dement 13:572

Finch J (2007) Displaying families. Sociology 41(1):65–81. https://doi.org/10.1177/0038038507072284

Fine M, Glendinning C (2005) Dependence, independence or inter-dependence? Revisiting the concepts of 'care' and 'dependency'. Ageing Soc 25(4):601–621

Fleming P, McGilloway S, Hernon M, Furlong M, O'Doherty S, Keogh F, Stainton T (2019) Individualized funding interventions to improve health and social care outcomes for people with a disability: a mixed-methods systematic review. Campbell Syst Rev 15(1–2):e1008. https://doi.org/10.4073/csr.2019.3

Fyson R, Tarleton B, Ward L (2007) Support for living? The impact of the supporting people programme on housing and support for adults with learning disabilities. Policy Press, Bristol

Giddens A, Sutton PW (2017) Sociology, 8th edn. Polity Press, Cambridge

Gilbert A, Lankshear G, Petersen A (2008) Older family-carers' views on the future accommodation needs of relatives who have an intellectual disability. Int J Soc Welf 17(1):54–64

Gilligan C (2003) In a different voice. Psychological theory and women's development. Harvard University Press, London

Gorfin L, McGlaughlin A (2004) Planning for the future with adults with a learning disability living with older carers. Housing Care Support 7(3):20–24

Hatton C (2017) Day services and home care for adults with learning disabilities across the UK. Tizard Learn Disabil Rev 22:109

Health Service Executive (2011). Time to move on from congregated settings - a strategy for community inclusion: Report of the Working Group on Congregated Settings. Dublin: Health Service Executive.

Health Service Executive (2018) A national framework for person-centred planning in services for persons with a disability. Retrieved from: https://www.hse.ie/eng/services/list/4/disability/newdirections/framework-person-centred-planning-services-for-persons-with-a-disability.pdf

Heller T, Caldwell J (2006) Supporting aging caregivers and adults with developmental disabilities in future planning. Ment Retard 44(3):189–202

Heller T, Harris SP (2012) Disability through the life course. Sage, Thousand Oaks, CA

Heller T, Kramer J (2009) Involvement of adult siblings of persons with developmental disabilities in future planning. Intellect Dev Disabil 47(3):208–219

Heller T, Murthy S, Keiling Arnold C (2021) Family caregiving for adults ageing with intellectual and developmental disabilities. In: Putnam M, Bigby C (eds) Handbook on ageing with disability. Routledge, New York

Hewitt A, Lightfoot E, Bogenschutz M, McCormick K, Sedlezky L, Doljanac R (2010) Parental caregivers' desires for lifetime assistance planning for future supports for their children with intellectual and developmental disabilities. J Fam Soc Work 13(5):420–434

Hirst M (2005) Carer distress: a prospective, population-based study. Soc Sci Med 61(3):697–708

Hirvikoski T, Boman M, Tideman M, Lichtenstein P, Butwicka A (2021) Association of intellectual disability with all-cause and cause-specific mortality in Sweden. JAMA Netw Open 4(6):e2113014. https://doi.org/10.1001/jamanetworkopen.2021.13014

Hourigan S, Fanagan S, Kelly C (2018). Annual report of the National Intellectual Disability Database Committee 2017 main findings. Retrieved from Dublin

Hussain R, Wark S, Janicki MP, Parmenter T, Knox M (2020) Multimorbidity in older people with intellectual disability. J Appl Res Intellect Disabil 33(6):1234–1244. https://doi.org/10.1111/jar.12743

Irazabal M, Pastor C, Molina MC (2016) Family impact of care and respite service: life experiences of mothers of adult children with intellectual disability and mental disorders. Rev Cercetare Interv Soc 55:7

Kelly C, Craig S, McConkey R (2020) Supporting family carers of children and adults with intellectual disability. J Soc Work 20(5):639–656. https://doi.org/10.1177/1468017319860312

Kozma A, Mansell J, Beadle-Brown J (2009) Outcomes in different residential settings for people with intellectual disability: a systematic review. Am J Intellect Dev Disabil 114(3):193–222. https://doi.org/10.1352/1944-7558-114.3.193

Krahn GL, Fox MH (2014) Health disparities of adults with intellectual disabilities: what do we know? What do we do? J Appl Res Intellect Disabil 27(5):431–446

Landes SD, McDonald KE, Wilmoth JM, Carter Grosso E (2021) Evidence of continued reduction in the age-at-death disparity between adults with and without intellectual and/or developmental disabilities. J Appl Res Intellect Disabil 34(3):916–920. https://doi.org/10.1111/jar.12840

Liu W, Gallagher-Thompson D (2009) Impact of dementia caregiving: risks, strains, and growth. In: Aging families and caregiving. Wiley, pp 85–112

Lunsky Y, Tint A, Robinson S, Gordeyko M, Ouellette-Kuntz H (2014) System-wide information about family Carers of adults with intellectual/developmental disabilities—a scoping review of the literature. J Policy Pract Intellect Disabil 11(1):8–18

Lynch K (2007) Love labour as a distinct and non-commodifiable form of care labour. Sociol Rev 55(3):550–570. https://doi.org/10.1111/j.1467-954X.2007.00714.x

Lynch L, McCarron M, McCallion P, Burke E (2022) Sedentary behaviour levels in adults with an intellectual disability: a systematic review and meta-analysis [version 3; peer review: 2 approved]. HRB Open Res 4(69). https://doi.org/10.12688/hrbopenres.13326.3

McCarron M, Swinburne J, Burke E, McGlinchy E, Mulryan N, Andrews V, Foran S, McCallion P (2011) Growing older with an intellectual disability in Ireland 2011: first results from the intellectual disability supplement of the Irish longitudinal study on ageing. Retrieved from Dublin: https://www.tcd.ie/tcaid/assets/pdf/idstildareport2011.pdf

McCarron M, McCausland D, Keenan P, Griffiths C, Hynes G, McCallion P (2013a) A collaborative initiative to implement person centred practice. Retrieved from Dublin

McCarron M, Swinburne J, Burke E, McGlinchey E, Carroll R, McCallion P (2013b) Patterns of multimorbidity in an older population of persons with an intellectual disability: results from the intellectual disability supplement to the Irish longitudinal study on aging (IDS-TILDA). Res Dev Disabil 34(1):521–527

McCarron M, McCallion P, Reilly E, Dunne P, Carroll R, Mulryan N (2017) A prospective 20-year longitudinal follow-up of dementia in persons with Down syndrome. J Intellect Disabil Res 61(9):843–852. https://doi.org/10.1111/jir.12390

McCausland D (2016) Social participation for older people with an intellectual disability in Ireland. PhD, Unpublished thesis, Trinity College Dublin

McCausland D, McCallion P, Brennan D, McCarron M (2018a) The exercise of human rights and citizenship by older adults with an intellectual disability in Ireland. J Intellect Disabil Res 62(10):875–887. https://doi.org/10.1111/jir.12543

McCausland D, McCallion P, Brennan D, McCarron M (2018b) Interpersonal relationships of older adults with an intellectual disability in Ireland. J Appl Res Intellect Disabil 31(1):e140–e153. https://doi.org/10.1111/jar.12352

McCausland D, Brennan D, McCallion P, McCarron M (2019) Balancing personal wishes and caring capacity in future planning for adults with an intellectual disability living with family carers. J Intellect Disabil 23(3):413–431. https://doi.org/10.1177/1744629519872658

McCausland D, McCallion P, McCarron M (2021a) Health and wellness among persons ageing with intellectual disability. In: Putnam M, Bigby C (eds) Handbook on ageing with disability, 1st edn. Routledge, New York

McCausland D, Murphy E, McCarron M, McCallion P (2021b) The potential for person-centred planning to support the community participation of adults with an intellectual disability. J Intellect Disabil. https://doi.org/10.1177/17446295211022125

McConkey R, McConaghie J, Barr O, Roberts P (2006) Views of family carers to the future accommodation and support needs of their relatives with intellectual disabilities. Ir J Psychol Med 23(04):140–144

McConkey R, Kelly F, Craig S (2011) Access to respite breaks for families who have a relative with intellectual disabilities: a national survey. J Adv Nurs 67(6):1349–1357. https://doi.org/10.1111/j.1365-2648.2010.05586.x

McGlinchey E, McCallion P, McDermott S, Foley M, Burke EA, O'Donovan MA, McCausland D, Gibney S, McCarron M (2019) Positive ageing indicators for people with an intellectual disability 2018. Retrieved from Dublin: https://assets.gov.ie/9674/abcdfeef1474423b983e531d2bde645d.pdf

Milne A, Larkin M (2015) Knowledge generation about care-giving in the UK: a critical review of research paradigms. Health Soc Care Community 23(1):4–13. https://doi.org/10.1111/hsc.12143

Morgan DHJ (2011) Rethinking family practices. Palgrave Macmillan, London

Mortimer JT, Shanahan MJ (2003) Preface. In: Mortimer JT, Shanahan MJ (eds) Handbook of the life course. Kluwer Academic Publishers, New York, pp xi–xvi

Nirje B (1973) The normalization principle—implications and comments in advances in the care of the mentally handicapped

Noddings N (1984) Caring: a feminist approach to ethics and moral education. University of California Press, Berkeley, CA

O'Donovan MA, Byrne E, McCallion P, McCarron M (2017) Measuring choice for adults with an intellectual disability–a factor analysis of the adapted daily choice inventory scale. J Intellect Disabil Res 61(5):471–487. Retrieved from: http://onlinelibrary.wiley.com/store/10.1111/jir.12364/asset/jir12364.pdf?v=1&t=jcbxsjja&s=4480170d0fc11c6c654d837ed668a8735cff2927

O'Donovan M-A, McCausland D, McCallion P, McCarron M (2020) Choice as people age with intellectual disability—an Irish perspective. In: Stancliffe MLWRJ, Shogren KA, Abery BH (eds) Choice, preference, and disability: promoting self-determination across the lifespan. Springer Books, New York

O'Leary L, Cooper S-A, Hughes-McCormack L (2018) Early death and causes of death of people with intellectual disabilities: a systematic review. J Appl Res Intellect Disabil 31(3):325–342. https://doi.org/10.1111/jar.12417

Oliver M (1990) The politics of disablement. Macmillan, Basingstoke

Parsons T, Bales RF (1956) Family socialization and interaction process. Routledge and Kegan Paul, London

Peterson JJ, Lowe JB, Peterson NA, Nothwehr FK, Janz KF, Lobas JG (2008) Paths to leisure physical activity among adults with intellectual disabilities: self-efficacy and social support. Am J Health Promot 23(1):35–42. https://doi.org/10.4278/ajhp.07061153

Priestly M (2001) Epilogue. In: Priestly M (ed) Disability and the life course: global perspectives. Cambridge University Press, Cambridge, pp 240–248

Prosser H (1997) The future care plans of older adults with intellectual disabilities living at home with family carers. J Appl Res Intellect Disabil 10(1):15–32

Pruchno RA, Patrick JH (1999) Effects of formal and familial residential plans for adults with mental retardation on their aging mothers. Am J Ment Retard 104(1):38–52

Pryce L, Tweed A, Hilton A, Priest HM (2017) Tolerating uncertainty: perceptions of the future for ageing parent carers and their adult children with intellectual disabilities. J Appl Res Intellect Disabil 30(1):84–96

Ratti V, Hassiotis A, Crabtree J, Deb S, Gallagher P, Unwin G (2016) The effectiveness of person-centred planning for people with intellectual disabilities: a systematic review. Res Dev Disabil 57:63–84

Ray M, Bernard M, Philips J (2009) Critical issues in social work with older people. Palgrave Macmillan, Basingstoke

Reppermund S, Trollor JN (2016) Successful ageing for people with an intellectual disability. Curr Opin Psychiatry 29(2):149–154

Rowe JW, Kahn RL (1997) Successful aging. The gerontologist 37(4):433–440

Rutter M (1995) Clinical implications of attachment concepts: retrospect and prospect. J Child Psychol Psychiatry 36(4):549–571. https://doi.org/10.1111/j.1469-7610.1995.tb02314.x

Ryan A, Taggart L, Truesdale-Kennedy M, Slevin E (2014) Issues in caregiving for older people with intellectual disabilities and their ageing family carers: a review and commentary. Int J Older People Nursing 9(3):217–226. Retrieved from: http://onlinelibrary.wiley.com/store/10.1111/opn.12021/asset/opn12021.pdf?v=1&t=j14vmupe&s=cf361663c2c6588661f478067c14d6d67aad6822

Schaffer HR (2004) Introducing child psychology. Blackwell Publishing, Oxford

Schalock RL, Brown I, Brown R, Cummins RA, Felce D, Matikka L, Keith KD, Parmenter T (2002) Conceptualization, measurement, and application of quality of life for persons with intellectual disabilities: report of an international panel of experts. Ment Retard 40(6):457–470

Scott HM, Havercamp SM (2014) Mental health for people with intellectual disability: the impact of stress and social support. Am J Intellect Dev Disabil 119(6):552–564. https://doi.org/10.1352/1944-7558-119.6.552

Shogren KA (2013) A social-ecological analysis of the self-determination literature. Intellect Dev Disabil 51(6):496–511

Shogren KA, Wehmeyer ML, Lassmann H, Forber-Pratt AJ (2017) Supported decision making: A synthesis of the literature across intellectual disability, mental health, and aging. Educ Training Autism Dev Disabil 52(2):144–157. Retrieved from: https://www-jstor-org.elib.tcd.ie/stable/26420386

Slota N, Martin D (2003) Methodological considerations in life course theory research. Disabil Stud Quart 23(2):19

Snow J (1998) What's really worth doing and how to do it—a book for people who love someone labelled disabled (possibly yourself). Inclusion Press, Ontario

Solomon J, George C (1996) Defining the caregiving system: toward a theory of caregiving. Infant Ment Health J 17(3):183–197

Southby K (2017) Barriers to non-residential respite care for adults with moderate to complex needs: a UK perspective. J Intellect Disabil 21(4):366–386. https://doi.org/10.1177/1744629516658577

Stainton T (2016) Supported decision-making in Canada: principles, policy, and practice. Res Pract Intellect Dev Disabil 3(1):1–11. https://doi.org/10.1080/23297018.2015.1063447

Taggart L, Truesdale-Kennedy M, Ryan A, McConkey R (2012) Examining the support needs of ageing family carers in developing future plans for a relative with an intellectual disability. J Intellect Disabil 16(3):217–234

Tatlow-Golden M, Linehan C, O'Doherty S, Craig S, Kerr M, Lynch C, McConkey R, Staines A (2014) Living arrangement options for people with intellectual disability: a scoping review. Retrieved from: https://oro.open.ac.uk/55665/1/Living%20FINAL%20Moving%20Ahead%20Research%20Synthesis%20Report%207th%20November%202014.pdf

Tichá R, Hewitt A, Nord D, Larson S (2013) System and individual outcomes and their predictors in services and support for people with IDD. Intellect Dev Disabil 51(5):298–315

Timmons JC, Hall AC, Bose J, Wolfe A, Winsor J (2011) Choosing employment: factors that impact employment decisions for individuals with intellectual disability. Intellect Dev Disabil 49(4):285–299. https://doi.org/10.1352/1934-9556-49.4.285

Tisdall K (2001) Failing to make the transition? Theorising the 'transition to adulthood' for young disabled people. In: Priestly M (ed) Disability and the life course: global perspectives. Cambridge University Press, Cambridge, pp 167–178

Trip H, Whitehead L, Crowe M, Mirfin-Veitch B, Daffue C (2019) Aging with intellectual disabilities in families: navigating ever-changing seas—A theoretical model. Qual Health Res 29(11):1595–1610. https://doi.org/10.1177/1049732319845344

Tronto J (1993) Moral boundaries: a political argument for an ethic of care. Routledge, New York

Tronto J, Fisher B (1990) Toward a feminist theory of caring. In: Abel E, Nelson M (eds) Circles of care: work and identity in women's lives. SUNY Press, Albany, NY, pp 35–62

United Nations (2006) Convention on the rights of persons with disabilities. United Nations, New York

UPIAS (1975) Fundamental principles of disability. Retrieved from: http://disability-studies.leeds.ac.uk/library/author/upias/

Verdonschot MML, De Witte LP, Reichrath E, Buntinx WHE, Curfs LMG (2009) Community participation of people with an intellectual disability: a review of empirical findings. J Intellect Disabil Res 53(4):303–318. https://doi.org/10.1111/j.1365-2788.2008.01144.x

Walker R, Hutchinson C (2018) Planning for the future among older parents of adult offspring with intellectual disability living at home and in the community: a systematic review of qualitative studies. J Intellect Develop Disabil 43(4):453–462. https://doi.org/10.3109/13668250.2017.1310823

Walker R, Hutchinson C (2019) Care-giving dynamics and futures planning among ageing parents of adult offspring with intellectual disability. Ageing Soc 39(7):1512–1527. https://doi.org/10.1017/S0144686X18000144

Wark S, Hussain R, Edwards H (2015) Assisting individuals ageing with learning disability: support worker perspectives. Tizard Learn Disabil Rev 20(4):213–222. https://doi.org/10.1108/TLDR-02-2015-0008

Weeks LE, Nilsson T, Bryanton O, Kozma A (2009) Current and future concerns of older parents of sons and daughters with intellectual disabilities. J Policy Pract Intellect Disabil 6(3):180–188

Wehmeyer ML (2003) Self-determination: a review of the construct. In: Wehmeyer ML, Abery BH, Mithaug DE, Stancliffe RJ (eds) Theory in self-determination. Charles C. Thomas Publishers Ltd., Springfield, IL, pp 5–24

Wennberg B, Kjellberg A (2010) Participation when using cognitive assistive devices—from the perspective of people with intellectual disabilities. Occup Ther Int 17(4):168–176. https://doi.org/10.1002/oti.296

WHOQOL Group (1998) The World Health Organization quality of life assessment (WHOQOL): development and general psychometric properties. Soc Sci Med 46(12):1569–1585

Wolfensberger W, Thomas S, Caruso G (1996) Some of the universal "good things of life" which the implementation of social role valorization can be expected to make more accessible to devalued people. Int Soc Role Valoriz 2(2):12–14

World Health Organization (2001) International classification of functioning, disability and health (ICF). World Health Organization, Geneva

Wos K, Kamecka-Antczak C, Szafrański M (2021) Remote support for adults with intellectual disability during COVID-19: from a caregiver's perspective. J Policy Pract Intellect Disabil 18(4):279–285. https://doi.org/10.1111/jppi.12385

Zhang D (2005) Parent practices in facilitating self-determination skills: the influences of culture, socioeconomic status, and children's special education status. Res Pract Persons Severe Disabil 30(3):154–162

Social Integration and Inclusion

14

Maria Paiewonsky, Annie Gomes Redig, and Kerry Watson (ID)

Chapter Topics

- Innovative government guidelines that guide inclusive policies and practices.
- Updated teacher training programs that reflect inclusive education.
- Inclusive postsecondary education for individuals with intellectual disabilities.
- Advancing policies that advance the rights of individuals to make their own decisions and direct their own lives.

Introduction

The United Nations Salamanca Statement (UNESCO 1994) stands out as one of the most important international responses to education for individuals with disabilities. With a commitment from 92 member countries and 25 international organizations at the World Conference on

M. Paiewonsky (✉)
University of Massachusetts, Boston, MA, USA
e-mail: maria.paiewonsky@umb.edu

A. G. Redig
State University of Rio de Janeiro,
Rio de Janeiro, Brazil

K. Watson
NSW Council for Intellectual Disability,
Surry Hills, NSW, Australia
e-mail: kerry@cid.org.au

Special Needs to promote and enact on inclusive education policies, the responsibility is now on governments, educators, and school systems rather than on the individual (Hernandez-Torrano et al. 2022). Equally important, the corresponding Framework for Action makes clear that "ordinary" and "neighborhood" schools should accommodate all children, regardless of disability. The United Nations Convention on the Rights of Persons with Disabilities (United Nations 2006) secured commitment from 164 signatories to support this move toward inclusion, marking a global commitment to inclusive education and signaling a shift in expectations for individuals with disabilities. It is, in fact, meant to serve as a lever for change and speed up reform processes (Buchner and Thompson 2021).

Systemic change can be slow, and the adoption of inclusive practices can be challenging and uneven due to competing discourses (Slee 2011). Yet, innovative policy and practices supported by strong advocacy and a coherent focus on inclusion, as laid out in the Salamanca Statement and the United Nations Convention on the Rights of Persons with Disabilities, can frame and influence transformation.

With the advancement of disability advocacy, research, and policies that reflect raised expectations for individuals with intellectual disabilities, universities and advocacy organizations have an obligation to retool special education and disability services for inclusion. At the university level,

© The Author(s), under exclusive license to Springer Nature Switzerland AG 2023
F. Sheerin, C. Doyle (eds.), *Intellectual Disabilities: Health and Social Care Across the Lifespan*,
https://doi.org/10.1007/978-3-031-27496-1_14

existing preservice preparation and training must be updated to reflect teacher practices that better prepare young people for inclusive lives. Training must be framed around self-determination, inclusive education, integrated and competitive paid work, and supported community living that aligns with more inclusive policies. In the United States and Brazil, federal and state policies provide guidance on these life domains that teacher educators can use to frame teacher practices. In Australia, moral obligations to international conventions and treaties guide a vision for inclusion with community-level organizations, often leading to systemic advocacy efforts for real practice change that reflect disability rights on the ground. Change led by and for individuals with intellectual disabilities will lead to more inclusive and responsive supports and services. Advancing policies regarding the rights of individuals with disabilities to make decisions and receive supports to make decisions with respect to their own will and preferences reflect a philosophy of self-determination and enable federal self-directed support systems to be implemented with integrity as intended.

In the United States, Brazil, and Australia, federal guidelines promote a framework of self-determination, inclusive education, career development, and integrated paid employment. In this chapter, each author describes policy-to-practice efforts that support preservice educators to prepare young people with disabilities for inclusive experiences and to advocate for them as adults. Each author will provide a summary of policies that influence their work, describe their projects, and share a vignette.

United States

In the United States, national trends to support individuals with intellectual disabilities are most evident in policies related to self-determination, inclusive education, and career development that leads to integrated and paid employment. Self-determination, defined as people's basic needs for competence, autonomy, and relatedness that drives them toward action (Shogren et al. 2015),

is supported through self-directed services, an approach that aims to provide greater control for individuals with disabilities. Beginning with federally funded projects in the 1990s, policy experts and disability advocates moved away from traditional "agency-directed" supports and in its place created a system of self-direction policy innovations (DeCarlo et al. 2019). Instead of providing eligible individuals with disabilities, a small menu of pre-determined services, self-directed services centers structure planning and control over services with the person with a disability and their family. This approach is responsive to the ideas of the self-determination movement (Wehmeyer 1992) and individualized models of support (Thompson and DeSpain 2016). Specifically, participants should have the right to control their daily life activities and are often the best monitors of service quality, particularly when they receive adequate training to do so (Nadash and Crisp 2005). Self-direction facilitates self-determination through services that provide individuals with opportunities to control aspects of their lives they consider to be important (DeCarlo et al. 2019).

Framing inclusive education at the secondary level in the United States is the Individuals with Disabilities Education Act (IDEA 2004), which provides regulations and guidance to support students with disabilities to gain access to general education in public schools. IDEA also provides guidance on creating opportunities for students to prepare for their post-school goals through transition services while they are still eligible for special education. Secondary transition services should be designed with a results-oriented process and be based on students' individual interests and preferences. The Higher Education Opportunities Act of 2008 (HEOA 2008) recognized that with increasing opportunities, students with disabilities and their families had more interest in higher education. HEOA authorized funds to create high-quality, inclusive postsecondary models on college and university campuses for students with intellectual disabilities (Grigal et al. 2019). As of 2022, the number of inclusive postsecondary education programs that support individuals with intellectual and developmental disabilities has grown to 310 across the United States (Think College 2022).

The Workforce Innovation and Opportunity Act (WIOA) of 2014 contains several features that address career development for youth with disabilities. One primary feature is the requirement that state vocational rehabilitation agencies (VR) set aside at least 15% of their federal funds to provide pre-employment transition services (pre-ETS) to all students with disabilities who are eligible or potentially eligible for VR services who could potentially benefit from these services. These agencies are required to make five pre-ETS services available, including job exploration counseling, work-based learning experiences, counseling on postsecondary opportunities, workplace readiness training, and instruction in self-advocacy, which may include peer mentoring. WIOA also requires increased coordination between VR area offices and local schools, including attendance at education planning meetings and person-centered planning meetings when invited (WINTAC 2016). This is a significant shift from previous policies that withheld important career services until students aged out of special education services.

Despite these innovative policies, a misalignment exists between transition laws and regulations and preservice teacher training. The course of study for teacher trainees in special education is predominately focused on academic content as guided by federal and local education guidelines. However, there is less often content related to transition research, policies, and services planning that education teams should be including in student services. A review of teacher training programs in the United States found that most special education training programs either do not offer any courses related to transition or they offer just one course (Morningstar et al. 2018).

One State's Systems Change Efforts

In the state of Massachusetts, grassroots legislative advocacy led to the passage of H.3720 (formerly H.159), An Act to Promote the Successful Transition of Students with Disabilities to Postsecondary Education, Employment, and Independent Living, codified as Chapter 51 of the Acts of 2012 (Commonwealth of MA 2012b). The law, also known as the "Transition bill," aligns with several other Massachusetts policies and practices that promote inclusive education, integrated paid employment, and self-determination for students with disabilities. Another bill, the Massachusetts Inclusive Concurrent Enrollment Initiative (MAICEI), supports public institutes of higher education in the state to partner with local school districts to create inclusive dual enrollment opportunities for students with intellectual disabilities (Commonwealth of MA 2012a). MAICEI serves up to 200 eligible students each year to include college in their transition services. Their college-based transition services include person-centered planning, which informs their course of study; enrollment in typical college classes, which they either audit or take for credit, access to accommodations through the college's disability services, and career development activities including work-based learning and paid employment (Igdalsky et al. 2020).

Massachusetts is also an Employment First state. In 2010, the Massachusetts Department of Developmental Services (DDS) issued an Employment First policy that established that integrated paid employment is the preferred service option and should be prioritized for working-age adults served by DDS. They outlined that service priorities for eligible individuals should lead to optimal goals, including being hired and directly paid by an employer, working in the community, and being hired individually, not as part of a group (MA DDS 2010). To support students while they are still in high school, the vocational rehabilitation agency, Massachusetts Rehabilitation Commission, began offering pre-ETS to students with disabilities who are still in high school through agreements with local provider agencies. These services include job exploration counseling, work readiness training, work-based learning experiences, counseling in postsecondary education, and self-advocacy and mentoring services (MA DESE 2020). Local school districts offer pre-ETS to students at school or in the community. If these innovative policies are going to be successful, educators must not only be aware of them but also integrate the related practices and opportunities into their work.

Establishing a Preservice Training Program

The University of Massachusetts Boston (UMass Boston) was one of the first universities to gain approval from the MA Department of Elementary and Secondary Education to offer a course of study for Massachusetts licensed special education teachers and rehabilitation counselors who want to pursue the state transition specialist endorsement. To ensure the most positive outcomes for students with intellectual disabilities, the UMass Boston Transition Leadership program is designed to teach MA educators a wide range of complex skills (e.g., person-centered planning, teaching functional skills within the general curriculum, collaborative teaming and community building, college career readiness, supported decision making). The course of study is designed to provide scholars with tools and applied learning assignments that will empower students with intellectual disabilities to articulate their vision of the future and then learn how to support students in achieving this vision (e.g., accessing community resources, including postsecondary education, pre-ETS, VR, workforce development, and public benefits planning). These innovative practices go beyond writing individual education plans (IEPs) or offering a handful of traditional vocational "readiness" activities (Morningstar et al. 2018). The program expects scholars to understand the unique challenges that students with intellectual disabilities from culturally and linguistically diverse backgrounds face in pursuance of satisfactory postsecondary outcomes (Cheng and Shaewitz 2020) and integrate opportunities students have for supported decision making (Jameson et al. 2015). Each course requires applied learning assignments, providing scholars with hands-on experience to implement transition services. Examples of these assignments include facilitating person-

centered planning, overseeing transition assessments to determine what skills students need to develop and pursue their goals, providing college and career development experiences in the community, and promoting ongoing opportunities for self-determination and self-advocacy. Scholars also form interagency transition teams to enhance transition services for a greater number of students.

With trained teachers, Massachusetts is better positioned to systematically develop effective transition services that will contribute to the vision that all students have "…the opportunity to reach their full potential and to lead lives as participants in the political and social life of the commonwealth and as contributors to its economy" (Commonwealth of MA 2012b).

Vignette: How One Transition Services Team Is Preparing a Student for Her Postsecondary Goals

The Bradley High School Transition Program in Massachusetts was established 4 years ago to support the transition needs of students with intellectual and developmental disabilities and autism, whose education teams determined they are eligible for services beyond the typical 4 years of high school. To implement high-quality services, they hired a transition specialist with the state transition specialist endorsement, who in turn hired a community job developer and three transition coaches. The program supports 6–10 students every year.

Over the last 4 years, the team has established a transition services protocol that includes facilitating person-centered planning with each student and individualizing their schedules based on their postsecondary goals. The team has also joined an inclusive postsecondary education partnership with a local community college and has partnered with the local workforce development office to establish paid internships and jobs for each student.

One 19-year-old Bradley High School student, Carmen, has received transition services from the team. She has intellectual disabilities and has received special education services in special programs for her entire education. As a result of participating in person-centered planning, Carmen identified two important goals: going to college and writing children's books. The transition team worked with Carmen to visit the college where they have a partnership to offer students an inclusive college experience. The college program advisor helped Carmen enroll in a children's literature course and register for disability services to access academic accommodations and take advantage of tutoring for her writing assignments. On the days when Carmen is not at college, she works in the children's section of the town library. Her team taught her how to use a public bus to get to college and work. This is an example of the high-quality transition services the Bradley High School Transition Program offers to students.

Brazil

Brazil has several national laws that promote employment and inclusive education for individual with disabilities. Regarding employment hiring practices, the Brazilian Constitution of 1988 (Brazil 1988) stipulates that job opportunities for people with disabilities must be reserved. The Constitution also prohibits any discrimination in relation to the salary and admission criteria of employees with disabilities. This provision of the Magna Carta was later ratified in follow-up legislation. In 1990, Law 8.112 (Brazil 1990) was enacted, which obliges employers to reserve up to 20% of job vacancies in public tenders to individuals with disabilities. This was followed by Law 8.213/91 (Brazil 1991), known as the "Quotas Law," which stipulates that companies with more than 100 employees must reserve vacancies for this population.

Brazil follows the principles of the Inclusive Education policy since the ratification of the Brazilian Constitution of 1988 (Brazil 1988). Since the Salamanca Declaration (UNESCO 1994), the Brazilian educational system has undergone increasing changes, promoting inclusive education for all students regardless of social, economic, and cultural status or abilities. The focus is on students' social and academic development through access to general education classes. In 2006, the signatory countries of the United Nations Convention on the Rights of Persons with Disabilities, including Brazil, made a commitment that "persons with disabilities can access an inclusive, quality, and free primary education and secondary education on an equal basis with others in the communities in which they live" (United Nations 2006). In 2008, the National Policy on Special Education in the Inclusive Perspective further reinforced inclusive practices (Alana 2019).

The Inclusive Education policy recommends that students with disabilities be included in inclusive classes that have an adequate structure for the teaching-learning process for student success. In the Law of Directives and Bases (LDB) 9394 (Brazil 1996), a chapter on special education specifies the enrollment of students with disabilities, preferably in typical schools, with trained professionals and with the support of specialist teachers. The National Policy on Special Education from the perspective of Inclusive Education (Brazil 2008) aims to ensure that all students with disabilities are enrolled in general education classes with support from specialized teachers. This acknowledgement of specialized teachers supports training for all teachers.

In 2015, the Brazilian Law for the Inclusion of Persons with Disabilities (Brazil 2015) facilitated the provision of subsidies for the enrollment and placement of individuals with disabilities in schools, in the workforce, in housing, and in all other aspects of society. Reflected in this law are principles of the Inclusive Education policy, which frames special education.

Teacher Training to Support Postsecondary Education for Young People and Adults with Intellectual Disabilities

The National Policy on Special Education from the perspective of inclusive education (Brazil 2008) infers that special education in Brazil is no longer a substitute for general education and that it should be considered complementary and/or supplementary to educating students with disabilities. Furthermore, eligible students, including those identified with physical, sensory, or intellectual disability, autism, or high incidence disabilities, should be offered specialized and inclusive educational services (SES) that preferably take place in the regular education setting. SES is intended to assure student success in the regular classroom by promoting physical access, architectural adaptations, and the provision of transportation and adaptive equipment. SES also aims to promote universally accessible teaching and learning experiences, including differentiated instruction and assessment instruments suited to students' needs. With these practices in place, schools can provide students with academic and social development.

In contrast to these policies and practices, professional development for teachers in Brazil remains challenging (Kiru and Cooc 2018). Chakraborti-Ghosh et al. (2014) note that teachers in Brazil feel ill-equipped and less confident about teaching students with disabilities. Although the Brazilian government has passed federal laws on inclusion services for students with disabilities, the financial investment in teacher training has been minimal (Kiru and Cooc 2018). Despite some discussion and research on the school inclusion of students with disabilities, little attention has been paid to teacher preparation to support students with disabilities for post-school outcomes. This contributes to the limited preparation students with disabilities have to prepare for their post-school lives in the community.

Ideally, Brazilian schools should be assuming the responsibility of preparing students with disabilities for adult life, especially at the secondary level. This work should start at school through a service that provides students opportunities for postsecondary education, work experiences, and social skills development. This process can be organized and structured based on the development of an Individualized Transition Plan (ITP). This process organizes a student's postsecondary aspirations into goals and a strategic plan, making it possible for students to dream about and prepare for inclusive adult lives (Redig 2021).

With a trained team of school professionals, it would be possible to implement the ITP process to identify students' individual goals and develop action plans to support their movement to postsecondary education or training, enter the workforce, and prepare for adult life. In Brazil, where there are no plans to help students with disabilities transition from school to independent life and no educators designated to support this work, we believe that a trained special education teacher who provides SES could oversee these transition plans.

With this transition services goal in mind, the research group "School Inclusion of Students with Special Educational Needs in Regular Education: Pedagogical Practices and School Culture" was established at the Graduate Program in Education at the State University of Rio de Janeiro (UERJ). Faculty offered four free teacher training courses related to postsecondary planning for students with intellectual disabilities from 2019 to 2020. The research group chose to narrow the focus on students with intellectual disabilities because they are the students with disabilities we find in Brazilian schools with the greatest demand for support and who need individualized transition planning. These were the first courses ever offered on this subject in Brazil.

The four teacher training courses covered content on inclusive education policies, the basic understanding of intellectual disabilities, Individualized Educational Plans (IEPs), Individual Transition Plans (ITP), transition planning and programs, self-management, and preparing students for the workforce. The teacher participants' course evaluations were very positive, highlighting: (1) the ITP as an important tool to standardize transition services for students with intellectual disabilities; (2) increased understanding of transition education; and (3) raised expectations for students with intellectual disabilities. The course participants/teachers also developed an understanding of the importance of working together with students to promote their self-determination skills, especially skills aimed at self-management that enables them to be the protagonists of their own lives (Pinheiro 2020; Redig and Santos 2020).

Vignette: Piloting Postsecondary Education for Individuals with Intellectual Disabilities

Since 2019, we have developed a secondary research project in the form of an extension project, uniting university and community. The goal is to provide a university experience at UERJ to local students and adults with intellectual disabilities and/or autism. Specifically, we offered the experience to individuals who are attending or who have finished high school and were interested in developing skills through academic and social experiences at the college. The research, still in progress, consists of two phases. The first phase was implemented in 2019 and offered 11 students with intellectual disabilities and autism a course that included topics in self-management, self-advocacy, social interaction, career awareness, emerging sexuality, social skills development, everyday English, and academic content. In the second phase, delayed until spring 2022 due to COVID-19 precautions, students take courses together with matriculated UERJ students.

In the 2019 course, which extended over 3 months, students participated in lectures, group work, and a culminating academic event organized and taught by them. Students identified lecture topics and discussions based on their interests. Specialists and/or young people with disabilities co-presented the lectures to broaden perspectives. In evaluating the course, the students

reported that they made friends through the experience and, equally important, recognized themselves as young people capable of working and attending a university. They also expressed interest in knowing more about UERJ, its course offerings, and the potential they had to improve their work skills. Parents reported that their children were more confident and independent because of this opportunity (Silva 2021; Silva and Redig 2021).

Australia

On the back of the global disability rights movement, a social shift in 1981 moved Australia to start viewing disability through a social model lens. The Disability Services Act 1986 assisted people with disability to receive the services necessary to enable them to work toward full participation as members of the community (Disability Services Act 1986). This included a framework for advocacy funding to sustain focus on disability self-determination. It was around this time that the establishment of "public advocates" and guardianship boards across Australia occurred.

In 1992, the Australian Government passed the Disability Discrimination Act to protect any person in Australia from disability discrimination. The Federal Parliament enacted the Disability Standards for Education (DSE) 2005 (Australian Government 2005) to strengthen education providers' compliance with their obligations toward persons with disabilities and their families, as mandated by the Disability Discrimination Act. In March 2007, Australia was one of the original state signatories to the United Nations Convention on the Rights of Persons with Disabilities (CRPD). In July 2008 and July 2009 sequentially, Australia ratified the CRPD and the Optional Protocol. The Optional Protocol makes Australia more accountable, ensuring CRPD obligations are achieved, and promotes Australia as an international leader in disability rights. Only 4 years after ratifying the

CRPD, Australia introduced the National Disability Insurance Scheme Act (NDIS), a major reform of disability support in Australia using an insurance-based approach to provide person-centered support for individuals with disabilities throughout their life span (Commonwealth of Australia 2013). Despite this apparent move toward community inclusion, legislation and policy did not lead to implementation or better lived experiences for people with disability.

In theory, the NDIS is an enabling structure to foster self-determination in people with disability. However, the lack of mandated Individual Education Plans (IEPs) for students with disability (Cumming et al. 2014) eliminates opportunities for students to develop self-determination skills (Wagner et al. 2012) and for schools to deliver evidence-based, student-centered transition practices (Kohler et al. 2016). In addition, Australia continues to grow its established two-track system of mainstream schooling and segregated specialist schooling to cater to students with specific disabilities, despite its international obligation to the CRPD that asserts that states must not exclude persons with disabilities from the general education system based on disability, and that general education systems must provide the resources required for genuine inclusion (United Nations 2006). Despite the existence of updated national policy about educational provision regarding inclusive education for students with disability, many students with intellectual disabilities are still excluded today. Policy is not enough to achieve inclusion (Slee 2013) and the current mechanisms in place are leaving individuals and families scrambling for resources in disjointed systems, often relying on disability organizations to advocate on their behalf.

Systemic Advocacy Led by People with Intellectual Disability

The Council for Intellectual Disability (CID) is a systemic advocacy organization, established nearly 70 years ago by a group of parents of children with intellectual disabilities. It is an organization for people with intellectual disabilities, led by people with intellectual disabilities. More than half of the board is made up of individuals with intellectual disabilities. CID's inclusive model, along with myriad Easy Read policies and procedures that support CID's open employment, leadership, and advocacy work, is clearly described in their constitution. Each project team and business area includes a combination of employees with and without intellectual disabilities.

As a disability rights organization, advocating for the human rights of people with disability is CID's core mission. CID often applies for funding directly through the NDIS' Information, Linkages, and Capacity (ILC) program. The intent of ILC projects is to build the knowledge, skills, and confidence of people with disability and improve their access to community and mainstream services (Australian Government 2022).

A recent strategic priority for CID, in alignment with an emerging national movement, is to promote the understanding and application of supported decision-making principles and practices in Australia. In 2014, the Australian Law Reform Commission (ALRC) recommended the adoption of Nationally Consistent Supported Decision-Making Principles (Australian Law Reform Commission 2014) that reflect this paradigm shift signaled in the CRPD to recognize people with disabilities as persons before the law and their rights to make choices for themselves. However, the Australian Government is yet to make a commitment to act on the ALRC's recommendation. To achieve this, CID secured funding and designed a new project with a direct goal to provide information and training, and systemic advocacy to provoke reform of the existing Guardianship Law (1987) in New South Wales that still allows substitute decision making into a legislative piece that clearly reflects the supported decision-making framework.

Within Australia, Victoria is the only state or territory that has a newly reformed and updated Guardianship and Administration Act (State of Victoria 2019). It ensures that people with disability are provided with a modern framework for guardianship and financial management and have statutory recognition for supported decision making (State of Victoria 2019). This progressive reform in Victoria is aligned with Australia's commitment to the CRPD, which states in Article 12 that there must be ongoing emphasis on the autonomy and independence of persons with a disability who may require support in making decisions in respect of their will and preferences (United Nations 2006), and not based on outdated paternalistic "best interests" considerations that were once applauded.

Vignette: Stan's Big Life of Working

Stan decided he "wanted a big life of working" in open employment, where people with and without intellectual disabilities work in the same workplace, after many years of working at a local Australian Disability Enterprise (ADE). Stan is a man in his early 60s late in his career. He was institutionalized as a child, has no family to support him, and spends his days at the ADE under a Supported Wage Scheme (i.e., a process that allows employers to pay a productivity-based wage for people with disability) topping milk bottles. Now Stan earns industry award wages working in open employment at CID.

The ADE where Stan worked is a segregated, sheltered workshop that pays poorly based on limited capability to produce, and often adds to a lifetime of negative experiences for people with intellectual disabilities. There is no special law protecting the rights of workers in these settings, and the legal status of workers revolves around the question as to whether they are employees or consumers of a service, such as a Disability Employment Service (DES) provider. In theory, DES providers are designed to provide a step toward open employment, providing people with disability with work and opportunity to gain skills. In practice, people with disability remain excluded or stuck in poorly paid work conditions and have no clear path to open employment.

Stan often reflects on the differences between the ADE and CID, commenting on his experiences of being exposed to dangerous objects and matter while working long hours for little money. Stan now spends his days developing and delivering training to local businesses, councils, schools, and organizations on how to improve disability inclusion policies and practices. He uses his lifetime of lived experiences to inform and provoke reform in the use of supported decision making as an alternative to guardianship and everyday practice. He uses his early experiences as a youth institutionalized and his working life stories when he gives presentations to individuals with disability, their supporters, and other organizations. Stan reflects on having no family to support him in his decision-making experiences, leaving him with a lifetime of decisions made for him by others. Stan wishes he graduated from school and was able to choose his own path. Therefore, he speaks up and encourages others to know their rights to make their own decisions and their rights to receive support to make decisions.

Recommendations

International commitment to the rights of individuals with disabilities to a fully accessible life and the national laws and regulations that support these rights are important for inclusion. The examples shared in this chapter from the United States, Brazil, and Australia highlight a common thread – recognizing the values of the Salamanca Declaration and having a commitment to inclusion. How each advanced the principles of inclusion differed based on the policies and priorities of their countries as well as the opportunities available to them. As pointed out earlier in this chapter, policy is not enough to achieve inclusion (Slee 2013). It takes initiative from practitioners as well as collaboration, training, persistence, and ongoing reflection to establish and advance opportunities for inclusion. Recognizing the wide-ranging opportunities for inclusion is an important first step. At the school level, an obvious first step is advocating for full inclusion in general education classrooms. This includes developing educational plans with students and parents that reflect high educational expectations. It also means considering accommodations that will promote students' educational success. Equally important is that students with intellectual disabilities have early instruction and opportunities to build their skills in directing their supports and make decisions that reflect their preferences in and out of school settings. The efforts to update university preservice programs to align policies with practices are imperative, especially for educators of students with intellectual disabilities so that individuals with disabilities have the skills and opportunities to direct their services and make decisions that reflect their preferences.

Key Concepts Discussed

1. International government guidelines that guide inclusive policies and practices
2. Updated teacher training programs that reflect inclusive education
3. International initiatives that provide inclusive postsecondary education for individuals with intellectual disabilities
4. Promoting supported decision making

References

Alana Institute (2019) What Brazilians think about inclusive education. Available at: https://alana.org.br/wp-content/uploads/2021/01/relatorio_educacao_inclusiva_INGLES.pdf

Australian Government (1986) Disability Services Act. Available at: https://www.legislation.gov.au/Details/C2013C00015

Australian Government (1992) Disability Discrimination Act. Available at: http://www.legislation.gov.au/Details/C2018C00125

Australian Government (2005) Disability Standards for Education 2005. Available at: http://www.legislation.gov.au/Details/F2005L00767

Australian Government (2022) Disability and careers. Information, Linkages and Capacity Building (ILC)

program. Available at: https://www.dss.gov.au/disability-and-carers-programs-services-for-people-with-disability/information-linkages-and-capacity-building-ilc-program

Australian Law Reform Commission (2014) Equity, Capacity and Disability in Commonwealth Laws (ALRC Report 124). National Decision-Making Principles-Recommendation 3. Available at: http://www.alrc.gov.au/publication/equality-capacity-and-disability-in-commonwealth-laws-alrc-report-124/3-national-decision-making-principles-2/national-decision-making-principles-2/

Brazil (1988) Constitution of the Federative Republic of Brazil: Constitutional text of October 5, 1988

Brazil (1990) Law No. 8,112 of December 11, 1990. Available at: http://www.planalto.gov.br/ccivil_03/leis/l8112compilado.htm

Brazil (1991) Law No. 8,213 of July 24, 1991. Available at: http://www.planalto.gov.br/ccivil_03/leis/l8213cons.htm

Brazil (1996) Law on National Education Guidelines and Bases 9394. Brasília

Brazil (2008) National policy on special education from the perspective of inclusive education. Brasilia

Brazil (2015) Law No. 13,146 of July 6, 2015. Brazilian law for the inclusion of persons with disabilities statute of persons with disabilities. Brasilia

Buchner T, Thompson SA (2021) From plot twists, progress, and the persistence of segregated education: the continuing struggle for inclusive education in relation to students with intellectual disabilities. J Pol Pract Intellect Disabil 18(1):4–6

Chakraborti-Ghosh S, Orellana K, Jones J (2014) A cross-cultural comparison of teachers' perspectives on inclusive education through a study abroad program in Brazil and in the US. Int J Special Educ 29(1):4–13

Cheng L, Shaewitz D (2020) The 2020 youth transition report: outcomes for youth and young adults with disabilities. Institute for Educational Leadership, Washington, DC

Commonwealth of Australia (2013) National Disability Insurance Scheme. Available at: http://www.ndis.gov.au

Commonwealth of Massachusetts (2012a) Inclusive concurrent enrollment partnership programs for students with disabilities pursuant to Chapter 139 of the Acts of 2012, line item 7061–9600

Commonwealth of Massachusetts (2012b) An act relative to student with disabilities in post-secondary education, employment, and independent living. Chapter 51 of the Acts of 2012. Retrieved at: https://malegislature.gov/Laws/SessionLaws/Acts/2012/Chapter51

Cumming TM, Strnadova I, Dowse L (2014) At-risk youth in Australian schools and promising models of intervention. Int J Special Educ 29(3):16–25

DeCarlo MP, Bogenschutz MD, Hall-Lande JA, Hewitt AS (2019) Implementation of self-directed supports for people with intellectual and developmental disabilities in the United States. J Disabil Policy Stud 30(1):11–21

Grigal M, Hart D, Papay C (2019) Inclusive higher education for students with intellectual disability in the United States: overview of policies, practices, and outcomes. In: O'Brien P, Bonati M, Gadow F, Sleeeds R (eds) People with intellectual disability experiencing university life: theoretical underpinnings, evidence, and lived experience, Studies in inclusive education, vol 42. Sense Publications, Boston, MA

Hernández-Torrano D, Somerton M, Helmer J (2022) Mapping research on inclusive education since Salamanca Statement: a bibliometric review of the literature over 25 years, Int J Incl Educ 26:9, 893–912

Igdalsky L, Gabbard G, Price M (2020) Report to the Legislature. Massachusetts Inclusive Concurrent Enrollment. MA Department of Higher Education. Available at: https://www.mass.edu/strategic/maicei/documents/report-to-the-legislature-FY19.pdf

Jameson JM, Riesen T, Polychronis S, Trader B, Mizner S, Martinis J, Hoyle D (2015) Guardianship and the potential of supported decision-making with individuals with disabilities. Res Pract Persons Severe Disabil 40(1):36–35

Kiru E, Cooc N (2018) A comparative analysis of access to education for students with disabilities in Brazil, Canada, and South Africa. J Int Special Needs Educ 21(2):34–44

Kohler PD, Gothberg JE, Fowler C, Coyle J (2016) Taxonomy for transition programming 2.0: a model for planning, organizing, and evaluating transition education, services, and programs. Western Michigan University. Available at: www.transitionta.org

Massachusetts Department of Elementary and Secondary Education (2020) Massachusetts Rehabilitation Commission Pre-Employment Transition Services (Pre-ETS) Technical Assistance Advisory SPED 2020-1. Available at: https://www.doe.mass.edu/sped/advisories/2020-1ta.html

Massachusetts Executive Office of Health and Human Services (2010) Department of Developmental Services employment first fact sheet. Available at: https://search.mass.gov/?q=employment%2Bfirst

Morningstar M, Hirano K, Roberts-Dahm D, Teo N, Kleinhammer-Tramill PJ (2018) Examining the status of transition-focused content within educator preparation programs. Career Dev Transit Except Individ 41(1):4–15

Nadash P, Crisp S (2005) Best practices in consumer direction. Centers for Medicare and Medicaid Services, Washington, DC. Available at: https://aspe.hhs.gov/sites/default/files/private/pdf/177236/CMS-CDBestPractices.pdf

Pinheiro VC (2020) Individualized transition plan: pedagogical strategy for students with intellectual disabilities to achieve an independent life. Master's thesis in education. Graduate Program in Education, University of the State of Rio de Janeiro (UERJ)

Redig AG (2021) Academic education and independent living: a dialogue to be built. Education 46(1):59, 1–26. https://doi.org/10.5902/1984644443012

Redig AG, Santos MP (2020) Continued teacher education: people with intellectual disabilities

at work. Educação em Foco 25(3). https://doi.org/10.22195/2447-524620202532902

Shogren KA, Wehmeyer ML, Palmer SB, Forber-Pratt A, Little TJ, Lopez SJ (2015) Causal agency theory: reconceptualizing a functional model of self-determination. Educ Train Autism Dev Disabil 50(3):251–263

Silva IF (2021) Weaving networks: university experience of students with intellectual disabilities and autism spectrum disorder. Dissertação de Mestrado em Educação. Programa de Pós-Graduação em Educação, Universidade do Estado do Rio de Janeiro (UERJ)

Silva IF, Redig AG (2021) University experience of students with intellectual disabilities and/or autism at the State University of Rio de Janeiro. Educ Soc Cult 58:97–115. https://doi.org/10.24840/esc.vi58.143

Slee R (2011). The irregular school: exclusion, schooling and inclusive education. The irregular school: exclusion, schooling and inclusive education. 1–220. https://doi.org/10.4324/9780203831564

Slee R (2013) How do we make inclusive education happen when exclusion is a political predisposition? Int J Incl Educ 17(8):895–907

State of Victoria (2019) Guardianship and Administration Act 2019. Available at: http://www.justice.vic.gov.au/justice-system/laws-and-regulation/guardianship-and-administration-act-2019

Think College (2022) College Search Directory. Available at: https://thinkcollege.net/college-search

Thompson JR, DeSpain SN (2016) Community support needs. In: Singh NN (ed) Handbook of evidence-based practices in intellectual and developmental disabilities. Springer, New York, pp 137–168

UNESCO (1994) The Salamanca statement and framework for action on special needs education. Adopted by the world conference on special needs education: access and quality. UNESCO, Salamanca

United Nations (2006) Convention on the Rights of Persons with Disabilities, Article 12: Equal recognition before the law

United States (2004) Individuals with Disabilities Education Act, 20 U.S.C. § 1400

United States (2008) Higher Education Opportunities Act (HEOA). Public Law 110-315

United States (2014). Workforce Innovation and Opportunity Act (WIOA). Public Law 113-128. (29 USC 3101)

Wagner M, Newman L, Cameto R, Javitz H, Valdes K (2012) A national picture of parent and youth participation in IEP and transition planning meetings. J Disabil Policy Stud 23:140–155. https://doi.org/10.1177/1044207311425384

Wehmeyer ML (1992) Self-determination and the education of students with mental retardation. Educ Train Ment Retard 27:302–314

WINTAC (2016) Preamble: final VR regulations at 81 FR 55685. Transition services (§ 361.5(c)(55)) scope of "Pre-Employment Transition Services" and "Transition Services"

Supporting Transitions

15

Michael Brown and Juliet MacArthur

Chapter Topics

- The term transition will be defined.
- Transitions theory will be explored.
- Detail will be provided on the research evidence regarding transitions across the lifespan.
- A discussion of transitions and people with intellectual disabilities will be presented.
- In applying learning, a transition case study regarding the needs of people with intellectual disabilities and complex needs will be presented.
- Details will be offered on the supports required to enable effective transitions across the lifespan required by people with intellectual disabilities.

Introduction

This chapter presents and explores definitions and theories related to transitions and the policy and practice responses necessary to ensure the needs of individuals at different transition points are identified and met effectively. The complexities of different transition processes and the implications on the care and support of people with intellectual disabilities are considered with a specific focus on healthcare that is linked to a research study undertaken in Scotland. A case vignette of the transition needs of Sarah, a young adult with intellectual disabilities, will be presented, highlighting the care and support needs necessary to ensure her effective transition.

Throughout life everyone goes through multiple transitions, involving a move from one state to another. There are numerous examples of transitions across the lifespan, such as transitioning from pre-school to primary education, transitioning from primary to secondary education and transitioning into the workplace or further education and then to retirement. The transition from child to adulthood is often viewed as the most significant transition, as young adults assume a wide range of legal, personal and social responsibilities as they become adults. Another important age-related transition relates to the move to requiring care and support from care services for older people either at home or in an institutional setting. There may also be a transition into end-of-life care and the need to access palliative care and support. Whatever the transition, it is important to recognise and appreciate the full range of life course transitions that are experienced and their potential impact and consequences.

M. Brown (✉)
Queen's University, Belfast, Northern Ireland, UK
e-mail: m.j.brown@qub.ac.uk

J. MacArthur
NHS Lothian and Queen's University,
Belfast, Northern Ireland, UK
e-mail: juliet.macarthur@nhslothian.scot.nhs.uk

© The Author(s), under exclusive license to Springer Nature Switzerland AG 2023
F. Sheerin, C. Doyle (eds.), *Intellectual Disabilities: Health and Social Care Across the Lifespan*,
https://doi.org/10.1007/978-3-031-27496-1_15

Defining Transitions

Within the context of health and social care, there are a number of policy documents and directives that focus on transitions and provide useful definitions. The Department of Health in England defines the transition from child to adult services as the

> *purposeful, planned process that addresses the medical, psychosocial and educational and vocational needs of adolescents/young adults with chronic physical and medical conditions as they move from child-centred to adult-oriented health care systems.* (Department of Health 2006, p. 14)

The National Institute for Health and Care Excellence (NICE) defines transition as:

> *the process of moving from children's to adults' services. It refers to the full process including initial planning, the actual transfer between services, and support throughout.* (NICE 2016, p. 18)

From a health perspective, the WHO states that:

> *the transitions of care refer to the various points where a patient moves to, or returns from, a particular physical location or makes contact with a health care professional for the purposes of receiving health care.* (WHO 2016, p. 3)

From these definitions it is apparent that to be safe, effective and person-centred, transitions involve:

- Purposeful activities
- Planning and coordination
- Clear processes
- Moves from one set of services and supports to another

In the context of healthcare for young people with an intellectual disability, this usually means leaving child health services that are often based in a specific specialist children's hospital and moving to care and support from a wide range of adult health services that can be provided in different hospitals as well as in primary and community health services. Young people with intellectual disability will also encounter many other types of transition, often occurring at the same time as a health transition. These may include personal and social transitions such as leaving home, which may involve going into supported living, developing more of an independent social life and finding suitable employment or training opportunities.

Transitions Theory

The terms 'transition' and 'transitioning' are often used in human services, such as education, social care and health services, referring to the process of moving, or being moved, from one group of services to another. To assist with understanding the issues related to moving services, *transitions theory* (Meleis 2010) identifies the complexities of the process and the need for a lifespan approach that adapts to changing needs at different times and at critical points in the transition process. To ensure care needs are effectively identified and met, *transitions theory* highlights the importance of proactive engagement, planning, communication and care coordination required by young adults with complex care and support needs (Li et al. 2022). To help develop the understanding of this often-complex process, there has been a sustained and developing focus on the concept of 'transition' in policy directives.

Transitions and Policy Initiatives

The Department of Health (DoH) and the Department for Education and Skills (DES) in England published *Transition: getting it right for young people Improving the transition of young people with long term conditions from children's to adult health services*, working with health professions and other services to promote collaboration across and between agencies to enable effective transition of young adults with long-term health condition from child to adult health services (DoH 2006). The policy articulates the key issues that need to be addressed to facilitate and enable the transition from child to adult health services for young adults with complex health conditions. Planning the transition before, during and after is central to the process and should be centred around models of care and support. The policy highlights that transitioning from child to adult services is a process and not a single event, with a need for early consultation involving the young adult and their family and the professionals from current services and those required in the future to provide care and support. There is no specific time when the transition process should commence; however, 14 years of age has been highlighted as a good time to start, with a need for flexibility. Flexibility is necessary to ensure that the young adult and their family is supported and prepared for the transition, with person-centred information provided for the young adult and their family. Supports need to be made available to the young adult and their family until fully established in adult health services.

The WHO highlights the need to focus on patient safety issues and the potential vulnerabilities of young adults at the point of transition from child to adult health services, with a particular focus on the key role of primary care services (WHO 2016). During the journey through healthcare systems, there are key roles for community services, primary care and acute hospitals to ensure that needs are identified and met and care effectively coordinated. The WHO report identifies and articulates the central role of the individual experiencing the transition and the important contributions required from their families and those involved in their care and support. The role of families and carers is vital as they are constant throughout the transition process, possessing essential information necessary to ensure it is smooth and effective, thereby minimising the risk of adverse events and harm.

In 2016, NICE published the *Transition from children's to adults' services for young people using health or social care services*. The NICE guidelines focus on the transition before, during and after the move from child to adult services. The primary purpose of the guidelines is to enable the effective transition across health and social care services that places the young adult at the centre of the process and involves their family and those involved in their care and support. The guidelines are set around overarching principles to shape and inform the transition process:

- Involving the young adult, their family and carers in service design, delivery and evaluation
- Early transition planning
- A named transition worker throughout the transition process
- Involving the young adult throughout the transition process
- Building independence
- Involving parents and carers
- Support before transition
- Support during the transition
- Support after the transition
- Supporting the infrastructure
- Planning and developing transition services

Transitions and People with Intellectual Disabilities

There is an increasing and ageing population of people with intellectual disabilities, with many experiencing a range of complex health needs requiring access to a diverse range of supports and services, including healthcare (Bélanger and Caron 2018). Families of people with intellectual disabilities experience a number of transitions across the lifespan. The first transition involves the diagnosis of cognitive and intellectual impairment with the issues that arise as they move from having the 'normal' expected child (Brown 2016). A further transition experienced by parents involves decisions regarding education and the best option to meet the needs of their child with intellectual disabilities. Some may opt for inclusive pre-school and school education, while others, often due to the range of complex support needs, choose specialist education for their child (Smogorzewska et al. 2019). The most common transition relates to the move from child to adult services. This transition may be viewed as the most significant for young adults with intellectual disabilities and their family as it involves a move from all familiar and known services, supports and personnel (Jacobs et al. 2018; Malapela et al. 2020). There is a growing evidence of the impact of this particular transition, notably the consequences on the young adult and their family when the process is not well coordinated and facilitated (Leonard et al. 2016; Brown et al. 2019). Therefore, it is necessary to ensure that there is effective early planning and coordination and information sharing with young adults with intellectual disabilities, their families and professionals involved (Young-Southward et al. 2017a).

There are multiple consequences of the transition from child to adult services, including decisions regarding further education, employment and day-care options. Further changes may include a move from child and family to adult social work which may also involve respite and short-break services (Redgrove et al. 2016). From a health perspective, the transition may have significant implications and consequences for young adults with intellectual disabilities, their family and carers. Long-established relationships with child services, including healthcare, will cease as the young adult moves into adult health services (Brown et al. 2020a). This can create gaps in provision that impacts negatively on the health and wellbeing of the young adult with intellectual disabilities as there are often no parallel adult health services (Young-Southward et al. 2017b). A further transition that also needs to be considered and planned for is the move from adult to services for older people and retirement (Stancliffe et al. 2015) This is an area that has not attracted the same attention as the transition from child to adult services and with the ageing population of older adults with intellectual disabilities is one that requires development and attention (Baumbusch et al. 2017; Egan et al. 2021). Following on from the ageing population of older adults with intellectual disabilities is the transition into palliative and end-of-life care, who may lack experience providing care and support for those with more complex needs, with a need for planning and coordination (Bekkema et al. 2015; Todd et al. 2021).

Facilitating Effective Transitions

During the transition between childhood and adulthood, young adults experience a range of physical, psychological, intellectual, personality and social developments (Kerckhoff 2019). At this time, transitions involve moving from child to adult-orientated services, including education, social care and healthcare. The transition from child to adult health services usually involves the transfer of care and support between various health teams (Stroud et al. 2015). At the same time, many young adults transition on to other services, such as adult social work and respite care to meet their ongoing care and support needs. It can therefore be seen that the transition process requires purposeful and interrelated activities, necessary to ensure the smooth transfer between services (Betz et al. 2016). Due to the often-complex needs of some young adults, it is necessary to ensure that the transition process is carefully planned and coordinated to ensure that ongoing care and support needs are fully identified and met (Schmidt et al. 2020).

Central to the planning and coordination of the transition is placing the young adult and their family at the centre of the decision-making process (Okumura et al. 2015). The co-production of assessment of needs and co-design of care plans are required to ensure care and support is reflective of the needs of the young adult (Hirano et al. 2018). As a consequence of the scope of their needs, young adults leave the familiarity of child services, moving to receive care and support from adult services. Some young adults due to the extent of their health needs require ongoing care and support from adult health services. Recognising the impact of the process on the young adult and their family is important as relationships that have been in place for many years will cease (Brown et al. 2020b).

From a transition perspective, young adults with health conditions that are ongoing and long-term will require involvement from adult health services to ensure their care and support needs are met (Gray et al. 2018). Examples of health conditions that may be lifelong, necessitating the transition into adult health care, include asthma, arthritis, congenital heart disease, diabetes, epilepsy, mental health and cystic fibrosis; there are many others (Schmidt et al. 2020). Other health-related concerns that may be lifelong, with the need for ongoing care and support from adult health services, include genetic conditions, such as Down syndrome, cerebral palsy and intellectual disability (VanZant and McCormick 2021).

As a consequence of their range of health conditions and complex needs, young adults require assessment, treatment, interventions, health education and care and support from a range of health services to ensure they are met safely and effectively (Borah et al. 2021).

It is apparent that for some, transitions are lifelong events, and for those with complex needs, they require detailed forward planning, with effective communication, coordination and collaboration with a range of stakeholders. When coordinated and planned for effectively, the transition process from child services is smooth and effective for the young adult and their family. However, for some, particularly those with multiple complex needs, the transition into adulthood and adult services can be poorly coordinated and stressful. Failure to recognise and ensure that the necessary services and care and support are in place throughout transitions can have significant negative consequences, including increased mortality, unmet health conditions, poor health outcomes, reduced quality of life and increased hospitalisation (Laski 2015; Jacob et al. 2017).

Researching the Experience of Health Transitions in Scotland

To understand the experiences of the health transition for young adults with complex intellectual disabilities when moving from child to adult health services, a 3-year research study was undertaken that involved all 14 NHS Health Boards across Scotland (Brown et al. 2020a, b). The study was undertaken in 2017–2020 to identify families' and nurses' experience of transition and identify the most effective ways of providing care and support before, during and after the process. The study involved qualitative data collection involving 10 parents of people with complex intellectual disabilities and 46 registered nurses and other practitioners with recent experiences of the transition process. Findings have been used to make recommendations for policy makers, health service leaders and educationalists (Brown et al. 2020b).

Case Study: The Story of Sarah's Transition

The different experiences of the families involved in this study have been captured in the story of Sarah, illustrating the range of issues that a young adult with complex intellectual disabilities and their family can experience during the transition process from child to adult health services.

Sarah is 15 years old and lives at home with her parents and two younger brothers. She is a sociable, content young girl who is non-verbal and can communicate in her own way. She has a rare genetic condition that has resulted in a number of complex health issues, and she has severe intellectual disability. Sarah is visually impaired, has epilepsy and has a chronic kidney disease. She has an established tracheostomy and a gastrostomy tube that is used for administering all nutrition and over 20 doses of daily medication. Sarah uses an adapted wheelchair and requires to be moved with a hoist.

The review and monitoring of Sarah's health conditions is coordinated by her paediatrician. She is also under the care of many specialist child health services including a neurologist and an epilepsy nurse specialist, a gastroenterologist, a respiratory nurse specialist, a nephrologist, a physiotherapist and a speech and language therapist. Sarah also has involvement from a community children's nurse who coordinates her medical supplies and provides ongoing assessment and support at home.

Sarah and her parents have an excellent relationship with child health services, who have been involved in her care and support since she was a baby. Sarah's parents feel safe in the children's services and know they can contact the paediatrician or specialist nurses if they have any concerns. They think that the professionals in child health services have a good understanding of Sarah's multiple health complexities, with well-established and trusted relationships.

Sarah will soon be 16 and the head teacher at her special school is organising a 'transition meeting' to commence planning for Sarah moving to adult services when she leaves at 19. Sarah's parents are very anxious about the process, as the 'transition' has not been discussed with them before and they do not know what to expect. They have heard negative stories from other parents, and this makes them not want to think about it. They would like Sarah to stay in child health services and have concerns they will be left with inadequate support, with their existing trusted services changing or removed.

Sarah is prone to respiratory infections and having open access to the paediatric ward where she is known well gives her parents confidence in the quality of care she receives. Sarah feels comfortable in the children's ward and the nurses know her well and understand her needs. The nurses know that loud noises can, for example, trigger spasms in Sarah and therefore try to provide a side-room in a quieter area of the ward. Due to Sarah's frequent admissions to the paediatric ward throughout her childhood, her parents are anxious about future adult hospital admissions. Sarah's older friend was recently admitted to an adult hospital and his parents felt isolated, excluded and not listened to.

Sarah's mother works part-time and her father full-time. Sarah will remain in full-time school education until she is 19. She has a complex care team delivering support four evenings a week and accesses respite regularly. Sarah's mother is concerned about changes in support when Sarah moves to adult day care, as well as the possible reduction in respite and complex care service provision. She is particularly concerned about the impact it will have on Sarah's mental and physical health. She feels she may have to give up her job to provide more of Sarah's care and day activities.

This Scottish study supported wider research findings that have shown that the transition from child to adult health services for young adults with complex intellectual disabilities like Sarah, their families and other professionals can be challenging and stressful (Camfield et al. 2011; Davies et al. 2011; Bindels-de Heus et al. 2013; Franklin et al. 2019). Although no consistent, well-established processes for transition in any of the health services across Scotland were found, there were many examples of good practice that made a real difference to the young person and their families. These positive experiences were used to propose a number of recommendations that were linked to a set of principles to underpin transition with clear management responsibilities and intended outcomes for young people and their families (Brown et al. 2020b).

The Transition Experience of Families

At the heart of the study was the experience of the ten parents who had all been through transition with their child in the previous few years. The following five themes identified, conveyed their experiences and revealed the magnitude of this transition process and many of the challenges they encountered: (1) a deep sense of loss, (2) an overwhelming process, (3) parents making transition happen, (4) a shock to the adult healthcare system and (5) unbearable pressure.

A Deep Sense of Loss

Parents talked about losing the sense of safety that they had felt throughout the years of accessing healthcare in child health services, where they and their child were often well known. This was often made more difficult as the transition to adult health services could be unexpected, as one parent described it 'all of a sudden it's like somebody taking a rug and just pulling it out'. Transition resulted in a move from a small group of doctors, nurses and allied health professionals who worked as an integrated team through to a range of specialists, sometimes in different hospitals. For the families in the study, it was a stressful time, with many expressing feelings of isolation, particularly when losing the emotional support they had received from professionals who had known their family for many years.

An Overwhelming Process

Transition involves establishing new care teams in adult services, which requires multiple meetings and a lot of new information. While this is perhaps an inevitable process, given the differences in the ways of delivering healthcare in adult services, it often felt overwhelming for the parents due to a lack of continuity or information sharing, which meant having to continually repeat the same information to multiple professionals. One parent described their sense of frustration: 'it's just the sheer fact that you almost have to start again with the referrals in many cases'. For many parents it felt that the transition was determined by the needs of the service, rather than being shaped around their child. However, some parents reported a positive experience, particularly when they were being supported by a 'transition nurse' who coordinated all appointments and explained what was involved and provided additional support throughout the process.

Parents Making Transitions Happen

Where there was a lack of coordination, parents frequently had to take responsibility for making sure that there were no gaps in their child's care and services. They often had to take a proactive approach and became the driving force behind the transition planning, something which required focus and perseverance. Some parents talked about a sense of having to 'battle' for services or for access to particular treatments or care provision, with one parent saying 'I've just come to the conclusion that everything is a struggle'. Despite this there were positive reports about the impact that a transition nurse made, with one mother appreciating the nurse's role in providing specialist care, organising training, liaising with hospital consultants, identifying appropriate adult health-

care services, advocating for the family and providing emotional support throughout the transition process.

A Shock to the Adult Healthcare System

Many of the parents in the study reported that their first encounters with adult healthcare services were difficult, with a sense that the extent of their child's health care needs was seen to be 'a shock' to the system. Many services lacked essential adaptations, including specific equipment, changing facilities and provision for parents to stay overnight if they did not feel confident leaving their child alone. These experiences often reinforced parent's perceptions that some adult healthcare professionals lacked essential knowledge of intellectual disabilities or the skills and experience to recognise and respond appropriately to the complex needs of their young adult. As one parent emphasised 'my 20-year-old doesn't speak, can't move, can't press buttons, can't get anybody's attention. She's not able to say that she needs changing or she's hungry or thirsty… and that really worries me'.

The change in legal status regarding consent and involvement in decision-making that comes when people reach adulthood can be quite complex for healthcare professionals and parents to negotiate. For some parents in this study, they felt excluded even when they had legal guardianship, or conversely healthcare staff sometimes did not know what was appropriate for the young person and would ask parents to make decisions that previously were made by the clinical team in the children's hospital.

While many parents reported a lack of continuity of care, which for some made them feel that they were 'falling between gaps', other families had positive experiences, which were often linked to an individual healthcare professional taking a particular interest and acting on the young adult's behalf. One parent described her confidence in a specialist nurse 'who is a lovely, lovely person. She has linked to the spasticity management consultant… and she can be contacted on our behalf. We don't see her every time, but she can be contacted'.

The Unbearable Pressure

Given the experiences that many parents reported, their sense of pressure increased significantly especially when they felt isolated trying to navigate unfamiliar healthcare environments. One parent's reflection on their child's first admission to the adult hospital was 'There was no help, no advice. I have never felt so isolated my entire life'. This increasing pressure was seen to impact on the mental and physical health of parents, which was also affected by issues such as a reduction in respite care provision, detailed as a common feature of transition to adult social care services. One mother described the reduction in support that was having a material impact on her own wellbeing: 'I get 42 nights respite a year, which is a hell of a drop-down. My children's hospice is gone, so I don't get my three weeks there, and complex care, rather than having three to four visits a week or someone helping out in the evenings for a few hours from half five to half nine, I'm lucky if I get one shift a week'.

There were also positive experiences with some parents reporting actions from healthcare professionals that helped reduce pressures. One example was a general practitioner taking on a lead role to provide continuity of care, with the parent reporting 'And now we just see him all the time and it's just ... the difference is huge'. Where intellectual disability liaison nurses were involved, parents highlighted their role in being an advocate for the family and helping adult healthcare staff make reasonable adjustments. For example, 'I was able to explain the situation to her, and obviously she had a better understanding than the actual doctors had, so she could go and speak to the doctors, and then obviously, things kind of relaxed a bit and they were a bit more helpful'.

The interviews with parents of young adults with complex intellectual disabilities confirmed previous findings about multiple challenges experienced during transition process to adult services and beyond. However, they also highlighted the opportunities for increased nursing involvement to help families navigate the transition process and minimise their anxiety. Families are not passive recipients of care and the reciprocal nature of the relationship among the health-care professionals, the young adult with complex intellectual disabilities and their family needs to be acknowledged and their needs addressed. This would help facilitate a more effective transition process and ensure families' health and wellbeing are not negatively affected.

Identifying Best Practices

As well as focusing on the experience of transition, the study aimed to identify examples of best practice, gathered from the perspectives of both parents and healthcare professionals, to inform those delivering, planning and leading services. Five main themes were identified, with 16 subthemes for the management of transition (Table 15.1). Each subtheme was further developed to identify potential outcome mea-

Table 15.1 Themes and related subthemes representing principles underpinning best practice strategies for improved transition care and associated elements of transition management

Principles underpinning improved transition care	Elements of transition management
1. Strategic level focus	• Strategic level commitment • Population projection and service planning • Transition education and training
2. Clear transition processes and pathways	• Transition pathway development • Cross health board transition practices
3. Proactive transition preparation	• Early preparation • Timely initiation of the transition planning process
4. Multiagency transition planning	• Collaborative working across services and agencies • Lead coordinator • Assessment and care planning • Emergency care planning
5. Continuity of care in adult services	• Coordinated handover of care • Holistic overview in adult health services • Access to services and quality care • Family carers as equal partners in care

sures that could be used by service providers to evaluate their own services or to inform parent feedback measures to understand local experiences (Brown et al. 2020b). Underpinning all the principles outlined below is that parents and families should be recognised as equal partners in care, who provide expertise on their children's complex needs as well as vital, unpaid support to the adult health service.

Principle 1: Strategic Level Focus

Supporting effective transitions relies on having the right resources and people in place to meet the needs of each young person and their families. This means each health board or authority and local council work together to identify the size of the local population of young people with complex intellectual disabilities on an annual basis. This should also be used to predict the actual numbers who will be transitioning to adult health services in any 1 year.

Principle 2: Clear Transition Processes and Pathways

Families need to know what to expect and where support will come from. While each young person will be different, there are common processes and pathways that can be identified and developed into clear information for all those involved. Transition pathways should be developed jointly by health and social work professionals, with clear involvement of the education providers who often initiate planning conversations with families. For some young people with very complex health needs, these pathways may involve care and treatment in different health boards and local authority areas.

Principle 3: Proactive Transition Preparation

It is the responsibility of all professionals to prepare the young person and their family for transition to adult health and social services. In this Scottish study parents and healthcare professionals felt that transition should be discussed from around the age of 14 and that families should be provided with reliable information on future care and their changing legal status with regard to their child. The findings also emphasised the importance that all professionals should recognise and acknowledge to the family that transition represents a major life change for the young person and their family and that this is often associated with feelings of fear and anxiety.

Principle 4: Multiagency Transition Planning

A young person's health needs must be recognised as a crucial aspect of the wider transition process and health professionals need to be involved in the multiagency meetings involving education and social work. In this study it was clear that having a named transition coordinator improved the quality of the process for families, the young person and other professionals. Nurses are very well placed to take on this role and to coordinate a detailed holistic assessment of needs, create a written plan, assign responsibilities to key professionals and recognise and mitigate the impact of the wider determinants of health, such as lack of meaningful day activities. Another priority should be preparing the young adult for any potential emergency care by developing an emergency support plan and summaries of their needs that can be presented to adult emergency departments and admission units, Where intellectual disability liaison nurses are available, the family and young person should be introduced to them.

Principle 5: Continuity of Care in Adult Services

A gradual handover of care should involve active engagement from child and adult health services as well as an opportunity for the person with intellectual disability and their family to meet and build trusting relationships with key professionals. Transition should be a person-centred, flexible process where care-planning decisions are based on the person with intellectual disabilities' needs and individuals should be followed up until all adult services are in place.

Recommendations for Transitions

Although this particular research study was mainly focused on the role of nurses, the experience of families was drawn from interactions with medical, allied health and social care professionals. The main recommendations are relevant for all professionals and can also be applied to different types of transitions and different stages of the life course. As well as there being important recommendations for health and social care planners, the key elements should be seen as the responsibility of individual practitioners and managers.

Central to all aspects is that young people with intellectual disabilities and their families need to be central to and fully involved in proactive transition preparation to ensure the process is effective and meets their needs. Education, health and social care services need to develop and implement clear transition processes and pathways that take account of and respond to the needs of young people with complex intellectual disabilities and their families. Education, health and social care services need to collaborate at an early stage in the transition from child to adult health services to ensure there is effective multiagency transition planning and service coordination.

Education and training are key elements to the achievement of these recommendations, and it is important that transition is seen as an integrated theme within all undergraduate programmes for health, education and social care professionals. Furthermore, there should be specific continuing professional development that focuses on specific areas of practice including the changes to welfare and legal systems that may affect issues including decision making and consent.

Conclusion

Transitions are a feature of life for all of us and can create both opportunity and uncertainty as individuals move from one stage to the next. For people with complex intellectual disability and their families, transition from child to adult services can be one of the most challenging periods of their lives. It is the responsibility of all policy makers, planners and professionals to be aware of the potential of this experience to have a profound impact on the wellbeing of the individual and their family members. The families' and nurses' accounts from the study undertaken in Scotland demonstrated that there is still considerable work to be done to make transition planning fit for increasingly complex needs of some individuals with complex intellectual disabilities. However, it was also evident that where there is commitment and appropriate allocation of resources transition services can be effectively developed, implemented and evaluated. This chapter has set out the key issues that need to be considered and addressed to improve transitions for people with intellectual disabilities.

Key Concepts Discussed

- Definitions of transitions
- Transitions theory and the relation to the needs of people with intellectual disabilities across the lifespan
- The research evidence regarding transitions and people with intellectual disabilities across the lifespan
- The transitions support needs of people with intellectual disabilities across the lifespan
- The application of learning from a transition case study regarding the needs of people with intellectual disabilities and complex needs
- The actions necessary required to enable effective transitions for people with intellectual disabilities across the lifespan

References

Baumbusch J, Mayer S, Phinney A, Baumbusch S (2017) Aging together: caring relations in families of adults with intellectual disabilities. J Gerontol B Psychol Sci Soc Sci 57(2):341–347

Bekkema N, de Veer AJ, Hertogh CM, Francke AL (2015) 'From activating towards caring': shifts in care approaches at the end of life of people with intellectual disabilities; a qualitative study of the perspectives of relatives, care-staff and physicians. BMC Palliat Care 14(1):1–10

Bélanger SA, Caron J (2018) Evaluation of the child with global developmental delay and intellectual disability. Paediatr Child Health 23(6):403–410

Betz CL, O'Kane LS, Nehring WM, Lobo ML (2016) Systematic review: health care transition practice service models. Nurs Outlook 64(3):229–243

Bindels-de Heus KG, van Staa A, van Vliet I, Ewals FV, Hilberink SR (2013) Transferring young people with profound intellectual and multiple disabilities from pediatric to adult medical care: parents' experiences and recommendations. Intellect Dev Disabil 51(3):176–189

Borah E, Cohen D, Bearman SK, Platz M, Londoño T (2021) Comparison of child and adult clinicians' perceptions of barriers and facilitators to effective care transition. Soc Work Ment Health 19(2):166–185

Brown JM (2016) Recurrent grief in mothering a child with an intellectual disability to adulthood: grieving is the healing. Child Fam Soc Work 21(1):113–122

Brown M, Macarthur J, Higgins A, Chouliara Z (2019) Transitions from child to adult health care for young people with intellectual disabilities: a systematic review. J Adv Nurs 75(11):2418–2434

Brown M, Higgins A, MacArthur J (2020a) Transition from child to adult health services: a qualitative study of the views and experiences of families of young adults with intellectual disabilities. J Clin Nurs 29(1–2):195–207

Brown M, Chouliara Z, Higgins A, MacArthur J, Truesdale M (2020b) Transition from child to adult health services for people with complex learning disabilities: learning from families and nurses. Final report. Queens University, Belfast. Available online Health transitions and young adults with complex learning disabilities | School of Nursing and Midwifery | Queen's University Belfast (qub.ac.uk)

Camfield PR, Gibson PA, Douglass LM (2011) Strategies for transitioning to adult care for youth with Lennox-Gastaut syndrome and related disorders. Epilepsia 52:21–27

Davies H, Rennick J, Majnemer A (2011) Transition from pediatric to adult health care for young adults with neurological disorders: parental perspectives. Can J Neurosci Nurs 33(2):32–39

Department of Health (2006) Transition: getting it right for young people improving the transition of young people with long term conditions from children's to adult health services. Department of Health, London

Egan C, Mulcahy H, Naughton C (2021) Transitioning to long-term care for older adults with intellectual disabilities: a concept analysis. J Intellect Disabil. https://doi.org/10.1177/17446295211041839

Franklin MS, Beyer LN, Brotkin SM, Maslow GR, Pollock MD, Docherty SL (2019) Health care transition for adolescents and young adults with intellectual disability: views from the parents. J Pediatr Nurs 47:148–158

Gray WN, Schaefer MR, Resmini-Rawlinson A, Wagoner ST (2018) Barriers to transition from pediatric to adult care: a systematic review. J Pediatr Psychol 43(5):488–502

Hirano KA, Rowe D, Lindstrom L, Chan P (2018) Systemic barriers to family involvement in transition planning for youth with disabilities: a qualitative metasynthesis. J Child Fam Stud 27(11):3440–3456

Jacob CM, Baird J, Barker M, Cooper C, Hanson M (2017) The importance of a life course approach to health: chronic disease risk from preconception through adolescence and adulthood. WHO, Geneva

Jacobs P, MacMahon K, Quayle E (2018) Transition from school to adult services for young people with severe or profound intellectual disability: a systematic review utilizing framework synthesis. J Appl Res Intellect Disabil 31(6):962–982

Kerckhoff AC (2019) Getting started: transition to adulthood in Great Britain. Routledge

Laski L (2015) Realising the health and wellbeing of adolescents. Br Med J 351:h4119

Leonard H, Foley KR, Pikora T, Bourke J, Wong K, McPherson L, Lennox N, Downs J (2016) Transition to adulthood for young people with intellectual disability: the experiences of their families. Eur Child Adolesc Psychiatry 25(12):1369–1381

Li L, Polanski A, Lim A, Strachan PH (2022) Transition to adult care for youth with medical complexity: assessing needs and setting priorities for a health care improvement initiative. J Pediatr Nurs 62:144–154

Malapela RG, Thupayagale-Tshweneagae G, Mashalla Y (2020) Transition of adolescents with intellectual disability from schools for learners with special educational needs: parents views for the preparedness. J Appl Res Intellect Disabil 33(6):1440–1447

Meleis AI (2010) Transitions theory: middle range and situation specific theories in nursing research and practice. Springer, New York

National Institute for Health and Care Excellence (2016) Transition from children's to adults' services for young people using health or social care services. NICE, London

Okumura MJ, Saunders M, Rehm RS (2015) The role of health advocacy in transitions from pediatric to adult care for children with special health care needs: bridging families, provider and community services. J Pediatr Nurs 30(5):714–723

Redgrove FJ, Jewell P, Ellison C (2016) Mind the gap between school and adulthood for people with intellectual disabilities. Res Pract Intellect Dev Disabil 3(2):182–190

Schmidt A, Ilango SM, McManus MA, Rogers KK, White PH (2020) Outcomes of pediatric to adult health care transition interventions: an updated systematic review. J Pediatr Nurs 51:92–107

Smogorzewska J, Szumski G, Grygiel P (2019) Theory of mind development in school environment: a case of children with mild intellectual disability learning in inclusive and special education classrooms. J Appl Res Intellect Disabil 32(5):1241–1254

Stancliffe RJ, Bigby C, Balandin S, Wilson NJ, Craig D (2015) Transition to retirement and participation in mainstream community groups using active mentoring: a feasibility and outcomes evaluation with a matched comparison group. J Intellect Disabil Res 59(8):703–718

Stroud C, Walker LR, Davis M, Irwin CE Jr (2015) Investing in the health and well-being of young adults. J Adolesc Health 56(2):127–129

Todd S, Brandford S, Worth R, Shearn J, Bernal J (2021) Place of death of people with intellectual disabilities: an exploratory study of death and dying within community disability service settings. J Intellect Disabil 25(3):296–311

VanZant JS, McCormick AA (2021) Health care transition for individuals with Down syndrome: a needs assessment. Am J Med Genet A 185(10):3019–3027

World Health Organisation (2016) Transitions of care: technical series on safer primary care. World Health Organisation, Geneva

Young-Southward G, Rydzewska E, Philo C, Cooper SA (2017a) Physical and mental health during transition to adulthood in young people with and without intellectual disabilities: analysis of a whole population of 815,889 young people in Scotland. J Intellect Disabil Res 61(10):984–993

Young-Southward G, Philo C, Cooper SA (2017b) What effect does transition have on health and wellbeing in young people with intellectual disabilities? A systematic review. J Appl Res Intellect Disabil 30(5):805–823

Sexuality, Gender Identity and Relationships

16

Jessica Mannion and Fintan Sheerin

Chapter Topics

- This chapter considers the importance of relationships in the lives of people with intellectual disabilities across the lifespan.
- The historical context of relationships and sexuality for people with intellectual disabilities is introduced.
- Key terms with regard to gender and sexuality are outlined.
- A discussion on diversity of sexual identity and binary understandings of gender in the lives of people with intellectual disabilities is presented.
- Challenges for society and services are addressed, and exemplars of best practices and approaches in sexual health are proffered.
- A vignette is presented addressing key issues discussed in the chapter.

Introduction

This chapter focuses on sexuality and gender in the lives of people with intellectual disabilities, and how practitioners can support the needs of the individuals they work with. Discussions pertaining to relationships and sexuality among people with intellectual disabilities have traditionally

been difficult ones and there has, perhaps, been a tendency to veer away from them as they have often been contextualised by concerns regarding risk, safety, choice and abuse. Whilst such concerns also exist in respect of the general (particularly younger) population, they tend to persist throughout the adult lives of people with intellectual disabilities, arguably framing the discussion and pre-determining the outcomes.

Thus, our knowledge of adults with intellectual disabilities' perspectives on relationships on sexuality and on their lived experiences is limited. This is concerning as sexuality is an important aspect of people's lives (Bathje et al. 2021; Lee and Lee 2019), and studies have found that intimacy, developing relationships (Council on Quality and Leadership 2017) and formation of sexual identity (Friedman 2019) are important to people with intellectual disabilities. Despite this, such importance is often not recognised by general society (McGrath and Sakellariou 2016), and people with intellectual disabilities frequently find themselves constrained by cultural, social and legal restrictions (AAIDD 2020).

Part of the reason for this may reside in the belief that these people are invariably vulnerable; a larger part may be joined to historically based perspectives on intellectual disability and mental disability which were significant contributors to the societal service response. Some of these historical perspectives have been addressed in Chap. 2 but it is important to note that the development

16

J. Mannion (✉) · F. Sheerin
Trinity College Dublin, Dublin, Ireland
e-mail: mannioje@tcd.ie; sheerinf@tcd.ie

© The Author(s), under exclusive license to Springer Nature Switzerland AG 2023
F. Sheerin, C. Doyle (eds.), *Intellectual Disabilities: Health and Social Care Across the Lifespan*,
https://doi.org/10.1007/978-3-031-27496-1_16

of institutionalised intellectual disability services, in many parts of the world, was premised on some form of eugenics, whether overt of otherwise, with a focus on controlling sexuality activity (Sheerin 2019); curtailment of sexuality, in this case, sought specifically to prevent sexual intercourse and procreation, hence the widespread use of sexual segregation and sterilisation. Eugenics was grounded in a mix of science, economics and sociology, with a fair injection of religion. It was this latter ingredient which brought a focus on women with intellectual disabilities and the specific suppression that they experienced, as they embodied the negative characteristics ascribed to women such as Eve (temptress) and the Magdalene (fallen women) in Christian writings (Rafter 1992). The segregation of people with intellectual disabilities in institutions also removed the relational context for developing and understanding one's sexual identity. Furthermore, that so many Irish institutions were run under a strongly religious ethos meant that the oppressive institutional voice that found its way into the consciousness of these people was one heavily imbued by religious perspectives (Sheerin 2021). This arguably supported the denial of adulthood and sexual maturity, through infantilisation and, consequently, the contextualising of any sexual behaviour as being unacceptable and inappropriate. The prevailing Roman Catholic ethos at that time, and well into the late twentieth century, supported a binary understanding of gender, a heteronormative perspective on orientation, an immutable alignment between physical and perceived gender and a clear delineation of male and female roles. The reality for people with intellectual disability was, however, that even such perspectives played no role in their lives.

Studies undertaken in the 1990s and early 2000s, particularly in the UK, exploring the staff attitudes in respect of relationships and sexuality almost invariably found that nurses' and other carers' views were quite conservative in nature and supported the *status quo*, whether actively or passively (Charitou et al. 2021). Attitudes of staff, carers, family and community are important, and, as others in mainstream society can expect to be able to explore their sexual identity in a climate of tolerance and acceptance, one would hope that decongregation and the ongoing move to community will bring similar openness to and acceptance of the diversity of sexuality and sexual identity among people with intellectual disabilities, and that they will experience the realisation of these aspects of personhood in their lives.

Background

Key Terms in Relation to Relationships and Sexuality

Before delving further into providing an understanding of the importance of relationships and sexuality for individuals with intellectual disabilities, it is important to break down some of the key terms related to these two broad concepts. These terms are sex, gender, gender roles, gender identity, sexuality, sexual identity and sexual orientation.

Sex is what makes us male or female, by our biological attributes (Zucker 2001), comprising possession of genitalia and organs that make the genitalia function (anatomical sex) as well as the sex chromosomes that influence the development of male and female body parts (genetic sex) (Hill 2008).

Gender refers to the cultural, social and psychological meanings attached to each sex in a society (Unger 1979). Gender can be constructed in many ways, such as through labelling and stereotyping (Hill 2008). This can lead to *gender roles*, which are cultural expectations of what a male and female should do and how they should act (Hill 2008). This can further be constructed by an individual's *gender identity*, which is how they understand themselves, and through their preferences, in how they want to behave (Hill 2008).

Sexuality includes a range of experiences relating to an individual's sexual nature, such as their physical, emotional, cognitive and behavioural experiences. Sexuality is necessary for reproduction, but sexual feelings and expression extend this (Hill 2008). This can be experienced through relationships, fantasies, attitudes, behaviours and roles (WHO 2006).

Sexual identity denotes how an individual understands their sexual characteristics and sexual behaviour (Hill 2008).

Sexual orientation moves beyond this understanding and refers to the individual's tendency to experience emotional or sexual attraction to females, males or both (Hill 2008).

There are many different aspects to sexuality and gender, with various terms used to describe sexual behaviour, attraction and orientation. Indeed, Abrams (2022) has identified 46 different terms relating to sexuality. LGBT, LGBTQ, LGBTQ+ and LGBTQIA+ (lesbian, gay, bisexual, transgender, queer or questioning, intersex, A-sexual), straight and gender fluid are used across different sources. However, the most frequently used in all the studies identified was LGBTQ, and as a result, this is the term that is used here. The + and IA additions are not used, as this chapter does not have the scope to cover all identities such as intersex, asexual and the range of identities covered under the +, such as pansexual. Like other writings in the disability field, asexuality is often not addressed due to people with intellectual disabilities having been wrongly labelled as either asexual or hypersexual (Whittle and Butler 2018). However, this is not to say that some people with intellectual disabilities are not asexual. There are many different gender identities which extend well beyond the historical definitions of female and male (Abrams and Ferguson 2022), and it is important to become familiar with terms that individuals identify with, in order to be best positioned to support individuals.

The Importance of Relationships and Sexuality to Adults and Young People with Intellectual Disabilities

Relationships and sexuality are important to people with intellectual disabilities, just as they are for everyone; people want to love and to be loved

(Bates et al. 2020). Research shows that many adults and adolescents with intellectual disabilities are in relationships, many are sexually active, and many others desire this. In a study focusing on adults, Gil-Llario et al. (2018) found that 96.4% of 360 participants with intellectual disabilities aged 19–55 had been in a steady relationship, and 84.2% had engaged in sexual intercourse. Another study focusing on adolescents found that 35% of the 31 participants were in a relationship and 85% of the single participants desired such (Heifetz et al. 2020). Out of the 42 young participants with intellectual disabilities aged 14–25 in yet another study, 34 reported having had a relationship, 12 had engaged in sexual intercourse, and a further 17 desired these in their lives (Retznik et al. 2021). Such relationships are often positive for people with intellectual disabilities, as reported by social care staff in Bates et al.'s (2020) work.

Whilst relationships and marriage offer potentially positive outcomes for people with intellectual disabilities, the rates of the same are much lower in this cohort than in the general population. This is despite their wish for love, companionship and friendship (Bates et al. 2017) and the desire to have relationships (Retznik et al. 2021), long-term commitment (Bates et al. 2017), marriage and children (Retznik et al. 2021; Azzopardi Lane et al. 2019).

Diversity of Sexual Identity

We will now explore sexual identity and behaviours in the context of individuals with intellectual disabilities. Much of the recent literature has focused, not on the opportunities but, rather, on the challenges that individuals face, resulting in a lack of opportunity for them to explore their sexuality and develop relationships.

One of the challenges expressed across studies with both adults and adolescents is that relationships are generally developed in segregated environments; integration into the mainstream population is poor (Bates et al. 2017). Bates et al.'s research on partner selection found that all participants had previously been in a relationship but had only dated other people with intellectual disabilities. Furthermore, they had met their partner in settings where people with intellectual disabilities congregated. Thus, the couples may have only been together due to availability as opposed to compatibility, as they did not all share the same life goals, and one third expressed loneliness within those relationships. The paucity of potential interactions with people from outside the cohort of people with intellectual disabilities is not limited to adults, and adolescents similarly have few opportunities to spend time with their peers outside of school (Heifetz et al. 2020), leaving them with less opportunities to create romantic relationships (Cheak-Zamora et al. 2019). They also have limited unsupervised time (Azzopardi Lane et al. 2019) with adolescents reporting only being able to meet their partner in a school/professional setting due to fewer opportunities to socialise outside those contexts. This meant that they could neither identify potential partners nor get periods alone with them. Whilst they saw their partners daily in school or work, the quality of the contact was poor as they seldom saw each other outside of these settings (Retznik et al. 2021). Sheltering and overprotection from parents and/or carers has been evident in several studies (Azzopardi Lane et al. 2019; Callus and Bonello 2017), leaving a lack of opportunity to socialise and build relationships (Azzopardi Lane et al. 2019). It is, therefore, not surprising that participants in this study indicated that living independently from parents, carers and institutions was important to them, if they were to be able to get married and have a family (Azzopardi Lane et al. 2019). However, with the lack of supported community living, personal assistants (Callus and Bonello 2017), physical support, transport and finance (Azzopardi Lane et al. 2019), this remains a challenge.

A further issue is that people with intellectual disabilities may have less knowledge regarding sex and any associated risks than their non-disabled peers (Baines et al. 2018; Cheak-Zamora et al. 2019). This could be due to a lack of appropriate sexual health education, with such education often reactive rather than proactive in character (Bates et al. 2020). One specific concern is the potential challenges for people with intellectual disabilities to be safe online, particularly if they have received no education on this (Bates et al. 2020).

Women with Intellectual Disabilities

Women with intellectual disabilities can be particularly disadvantaged. Socio-cultural assumptions and disablist practices are argued to have led to the exclusion of women in respect of their sexual lives (Reeve 2019). Global policy on human rights and equity has had little impact on their lives and women with intellectual disabilities are often not viewed as sexual citizens (Wiseman and Ferrie 2020). They must frequently hide sexual relationships due to strict rules, lack of privacy and negative attitudes in their group home or institution (Matin et al. 2021). Further to this, they are often scared about unwanted pregnancies and sexually transmitted infections and may be at a higher risk of these than non-disabled women (Matin et al. 2021). There is also a high prevalence of abuse experienced by women with intellectual disabilities (O'Shea and Frawley 2020).

Women with intellectual disabilities may also be more likely to experience unequitable healthcare and reproductive outcomes (Agaronnik et al. 2020). One study found that women's sexual relations, fertility and sterilisation are controlled much more than men (Björnsdóttir et al. 2017), such that they may have little control over their lives when it comes to decisions about their sexual lives (Matin et al. 2021). Gender is often silenced with women seen as unable to appropriately fit gender roles and the denial of related rights such as expressing their sexuality, forming relationships, getting married and having children (O'Shea and Frawley 2020). Mothers too are often not accepted as being capable parents (Wiseman and Ferrie 2020) and may be subject to arbitrary removal of their children (Sheerin et al. 2013; Mitra 2017). Reproductive rights are often denied (O'Shea and Frawley 2020) and controlled by family and government policy (Matin et al. 2021), with women experiencing a lack of access to health screening (Xu et al. 2017), enforced sterilisation to prevent pregnancy, coerced contraception or even abortion (Agaronnik et al. 2020). Moreover, women with intellectual disabilities are 1.5 times more likely to undergo sterilisation (Mosher et al. 2018) and 2.7 times more likely to undergo a hysterectomy without a medical cause (Li et al. 2018), in comparison to non-disabled women. One study found that even women's menstruation was managed by others, as the women had a lack of bodily autonomy and knowledge on menstruation, which impacted on their ability to self-care (Wiseman and Ferrie 2020). The 'problem' of menstruation has even prompted some carers to advocate for sterilisation as a solution (Patel 2017). Wiseman and Ferrie (2020) study also reported women had a lack of knowledge on breast health and cervical smears, resulting in some women never having a smear test and having to undergo a colposcopy to remove the affected cervical tissue. These women further voiced a lack of knowledge on vaginal care, sexually transmitted infections and menopause, the information reportedly withheld by family and carers. Finally, women have reported being too embarrassed to talk to male clinicians, as they were perceived to be in a position of power in respect to these health topics (Wiseman and Ferrie 2020). Despite these challenges, participants in O'Shea and Frawley's (2020) study on women, gender, sexuality and relationships found that where such barriers were not predominant, women with intellectual disabilities valued their roles as either girlfriend, fiancé, bride or wife, along with valuing their femininity.

Men with Intellectual Disabilities

Such assumptions and disablist practices are not isolated to women. There is also a tension between disability and hegemonic masculinity (Björnsdóttir et al. 2017), the societal expectation of what it is to be a 'real man' (Coston and Kimmel 2012). Such masculinity is dominated by a particular perspective of heterosexuality, which is associated with strength, independence and providing for a family (Björnsdóttir et al.

2017). Men with intellectual disabilities have been found to aspire to a normative heterosexual identity in order to fit in (Björnsdóttir et al. 2017; Wilton and Fudge Schormans 2020), and these studies have found that the participants held traditional views of gender and hegemonic masculinity associated with bravery and strength. However, they felt that staff and family threatened their autonomy in this regard, and societal perceptions on intellectual disability made it difficult for them to gain employment and so fulfil the 'masculine role' of provider. Many of the men in these studies wished to live independently as they saw it as a steppingstone to getting married, starting a family and having a normative heterosexual masculine identity. However, many held concerns about being able to provide for a family; they held the view that men are the breadwinners and women are the homemakers (Björnsdóttir et al. 2017; Wilton and Fudge Schormans 2020).

One Canadian study reported that men who lived in group homes were cared for in an over-controlling and paternalistic manner (Wilton and Fudge Schormans 2020). Domestic life was controlled by the staff and house rules, and the men had little voice in their daily routines, space and when they left the home and for how long. Many participants expressed a lack of independence. One man said he felt like a child due to the way he was controlled by the staff. He would be sent to his room for an hour so the staff could concentrate on administration work; he was not allowed to control his money and was only permitted 3 hours community time out of the house each day. Other male participants who lived in group homes could not go out alone and stated they had no choice but to go on scheduled supervised activities that they did not enjoy. Another participant who lived with his parents spoke about resisting their control by eating fast food, staying up late and going to bars and clubs. He may have been protesting his masculinity when he went to strip bars with his brother. This man wanted to live independently. Other participants who lived with their families, but had employment, were happier with their living situation. Although gendered expectations may have meant less to these men, it may have been because they had a valued social role and what they recognised as a more normative masculine identity.

Björnsdóttir et al. (2017) noted that men with intellectual disabilities did not know much about LGBTQ and did not see that as an option for them, believing gay men were not 'real men'. Some, particularly older, men displayed misogyny and sexism (Björnsdóttir et al. 2017). This may be due to the tension of not being able to reach the perceived idealised standard of what it means to be a man, being denied access to adult roles and treated as vulnerable and dependant (Shuttleworth 2000). It may also be linked to their lack of sexual health education and the influence of the media, where men with intellectual disabilities have reported learning about sex through pornography or from their peers. Schools and disability services may further contribute to this, especially when schools teach gendered subjects (e.g. woodwork for boys) and services offer gendered activities (e.g. bowling for men) or choose clothes they perceive to be suitable for the individuals' genders (Björnsdóttir et al. 2017).

Men can also often find themselves wrongly labelled as sexually deviant. Thus, for example, a man who enjoys masturbating or sex may be judged as being 'dirty' (Deffew et al. 2022); such negative labels can be harmful. Men can also be vulnerable to abuse as a result of social isolation and limited support (Bates et al. 2020). As a result of all these challenges, men may not have the opportunity to develop their sexual and gender identity (Björnsdóttir et al. 2017). That said, it has been found that men with intellectual disabilities will try to craft their gender identity, even though it is inconsistent with their everyday realities (Wilton and Fudge Schormans 2020).

LGBTQ People with Intellectual Disabilities

Further marginalisation exists for those who identify as LGBTQ, as people with intellectual disabilities are often sheltered from even talking about this (Toft et al. 2020). They may be perceived to be incapable of being LGBTQ and

viewed as immature due to their disability (Toft et al. 2020). Where their sexual identity is accepted, it is often labelled as a symptom of their disability (Toft et al. 2020) and parents may be disapproving of their LGBTQ identity (Schaafsma et al. 2017). The result is that people with intellectual disabilities may believe that these identities are unavailable to them (Zirnzak 2022). They may also be concerned of multiple stigmas, and associated jeopardy, and take the safe route of avoiding another minority label (Smith et al. 2021). This is a very real outcome, with research suggesting that dual marginalisation exists in relation to intellectual disability and gender expression or sexual orientation (Wilson et al. 2018). This layered stigma can lead to increased segregation and even more limited opportunities for both social and sexual relationships (McCann et al. 2016). People with intellectual disabilities have reported discrimination, abuse and lack of support from professionals and others in their community in relation to their sexual and gender identity (Dinwoodie et al. 2020). It has been found that within intellectual disability services, LGBTQ and gender diverse individuals experience exclusion (Smith et al. 2021) and discrimination, where their identified sexual orientation or gender diversity may be explained as a behavioural issue (Abbott 2013) or minimised as only a phase (Toft et al. 2020). Staff have also aired concerns regarding the risks of living with an LGBTQ identity in the reality of heteronormativity, homophobia, biphobia and transphobia (Wilkinson et al. 2015). People with intellectual disabilities often do not have access to the tools to express their sexuality, when they are living in restrictive and uneven environments, making coming out challenging (Toft et al. 2020). Furthermore, they often do not have access to LGBTQ spaces (Toft et al. 2020).

It is clear, therefore, that there are many barriers to sexual expression and to forming relationships in the lives of people with intellectual disabilities. These include issues around partner selection due to limited opportunities to meet people outside of segregated settings, and a lack of privacy with being constantly monitored by parents or staff. There is limited support, transport and finance for adults to live independently from their parents/carers or service providers, making it difficult to get married and start a family. Adolescents and adults with intellectual disabilities may also have inadequate knowledge on relationships and sexuality. There are further barriers for women, particularly pertaining to unequitable healthcare and reproductive outcomes. Men face different barriers, particularly in relation to forming a masculine identity, due to a lack of access to non-disabled experiences and spaces and by being controlled by staff and family members. Those that are LGBTQ experience further marginalisation, where it has been reported that many people experience multiple stigmas and, as a result, live with discrimination, abuse and a lack of support.

Binary Understandings of Gender

There is a limited understanding of and perspective on gender identity in disability research. Society has moved on in this regard, but this has not transferred to our understanding of people with intellectual disabilities. This is evident in the Health Research Board's annual reports on medical research in Ireland, which maintain limited definitions of gender. As stated earlier in this chapter, there are many definitions related to different gender terms. If a person is gender fluid, it means their gender identity is not fixed and can change (Maxwell Triska 2018). Non-binary is an umbrella term used when a person identifies with a gender that is neither a woman nor a man, a combination of both or something else (Abrams 2022). A transgender person is an individual who identifies as a gender other than their assigned birth gender (Maxwell Triska 2018). The few studies that exist on intellectual disability and transgender highlight transphobia and abuse. Participants reported exclusion and transphobia in disability services, where they were subjected to abuse by staff (Newman et al. 2018; Dinwoodie et al. 2020). This was particularly evident when trying to locate accommodation which would accept transgender individuals, being regularly mis-gendered by hospital staff (often intention-

ally) and finding transgender support needs unaddressed and actively avoided at times (Newman et al. 2018). One trans woman voiced how she did not get the opportunity to come out to staff as they were already told before they met her. Although the staff received specific training and the woman believed they were not transphobic, she felt that they did not get to know her, but focused on only her gender identity (Maxwell Triska 2018). In another study, a trans man reported confusion and dismay at being 'deadnamed' (being referred to by the name he used prior to transitioning, such as his birth name) by the professional he confided in (Toft et al. 2020).

There is often a lack of understanding on transgender issues in disability services (Smith et al. 2021). As people with intellectual disabilities are reliant on their services, they are at a higher risk of prejudice and abuse in comparison to non-disabled people (Latham 2017).

Challenges for Societal and Service Responses

People with intellectual disabilities can be vulnerable to abuse and exploitation, which is one of the reasons why parents and professionals express concern about autonomy in relationships and sexuality. One study found that 6.1% of the 360 participants reported having been sexually abused in the past (Gil-Llario et al. 2018). Professionals have voiced that there is a real challenge to finding a balance between supporting autonomy and protecting from harm (Wickström et al. 2020). With the right education and support, people can have healthy relationships and explore their sexuality. In fact, Dukes and McGuire (2009) have shown that when sexual health information is provided it can increase an individual's capacity, at least in the short term. Positive risk taking can enhance people's lives; however, if staff in disability services are to support individuals with relationships and sexuality, they need clear guidance, policy, training and supervision.

Views on people with intellectual disabilities' rights to develop relationships and express their sexuality have been influenced by a broader societal discourse which views people with intellectual disabilities as perpetual children requiring protection (infantilisation). They are conceptualised as prepubescent, asexual or hypersexual. If perceptions changed and people were viewed as the sexual beings which they often are, and if support and education were available, it stands to reason that the chance of risk would decrease and the capacity to make decisions in their relationships and sexuality would increase.

There has been a significant shift in the flavour of legislative change, influenced by international law and the adoption of the United Nations Convention on the Rights of Persons with Disabilities (UNCRPD) (2006). The Convention states that people with disabilities should have equal rights like everyone else regarding relationships, marriage, sexual health education, fertility, reproduction, family planning, parenthood and family life. As a result, many national policies changed, such as the Criminal Law (Sexual Offences) Act 2017 in Ireland (Government of Ireland 2017), which replaced previous legislation criminalising people with intellectual disabilities who had sex outside of marriage and independent living.

For service providers to move beyond risk, there are several approaches they could take. They need to move away from paternalistic, risk-averse attitudes and methods (Wilkinson et al. 2015) and recognise the dual marginalisation that exists, as well as the systematic and personal barriers that come with this (Wilson et al. 2018). This means taking a broader lens than the hetero- and cis-normative ones (Wilkinson et al. 2015). Professionals should be involved in advocacy and awareness-raising (Stoffelen et al. 2018) and services should have clear policy guidance for professionals to support sexual exploration and risk management (Wilkinson et al. 2015). Professionals' pre-service and in-service education should include supported supervision, the exploration of ethical dilemmas, knowledge on legal guidelines and networking among multi- and interdisciplinary professionals (Höglund and Larsson 2019; Wickström et al. 2020).

However, this change cannot happen in isolation, and the burden cannot be solely placed on service providers' shoulders. Governments need to support this through legislation and policy, ensuring that resources and funding are provided to allow this extra work to happen. Overall, there needs to be a societal shift in attitudes towards realising people with intellectual disabilities have rights to express their sexuality and form relationships. This does raise the question as to whether people with intellectual disabilities will ever achieve the right to gender and sexual identity, and to love on an equal basis to the rest of society. Although change has been so slow, there are several innovative practices happening that are pushing towards such an outcome. One example is the first author's PhD project, a co-operative inquiry group which supports people with intellectual disabilities to speak about relationships and sexuality. This group has been proactively presenting at conferences and publishing on this topic, to ensure that their voices and opinions are heard. It is hoped that approaches such as this will serve to educate others on the topic and challenge the ways that they may have been viewing people with intellectual disabilities.

Exemplars of Best Practice and Approaches

Despite the challenges and complexity involved in relationships and sexuality, there are many advancements in understandings about people with intellectual disabilities (Houtrow et al. 2021), as well as reconfigured, collaborative and normalised approaches to sexual health (Pariseau-Legault and Holmes 2017). Such approaches are considered health and human rights issues (Giami 2016). It has been found that, when provided, sexual health education provides a positive view on sexual relationships, increases decision-making capacity in relation to sexual life and raises self-esteem (McCann et al. 2019). It is vital to seek out evidence-based and informed programmes, as well as opportunities for real-life experiences whilst ensuring autonomy and privacy for the individual (Houtrow et al. 2021).

Developmentally appropriate sexual health education should begin in childhood and include families and carers (Houtrow et al. 2021). Sexual health programmes need to move beyond puberty, anatomy and reproduction. Topics that include body image, interpersonal relationships, sexual expression, gender identity, intimacy and sexual orientation (Wolfe et al. 2019), coming out, hate crime (Dinwoodie et al. 2020), sexual consent, safety, sexual pleasure, public and private behaviour, sexual self-advocacy and physical barriers need to be addressed (Maxwell Triska 2018). There needs to be a focus on supporting people with intellectual disabilities to express romantic feelings, engage in decision making and make choices in a healthy relationship (Chou et al. 2015), self-protecting, exploring and using contraception whilst being aware of sexually transmitted infections (Matin et al. 2021). Finally, women should be supported to navigate menstruation, menopause (Wiseman and Ferrie 2020) and parenthood (Wolfe et al. 2019) to the best of their abilities. All educational materials need to be presented in a variety of formats (Wilson et al. 2018), inclusive of sexual diversity (Abbott 2013) and incorporating pictures of disabled people (Bollinger and Cook 2019). Some specifically designed programmes and resources are available in the useful resources section below.

Vignette

Mannion's (2016–2023) PhD study is a co-operative inquiry group comprising six co-inquirers with intellectual disabilities, the PhD researcher and an assistant (both of whom are neuro-divergent and also co-inquirers). A co-inquirer is an individual who is a co-researcher and co-subject; they do research on their own lives collaboratively. This co-operative inquiry group did research on relationships and sexuality. The co-inquirers were actively involved in all decisions of the study: deciding what topics to research, what methods to use to explore the topics, applying for funding, co-creating the findings, co-creating the data analysis method, co-analysing the data, working through the actions of the study and disseminating the findings. They met fortnightly for research meetings for a

year and used creative methods such as art, rap and LEGO® to co-create and co-analyse the data. Some of the topics which the group discovered were important to them included sexual health education, online safety, LGBTQ and the rights to get married and have children: topics that have been raised in this chapter. What made this study unique is that the group had full control in its direction. The group also worked on agreed actions that arose from issues identified in the study. They collaboratively presented their research findings at an international action research colloquium. They then co-authored a publication together (Mannion et al. 2022) and in this voiced the power of researching collaboratively. The co-inquirers stated that it gave them a voice, an opportunity to speak and learn about relationships and sexuality and an understanding on their rights. Many of the group stated that, as a result of this experience, they loved themselves for who they were and accepted their disability for the first time in their lives. The group shared their experiences of growing up and being told that they could not do the things they wanted to do. As it can be seen in the literature, many people are concerned of vulnerability, lack of capacity and risk. This group learnt that they could achieve high goals and be researchers, public speakers and authors. They learnt skills such as group facilitation, data analysis, applying for funding, presentation skills and publishing. They are now educating others about relationships and sexuality for people with intellectual disabilities through their dissemination activities, and it is hoped that they are contributing to changing people's attitudes, a goal they are working towards. Inclusive and accessible projects like this will help move society forward regarding relationships and sexuality for people with intellectual disabilities.

Reflective Questions

1. Has this made you think differently about people with intellectual disabilities and their capabilities, and how you may approach your profession?
2. How would you feel about sharing power and decision making with individuals you support?
3. How can positive risk taking actively be supported by service providers? What barriers may you face as a professional and how may you overcome them?
4. How can an approach like this be applied to practice, to create a platform where individuals can explore what is important to them?
5. How may you support individuals to identify and develop their skills? How can you make advocacy work more accessible?

Conclusion

Relationships and sexuality for people with intellectual disabilities have traditionally been contextualised with concerns of risk, safety, choice and abuse. This is concerning, as expressing sexuality and developing relationships is important to people with intellectual disabilities. Research shows that adults and adolescents are in relationships, are sexually active or desire this. Their wish for love, marriage and starting a family is coupled with lower relationship and marriage rates than non-disabled people.

The barriers to sexual expression and forming relationships include limited opportunities to meet partners and sustain relationships in private and a lack of support to live indepen-

dently, get married and start a family. They also lead to inequitable healthcare access and reproductive outcomes for women and gender challenges for men, with marginalisation and a lack of support for those who are LGBTQ. There is a limited understanding and narrow perspective of gender identity. This can result in prejudice and abuse.

Although people with intellectual disabilities are at a higher risk of abuse, there are actions that can be taken from a societal, government and service provider level. If perceptions changed and support and education was available, it is likely that such risk could be mitigated and the capacity to make decisions in relationships and sexuality would be maximised. International and national legislation protect rights in this regard, so it is important to look at ways to support these rights.

Sexual health education provides many benefits, including increasing decision-making capacity in relation to sexual life. A range of specifically designed sexual health programmes and resources have been compiled (see below) that can be used to support individuals across the lifespan. By working in collaboration with people with intellectual disabilities to provide an equal space to talk about relationships and sexuality, and to find innovative ways to be heard by society, it may be possible to realise the much-needed shift in societal, government and service provision attitudes and change.

Key Concepts Discussed

- Gender identity
- Sexual identity
- Control of sexuality and relationships
- Eugenics
- Responses of governments, society and service providers
- Advocacy
- Positive risk taking

Useful Resources

Name of resource	Explanation of the resource	Where resource is available
Amaze	An online platform to provide sexual health education to children and young people, educators, healthcare providers, parents and guardians, mainly through the use of videos	https://amaze.org
Bodysense instructional dolls	Three dolls to assist teaching sexual health education to students with intellectual disabilities. Two of the dolls are anatomically correct adult dolls. To teach about the human body, hygiene and social interactions. The third doll has female genitalia and internal reproductive organs to teach anatomy, menstruation, hygiene, masturbation and reproduction	http://bodysense.org.uk/wordpress/
Change People UK	A range of accessible resources for people with intellectual disabilities are available to buy on friendships, relationships, sexuality, LGBTQ, sex, safe sex, contraception, masturbation, pregnancy, parenting and sexual abuse	https://www.changepeople.org/shop/products
Circles Social Skills Utility™	An app that simplifies sexuality by teaching about social relationships, intimacy and boundaries. A pilot study found an improvement in user's understanding of social boundaries after using the app, particularly where physical contact should be minimal or not at all (Faught et al. 2020)	https://www.circlesapp.com/
Puberty and Sexuality for Children and Young People with a Learning Disability (NHS, Leeds 2009).	A sexual health teaching pack for children and young people with disabilities aged 9–18 years including children with severe intellectual disabilities.	https://s3-eu-west-1.amazonaws.com/leedssexualhealth.com/downloads/Puberty-Sexuality-Pack.pdf
Sanctuary film, Blue Teapot Company, Galway, Ireland	A film made with actors and advocates with intellectual disabilities to highlight relationships and sexuality	http://blueteapot.ie/our_performances/sanctuary-film/
Sexuality and Intellectual Disability: A Guide for Professionals	A book on gender and sexuality for professionals working in the intellectual disability sector. Provides guidance and toolboxes on dating, sex education and LGBTQ inclusion	Maxwell Triska, A. (2018) Sexuality and intellectual disability: a guide for professionals. Oxfordshire: Routledge
Shepherd School, Nottingham, UK	A video of best practice showing the delivery of a sexual health education programme to young people with intellectual disabilities	https://online.clickview.co.uk/exchange/channels/32366675/teachers-tv/videos/36769760/sex-and-relationship-education
Sex and the 3Rs: Rights, Risks and Responsibilities: A Sex Education Pack for Working with People with Learning Disabilities	A resource that offers a framework for professionals to facilitate sexual health education to adults with intellectual disabilities that is inclusive of LGBTQ. Possible issues are identified, as well as suggestions on how to work around them. The topics include consent, safer sex, sexting, pornography and sexual abuse	McCarthy, M. and Thompson, D. (2016) Sex and the 3Rs: Rights, Risks and Responsibilities: a sex education pack for working with people with learning disabilities. West Sussex: Pavilion Publishing and media. https://www.pavpub.com/learning-disability/sexual-health/sex-and-the-3-rs-rights-risks-and-responsibilities

Name of resource	Explanation of the resource	Where resource is available
Supported Loving UK	A website advocating for the rights of people with intellectual disabilities to have relationships and provides a range of resources for people with intellectual disabilities, parents and staff.	https://www.choicesupport.org.uk/about-us/what-we-do/supported-loving
The Center for Parent Information and Resources	A website with a range of sexual health education resources for educators to use with children and adults with disabilities. This includes sexual development, sexuality, dating, healthy relationships, sexual self-advocacy and information for parents and resources for specific disabilities	https://www.parentcenterhub.org/sexed/
Things Ellie Likes and *Things Tom Likes*	Accessible books about sexuality and masturbation	Reynolds, K.E. (2015) Things Ellie likes. A book about sexuality and masturbation for girls and young women with Autism and related conditions. London: Jessica Kingsley. Reynolds, K.E. (2014) Things Tom likes. A book about sexuality and masturbation for girls and young women with Autism and related conditions. London: Jessica Kingsley

References

Abbott D (2013) Nudge, nudge, wink, wink: love, sex and gay men with intellectual disabilities—a helping hand or a human right? J Intellect Disabil Res 57(11):1079–1087

Abrams M (2022) 47 Terms that describe sexual attraction, behaviour, and orientation. Available at: https://www.healthline.com/health/different-types-of-sexuality. Accessed 10 Jun 2022

Abrams M, Ferguson S (2022) 68 Terms that describe gender identity and expression. Available at: https://www.healthline.com/health/different-genders. Accessed 10 Jun 2022

Agaronnik N, Pendo E, Lagu T, DeJong C, Perez-Caraballo A, Iezzoni L (2020) Ensuring the reproductive rights of women with intellectual disability. J Intellect Dev Disabil 45(4):365–376

American Association on Intellectual and Developmental Disabilities (2020) Definition of intellectual disability. Available at: https://aaidd.org/intellectual-disability/definition. Accessed 21 Sept 2022

Azzopardi Lane C, Cambridge P, Murphy G (2019) Muted voices: the unexplored sexuality of young persons with learning disability in Malta. Br J Learn Disabil 47:156–164

Baines S, Emerson E, Robertson J, Hatton C (2018) Sexual activity and sexual health among young adults with and without mild/moderate intellectual disability. BMC Public Health 18:667

Bates C, Terry L, Popple K (2017) Partner selection for people with intellectual disabilities. J Appl Res Intellect Disabil 30:602–611

Bates C, McCarthy M, Milne Skillman K, Elson N, Forrester-Jones R, Hunt S (2020) Always trying to walk a bit of a tightrope: the role of social care staff in supporting adults with intellectual and developmental disabilities to develop and maintain loving relationships. Br J Learn Disabil 48:261–268

Bathje M, Schrier M, Williams K, Olson L (2021) The lived experience of sexuality among adults with intellectual and developmental disabilities: a scoping review. Am J Occup Ther 75(4). https://doi.org/10.5014/ajot.2021.045005

Björnsdóttir K, Stefánsdóttir Á, Stefánsdóttir G (2017) People with intellectual disabilities negotiate autonomy, gender and sexuality. Sex Disabil 35(3):295–311

Bollinger H, Cook H (2019) After the social model: young physically disabled people, sexuality education and sexual experience. J Youth Stud 23(7):1–16

Callus A, Bonello I (2017) Over protection in the lives of people with intellectual disability in Malta: research findings. Available at: https://www.um.edu.mt/__data/assets/pdf_file/0020/337502/Reportonoverprotectionresearch.pdf. Accessed 10 Jul 2022

Charitou M, Quayle E, Sutherland A (2021) Supporting adults with intellectual disabilities with relationships and sex: a systematic review and thematic synthesis of qualitative research with staff. Sex Disabil 39:113–146

Cheak-Zamora N, Teti M, Maurer-Batjer A, O'Connor K, Randolph J (2019) Sexual and relationship interest, knowledge, and experiences among adolescents and young adults with autism spectrum disorder. Arch Sex Behav 48:2605–2615

Chou Y, Lu Z, Pu C (2015) Attitudes toward male and female sexuality among men and women with intellectual disabilities. Women Health 55(6):663–678

Coston BM, Kimmel M (2012) Seeing privilege where it isn't: marginalized masculinities and the intersectionality of privilege. J Soc Issues 68(1):97–111

Council on Quality and Leadership (2017) Let's talk about intimacy. Available at: https://www.c-q-l.org/resources/newsletters/lets-talk-about-intimacy/. Accessed 21 Sept 2022

Deffew A, Coughlan B, Burke T, Rogers E (2022) Staff member's views and attitudes to supporting people with an intellectual disability: a multi-method investigation of intimate relationships and sexuality. J Appl Res Intellect Disabil 35:1049–1058

Dinwoodie R, Greenhill B, Cookson A (2020) 'Them two things are what collide together': understanding the sexual identity experiences of lesbian, gay, bisexual and trans people labelled with intellectual disability. J Appl Res Intellect Disabil 33(1):3–16

Dukes E, McGuire B (2009) Enhancing capacity to make sexuality-related decisions in people with an intellectual disability. J Intellect Disabil Res 53(8):727–734

Faught BM, Moore G, Hande KA, Walker-Hirsch L. (2020) Social boundaries in young adult females with down syndrome as a foundation for sexuality education, Am J Sex Educ. 15:4:426–443. https://doi.org/10.1080/15546128.2020.1831677

Friedman C (2019) Intimate relationships of people with disabilities. Inclusion 7:41–56

Giami A (2016) De l'émancipation à l'institutionnalisation: santé sexuelle et droits sexuels [From emancipation to institutionalization: sexual health and sexual rights]. Genre Sex Soc 15:1–14

Gil-Llario M, Morell-Mengual V, Ballester-Arnal R, Díaz-Rodríguez I (2018) The experience of sexuality in adults with intellectual disability. J Intellect Disabil Res 62:72–80

Government of Ireland (2017) Criminal law (sexual offences act) 2017. Government of Ireland, Dublin

Heifetz M, Lake J, Weiss J, Isaacs B, Connolly J (2020) Dating and romantic relationships of adolescents with intellectual and developmental disabilities. J Adolesc 79:39–48

Hill C (2008) Human sexuality: personality and social psychological perspectives. Sage, California

Höglund B, Larsson M (2019) Ethical dilemmas and legal aspects in contraceptive counselling for women with intellectual disability: focus group interviews among midwives in Sweden. J Appl Res Intellect Disabil 32(6):1558–1566

Houtrow A, Elias E, Davis B, Council on Children with Disabilities (2021) Promoting healthy sexuality for children and adolescents with disabilities. Paediatrics 148(1):e2021052043. https://doi.org/10.1542/peds.2021-052043

Latham J (2017) Making and treating trans problems: the ontological politics of clinical practices. Stud Gend Sex 18(1):40–61

Lee G, Lee D (2019) Effects of a life skills-based sexuality education programme on the life-skills, sexuality knowledge, self-management skills for sexual health, and programme satisfaction of adolescents. Sex Educ 19(5):519–533

Li H, Mitra M, Wu J, Parish S, Valentine A, Dembo R (2018) Female sterilization and cognitive disability in the United States, 2011-2015. Obstet Gynaecol 132(3):559–564

Mannion J, Blee P, Gallagher R, Gallagher T, Higgins B, McHugh M, Mulligan J (2022) We are proud to be researchers with disabilities. Methodspace. Available at: https://www.methodspace.com/blog/we-are-proud-to-be-researchers-with-disabilities. Accessed 24 Jul 2022

Matin B, Ballan M, Darabi F, Karyani A, Soofi M, Soltani S (2021) Sexual health concerns in women with intellectual disabilities: a systematic review in qualitative studies. BMC Public Health 21:1965. https://doi.org/10.1186/s12889-021-12027-6

Maxwell Triska A (2018) Sexuality and intellectual disabilities: a guide for professionals. Routledge, New York

McCann E, Lee R, Brown M (2016) The experiences and support needs of people with intellectual disabilities who identify as LGBT: a review of the literature. Res Dev Disabil 57:39–53

McCann E, Marsh L, Brown M (2019) People with intellectual disabilities, relationship and sex education programmes: a systematic review. Health Educ J 78(8):885–900

McGrath M, Sakellariou D (2016) Why has so little progress been made in the practice of occupational therapy in relation to sexuality? Am J Occup Ther 70(1):1–5

Mitra M (2017) Postpartum health of women with intellectual and developmental disabilities: a call to action. J Womens Health 26(4):303–304

Mosher W, Hughes R, Bloom T, Horton L, Mojtabai R, Alhusen J (2018) Contraceptive use by disability status: new national estimates from the national survey of family growth. Contraception 97(6):552–558

Newman W, Barnhorst A, Landess J (2018) A transgender woman with intellectual disability and borderline personality disorder. Am J Psychiatr 175(11):1061–1063

NHS, Leeds (2009) Puberty and sexuality for children and young people with a learning disability. Puberty & Sexuality Pack (sexualhealthsheffield.nhs.uk)

O'Shea A, Frawley P (2020) Gender, sexuality and relationships for young Australian women with intellectual disability. Disabil Soc 35(4):654–675

Pariseau-Legault P, Holmes D (2017) Mediated pathways, negotiated identities: a critical phenomenological analysis of the experience of sexuality in the context of intellectual disability. J Res Nurs 22(8):599–614

Patel P (2017) Forced sterilization of women as discrimination. Public Health Rev 38:15. https://doi.org/10.1186/s40985-017-0060-9

Rafter N (1992) Claims-making and socio-cultural context in the first U.S. eugenics campaign. Soc Probl 39(1):1–34

Reeve D (2019) Psycho-emotional disablism: the missing link? In: Watson N, Roulstone A, Thomas C (eds)

Routledge handbook of disability studies. Routledge, Oxfordshire, pp 102–116

Retznik L, Wienholz S, Höltermann A, Conrad I, Riedel-Heller SG (2021) "It tingled as if we had gone through an anthill." Young people with intellectual disability and their experiences with relationship, sexuality and contraception. Sex Disabil 39:421–438

Schaafsma D, Kok G, Stoffelen J, Curfs L (2017) People with intellectual disabilities talk about sexuality: implications for the development of sex education. Sex Disabil 35(1):21–38

Sheerin F (2019) Leadership and intellectual disability services. In: Sheerin F, Curtis E (eds) Leadership for intellectual disability service. CRC Press, London, pp 1–17

Sheerin F (2021) Distributed leadership practices and interventions in intellectual disability services. In: Curtis E, Beirne M, Cullen J, Northway R, Corrigan S (eds) Distributed leadership in nursing and healthcare: theory, evidence and development. Open University Press, London, pp 109–120

Sheerin F, Keenan P, Lawler D (2013) Mothers with intellectual disabilities: interactions with children and family services in Ireland. Br J Learn Disabil 41:189–196

Shuttleworth R (2000) The search for sexual intimacy for men with cerebral palsy. Sex Disabil 18:263–282

Smith E, Zirnsak T, Power J, Lyons A, Bigby C (2021) Social inclusion of LGBTQ and gender diverse adults with intellectual disability in disability services: a systematic review of the literature. J Appl Res Intellect Disabil 35:46–59

Stoffelen J, Schaafsma D, Kok G, Curfs L (2018) Women who love: an explorative study on experiences of lesbian and bisexual women with a mild intellectual disability in the Netherlands. Sex Disabil 36(3):249–264

Toft A, Franklin A, Langley E (2020) You're not sure that you are gay yet': the perpetuation of the 'phase' in the lives of young disabled LGBT+people. Sexualities 23(4):516–529

Unger R (1979) Toward a redefinition of sex and gender. Am Psychol 34:1085–1094

United Nations Convention on the Rights of Persons with Disabilities (UNCRPD) (2006) Convention on the rights of persons with disabilities. United Nations, Geneva

Whittle C, Butler C (2018) Sexuality in the lives of people with intellectual disabilities: a meta-ethnographic synthesis of qualitative studies. Res Dev Disabil 75(2):68–81

Wickström M, Larsson M, Höglund B (2020) How can sexual and reproductive health and rights be enhanced for young people with intellectual disability? Focus group interviews with staff in Sweden. Reprod Health 17:86. https://doi.org/10.1186/s12978-020-00928-5

Wilkinson V, Theodore K, Raczka R (2015) 'As Normal as possible': sexual identity development in people with intellectual disabilities transitioning to adulthood. Sex Disabil 33(1):93–105

Wilson N, Macdonald J, Hayman B, Bright A, Frawley P, Gallego G (2018) A narrative review of the literature about people with intellectual disability who identify as lesbian, gay, bisexual, transgender, intersex or questioning. J Intellect Disabil 22(2):171–196

Wilton R, Fudge Schormans A (2020) 'I think they're treating me like a kid': intellectual disability, masculinity and place in Toronto, Canada. Gender Place Cult 27(3):429–451

Wiseman P, Ferrie J (2020) Reproductive (in)justice and inequality in the lives of women with intellectual disabilities in Scotland. Scand J Disabil Res 22(1):318–329

Wolfe P, Wertalik J, Domire Monaco S, Gardner S, Ruiz S (2019) Review of sociosexuality curricular content for individuals with developmental disabilities. Focus Autism Other Dev Disabil 34(3):153–162

World Health Organisation (2006) Sexual health definitions. Available at: https://www.who.int/health-topics/sexual-health#tab=tab_2 Accessed 24 Jul 2022

Xu X, McDermott S, Mann J, Hardin J, Deroche C, Carroll D, Courtney-Long E (2017) A longitudinal assessment of adherence to breast and cervical cancer screening recommendations among women with and without intellectual disability. Prev Med 100:167–172

Zirnzak T (2022) Commentary on: "Lost in the literature." People with intellectual disabilities who identify as trans: a narrative review. Tizard Learn Disabil Rev 27(1):53–56

Zucker K (2001) Biological influences of psychosexual differentiation. In: Unger R (ed) Handbook of the psychology of women and gender. Wiley, New York, pp 101–115